THE ROAD TO
OVERCOME
CANCER

AUTHORS:
XU ZE;
XU JIE;
BIN WU

authorHOUSE®

AuthorHouse™
1663 Liberty Drive
Bloomington, IN 47403
www.authorhouse.com
Phone: 1 (800) 839-8640

Published by AuthorHouse 12/06/2016

ISBN: 978-1-5246-4993-7 (sc)
ISBN: 978-1-5246-4992-0 (e)

Library of Congress Control Number: 2016919003

Contents

Section I   Seeking for the Road
Experimental Research

Section II   Footprint
Thinking and reform of traditional therapy

Section III Forward
To overcome cancer and to launch a general offensive

The introduction to this book

In China there is a proverb "The super doctor prevents the people from the disease before the disease happens". Many diseases can be prevented before they happen like Cancer and can be prevented before they cause damage to us. Cancer is human's disaster. We should attach importance to prevent Cancer. Cancer prevention should be paid attention to for everyone and should start from our daily life. Cancer prevention is extremely important and critical as its treatment. In this book based on all of our research and clinical practice, we summarized our previous results and further to discussing how to do well both treatment and prevention. In this book many contents were awarded in China as the following certificates of the awarded.

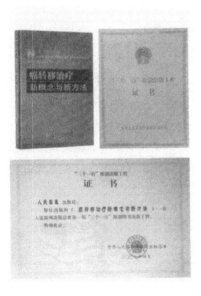

In addition, because we finished this book in such a short time and please be forgiven for any mistake and also welcome for your feedback.

Thanks again
Bin Wu
11-12-206, Baltimore in Maryland, U.SA

Brief Introduction to The first Author

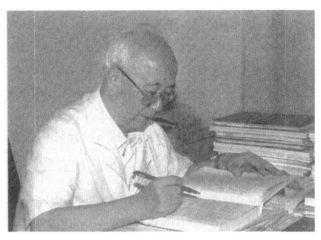

Xu Ze, male, born in Leping County of Jiangxi Province in Oct. 1933, gradated from Tongji Medical University in 1956, successively held the post of director of department of surgery of Affiliated Hospital of Hubei College of Traditional Chinese Medicine, professor, chief physician, tutor of postgraduate and doctoral student, President of Experimental Surgery Restitute Institute of Hubei College of Traditional Chinese Medicine, Director of Abdominal Tumor Surgery Research Room and Director of Anti Carcinomatous Metastasis and Reoccurrence Research Room. in addition, he held concurrent posts of Standing Director of China Medical Association Wuhan Branch, Vice President of Wuhan Micro-circulation Academy, Academic Member of International Liver Disease Research, Cooperation and Exchange Center, Member of International Surgeon Union, Standing Member of 1st, 2nd, 3rd and 4th Editorial Board of China Experimental Surgery Journal, Standing Member of 1st, 2dn and 3rd Editorial Board of Abdominal Surgery Journal. Enjoying Special Allowance of State Council.

He has been engaged in surgery work for 49 years and accumulated rich experience in radical operation of lung cancer, esophageal carcinoma, liver cancer, carcinoma of gallbladder, adenocarcinoma of pancreas, gastric carcinoma and intestinal cancer as well as in clinical therapy with Chinese Traditional Medicine combined with Western Medicine of prevention of reoccurrence and metastasis after operation.

He has been engaged in scientific research of surgery for 15 years and obtained many fruits, among which the task of Experimental Study and Clinical Application of Self-made Type Z-C1 Abdominal Cavity---Vein Flow Turning Unit in Therapy of Chronic Ascites of Hepatic Cirrhosis issued by Science Commission of Hubei Province was awarded Second Prize of Scientific Fruit by People's Government of Hubei Province and was popularized and applied in 38 hospitals in 12 provinces all over the country in

1982. The task "Experimental Study on Physiological Mechanism and Pathogenesis of Schistosome with Method of Experimental Surgery", issued by National Natural Fund Commission was awarded Second Prize of Scientific Fruit by People's Government of Hubei Province in 1986.

He began to study the tumor experience, established the tumor animal model and metastasis and reoccurrence animal model and probed into the mechanism and rules of carcinomatous metastasis and reoccurrence to find out the method to inhibit the metastasis. 48 kinds of Chinese traditional herbs that could counteract the intrusion, metastasis and reoccurrence were found and selected from a large number of natural herbs. Based on this, he invented and developed China Xu Ze (Z-C) Medicine Treating Malignancy, which had remarkable curative effects through over 10 years' clinical validation of many cases.

He has been engaged in teaching for 40 years and has cultivated many young doctors, 10 masters and 2 doctors. He has released 126 papers, published New Understanding and New Mode of Therapy of Cancer as the editor in charge, participate in writing 8 medical exclusive books including Therapeutics of Liver Disease, Surgery of Liver, Gallbladder and Pancreas and Surgical Operation of Abdomen.

A Brief Introduction to the Second Author

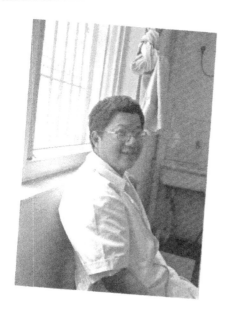

Xu Jie, male, graduated from Hubei College of Traditional Chinese Medicine in 1992, graduated from Hubei Medical University in 1996, Department of Clinical Medicine. Now He is chief physician in Hubei University of Traditional Chinese Medicine Hospital and Hubei Provincial Hospital of Surgery, engaged in experimental surgical tumor research and general surgery, urology clinical work.

Since 1992, he has been involved in the experimental tumor research of the Institute of Experimental Surgery of Hubei College of Traditional Chinese Medicine. He has carried out cancer cell transplantation and established a tumor animal model. He has carried out a series of experimental tumor research: exploring the mechanism of recurrence and metastasis of cancer and in vivo screening experiment of more than 200 kinds of Chinese herbal medicine in vivo tumor model of tumor inhibition s from a large number of natural medicine to find out, screening out of 48 kinds of anti-cancer invasion, metastasis, relapse traditional Chinese medicine

He participates in clinical validation and followed up for XZ - C immunoregulatory Chinese herbal medicine and completes the experimental research and clinical verification, data collection, collection and summary of this book.

A brief introduction to the third author and the main translator and one of the editors

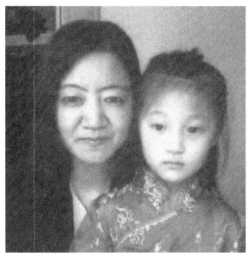

Bin Wu, MD, Ph.D., graduated from College of Yunyang of Tongji University of Medical Sciences for her MD degree; Studied her Master degree and her Ph. D degree in Sun Yat-Sen University of Medical Sciences. After she received her Ph.D., she worked as a Post-doctoral Follews in the Johns Hopkins Medical School and University of Maryland Medical School. She passed her USMLE tests and is going to do her residency training in America. She dedicated herself to oncology clinical and research. Her goal is to conquer cancer, which she believes this great contribuation to our health. She has a daughter, named Lily Xu.

The Summary of This Book

This book is the scientific summary of author 50 years of experience in tumor surgery and more than 20 years of cancer research results and clinical validation. The book is divided into three sections, 15 chapters; the first chapter "Pathfinder" from the beginning of the experimental study which introduced how to explore the etiology and pathogenesis of cancer and learned the new revelation from these and had the new discoveries and new knowledge; in section II or chapter "footprint", the author had the multi-angle analysis and comments about the traditional cancer therapy, proposed the suggestion of the cancer treatment as well as innovative results generated through laboratory research and clinical validation, including cancer initiation and metastasis, a new method of cancer treatment, both of which traditional radical surgery and radiotherapy and chemotherapy case review and reflection, and the experimental results and typical cases of clinical data of the applications of XZ-C anti-cancer Immune regulation drug treatment of malignant tumors ; the next "forward", mainly the author gives the suggestions and the general strategy of attacking the cancer. In this book the contents are initiative, the ideas are new, the theories are combined with practice and ideas, theory with practice, has a strong academic value and clinical practicality, suitable for hospitals at all levels oncology, cancer specialist clinic doctors, cancer researchers, cancer Patients and their families reading reference.

Preface

Recalling the history of cancer treatment, the three major traditional treatment methods: surgical treatment has been more than 100 years of history, 80-year history of radiotherapy, chemotherapy is also nearly 60 years of history. In 80 years of the 20th century biological therapy and immunotherapy rise. In the world the medical scientists work together, many tumor treatment has achieved good effect, but there are still many of the efficacy of cancer that is still in a very poor situation. In China, the high incidence of cancer is high; in recent years it also showed an upward trend, cancer has become the first cause of death among urban and rural residents. To reduce cancer mortality is an urgent desire; to overcome cancer is also a difficult task for the medical profession.

In order to overcome cancer, where is the road? How is this road found?

After 29 years of long process, the research direction and the main task in our Institute of Experimental Surgery is to overcome cancer. Around this major issue a new way worked out of overcoming which is the combination ways ; adhering to the characteristics and dvantages of Chinese medicine, adhering to the combination of Chinese and Western medicine methods, using reformation and innovation as the driving force to improve the effectiveness of cancer treatment, initially walking out a traditional Chinese medicine immune regulation and regulation of immune activity to prevent thymic atrophy and promote thymic hyperplasia, to protect bone marrow hematopoietic function, to improve immune surveillance, and thus to overcome the cancer of a new road.

This path is from the laboratory (a large number of animal experimental studies) to clinical practice validation, step by step walked out; is the combination of chinese and Western medicine at the molecular level. I think that the combination of Chinese and Western medicine is just a method, is a means. Why should the combination of Chinese and Western medicine be used? How should the combination of Chinese medicine and Western medicine be done?

What is the goal of combining medicine? Wu Xianzhong academician proposed: Chinese and Western medicine should be combined with the goal of innovation. Then, what is the goal of the combined innovation. I believe that: "cancer patients have long survival time, good quality of life, fewer complications" This is our goal!

In April 2014 Tang Zhaoyou Academician published a "Chinese-style anti-cancer" works, is about how the wisdom of the Art of War in the strategy of anti-cancer and tactical thinking. Inspired by Tang Yuanshi's word, recalling my decades of cancer treatment research and clinical work of the long experience, it is just to seek to overcome cancer and fight with cancer, then decided to publish this new work, whose name is "the road to overcome cancer."

This book is also in my edited publication of "cancer treatment new concept and new method" and three monographs on the basis of revision, which increased the new results from over the past five years we have studied and the new drugs of the development and many new cases of the tumor specialist outpatient treatment of; in the last section, we give out our ideas and proposals for cancer prevention and cancer treatment of overcoming cancer, as well as suggestions and hopes for the government.

Xu Ze
10-15-2015 In Wuhan in China
Tel: 027-88049526

Acknowledgements

This book is for all of people who concern human being health. We are deep grateful to all of people who like our new ways to improve our human being health.

My daughter Lily Xu gives me many smart and creative ideas while we sere finishing this book.

I would like to express our sincere gratitude to the following:

1. All of Authorhouse staffs

2. Dr. Xu Ze's family and Dr. Xu Jie's family

3. Mrs. Bo Wu's family and Mrs. Tao Wu's famly: espeicaly their daughters Chongshu Luo and Xunyue Wang

4. Medchi CEO: Gene Ransom III gives us great help

Bin Wu, M.D., Ph.D
In October, 2016 in Baltimore, Maryland in USA

Seeking for the Road

Experimental Research

Introduction

In 1985 I visited over 3000 patients after radical surgery treatment of the carcinomas in thoracic surgery department an general surgery department by me through letters and calls. Finally, I found that most of the patients experienced recurrence and metastasis within 2 to 3 years after the operation or even within several months for some patients, from which I deeply realized that the operation was successful and standard, but the long-term effect was unsatisfactory or even unsuccessful. It also suggested that to prevent from recurrence and metastasis is the key to prolong the survival period after the operation. Therefore, we must make clinical fundamental research in depth and it will be difficult to improve the clinical curative effect without the breakthrough in fundamental clinical research. As a result, we build the Institute of Experimental Surgery of anticancer recurrence and metastasis, and spent 24 years on doing a series of experimental research and clinical testifying work from the following aspects:

1. Following up on the results of our follow-up studies on cancer patients who had traditionally been treated, we had decided to find new ways to prevent recurrence and metastasis of cancer.

2. Through the results of the experimental study --- to find to prevent thymic atrophy, to promote thymic hyperplasia, and to increase immune path.

3. After the analysis of the effect of chemotherapy - must find the way of immune reconstruction.

4. Through animal studies and analysis there are new understandings of the concepts and theory of cancer recurrence - to find ways to eliminate the way of the metastasis of cancer cells.

5. Through the above research process: the initial explored out a new anti-cancer road --- gradually established the XZ-C immune regulation therapy.

We believe that this is the way to overcome cancer. We did a series of animal experiments in order to explore the cause of cancer, pathogenesis, pathophysiology. From the experimental results, new discoveries and new insights were found that : thymus atrophy and immune function decrease are one of the reasons for cancer etiology and pathogenesis. Therefore, at the international conference Dr. Xu Ze proposed that one of the etiology and pathogenesis of cancer may be the thymus atrophy, central immune organ damage, immune function decrease, immune surveillance capacity decrease and immune escape.

Irrespective of the complexity of the mechanisms underlying cancer, immune suppression is the key to cancer progression, and the removal of immunosuppressive agents and the restoration of immune system cells' recognition of cancer cells are likely to be effective against cancer.

The cancer treatment throughactivating the body's antitumor immune system is a promising breakthrough in the treatment of tumors, and immunotherapy is promising.

Chapter 1 The experimental research of exploring the etiology and pathogenesis of cancer

As a result of follow-up the questions were found -----postoperative recurrence, or metastasis is the key to determine the long-term efficacy of surgery.

Therefore, the problems are put forward - clinical surgeons should pay attention to and study the prevention measures of recurrence, or metastasis.

Therefore, we built our own experimental research laboratory to conduct the cancer research. First, to make the experiment tumor model, then to start the basic research from the clinical practice.

To look for the tumor pathogenic factors, pathogenesis and metastasis mechanism to search the preventive an treating methods through many steps of cancer cells metastasis. After seven years animal research, the author finished the following research work by steps and steps.

1. The experimental research of making cancer animal models

Why can human get cancer? Under what condition can cancer happen? Why can some get cancer and others can not get cancer under the same condition and the same environment? Are there intrinis or extrinis factors or both of them? Therefore, we should make the animal cancer models to study?

1). To make the cancer animal models in order to do tumor experimental research

The author was the chairman in Department of surgery in the affility hospital of Hubei traditional medical University so that he could do clinical work and do animal experimental together such as the tumor samples from the patients in operation room to place to the animal bodies after 30 minutes heat ischemia processes, however there were no tumor growth after 100 times experiment(more than 400 animals). After removing the thymus, then transplant the tumor again, the animal models were built up(210 animals models). Some of tumor animal models were set up by injection of steroid to reduce small animal immune function, then transplanted the tumor successfully. After removing thymus five days, the tumor were transplanted to the body, then after 5 or 6 days the lump would grow up to the yellow been-size, after 12-21 days the lump size will become thumb-size. The tumor can be alive three or four weeks, however it cannot be passed from generation to generation.

1>. It was found that after removing thymus, the tumor animal model can be set up. The steroid injection can assist to make the animal tumor models set up.

2>. The result showed that tumor growth and development are related to the host's immune response and has significant relation to host immune organs and immune tissue functions

3>. The result showed that thymus and immune system have certain/sure relations to the cancer growth. After removing host's thymus, the cancer animal models can be set up. If the thymus didn't be removed, the animal model cannot be built. Also injection steroid can decrease the host immune response, which is helpful to set up the animal model. If the immune system doesn't reduce, the animal models will not set up.

The research result showed that the correlation between the immune response and cancer cell growth is negative. When the immune response is dfficiency or decrease, the tumor can grow after transplantation, which will not be get rid of by hosts' immune response.

2). Which does the first happen: immune decrease first and causes the cancer or the cancer first happens and causes the immune response decrease?

There are 320 Quanming mice which are separated into A, B, C, D group. Each group has 80 mice. The methods of removing thymus and injection of tumor cells are the same as before.

In group A, first remove thymus, then five days later injection of 10^6 cancer cells; in group B, first inject the steroid, then seven day later injecting cancer cells; in group C, first inject the cancer cells, then 10 days later removing thymus; in group D, first injecting cancer cells, then 10days later inject steroid.

The result showed: the tumor growed in group A and B; There are only 18 mice which grew the green pea-size tumor in the 14day. This experiment implied that first the host's immune function decreased, or immune organ thymus has difficiency, then tumor can grow. If the host has good immune function, the tumors will not grow so that we get the conclusion: first immune function decrease, then cancer can develop and grow. If the immune system doesn't decrease, we can not build the cancer model successful.

From this research, to improve and to maintain good immune function and to keep the good immune organ function are the most important methods to prevent from cancer growth.

3). The research animal model of tumor metastasis:

In 1985 the author built his tumor metastasis animal models, which he injected human cancer cells into the mice whose thymus is removed. Later he built up tumor metastasis model through lymph system.

In 60 mice 0.2 ml / 10^6/ml H_{22} cells fuild was injected into animals' claw skin. After seven or eight days, a broad bean size tumor grew up and the whole foot and ankle started to swell. After 16 days there are 8 mice which the right inguinal lymph nodes started to enlarge so that the lymphatic drainage metastasis animal models were built. Later the author built blood metastasis animal models which 0.4ml 10^6/ml of H_{22} cell were injected into the vein, then caused multiple tumors growth in lungs. After that, the liver metastasis animal models were built. 80 Quanming mice are divided into two groups A and B. In A group, there are 40 mice. First inject steroid, seven days later 1% 75mg/kg xxxx was injected into abdominal cavity, then open it through cutting in with 0.5cm opening, expose spleen. 10ul H_{22} liver cells were injected to spleen capsule and presses 3-5min to prevent cells from flow out so that cells can flow into lymphatic system and blood system. After 11 days these animal were sacrified to get the liver and to count the tumor nodes in liver. The result show that in A, B groups, the tumors grew, however, the tumor number in A group are much more than those in B group. In A group there are 3-5 nodules which sizes are around 1mm. In B group there are 1-3 nodules.

The result showed us that metastasis is significantly related to immune systerm. When the immune system decrease s or when the medication inhibits the immune system, the tumors will grow up.

2. Experimental Study on Effects on the growth of tumor from spleen

In many years, effects of spleen on the anti-tumor immunity are receiving more and more attentions from people. Its anti-tumor effects are extremely complicated. At present there are many differences and doubts. For further investigating effects of spleen on the growth of tumor and understanding the relation between spleen and tumor immunity, the experimental surgical method is adopted to prepare Ehrlich ascites tumor model. Group without spleen should respectively remove spleen before and after the inoculation of cancer cells. Then by contrasting it to the group with spleen, we perform the following experiment to observe whether the splenectomy will affect tumor immune state.

[Material and Method]

1. Experimental Animal Grouping Kunming mice, no gender classification, mice age 50~60d, weight 15~20g, and quantity of 300. According to the group with or without spleen, different sequence of splenectomy and inoculation of cancer cells, they are divided into 5 groups. Then on the basis of various amounts of inoculated cells (1×10^4 ml or 1×10^7 ml) and different inoculated regions (abdominal cavity or subcutaneous), each group is further separated into subgroups A and B. The specific grouping is shown in the following table 1.

Table 1 Summary table of experimental animal grouping

Group Inoculation Method	cancer cells concentration 1×10^4/ml		cancer cells concentration 1×10^7/ml	
	percutaneous	transabdominal	percutaneous	transabdominal
Group I simulating spleen removal	I A$_1$ (15)	I A$_2$ (15)	I B$_1$ (15)	I B$_2$ (15)
Group II (spleen removal before inoculation)	II A$_1$ (15)	II A$_2$ (15)	II B$_1$ (15)	II B$_2$(15)
Group III (inoculation before spleen removal)	III A (30)		III B (30)	
Group IV (spleen removal before inoculation+ splenic cells)	IV A$_1$ (15)	II A$_2$ (15)	IV B$_1$ (15)	IV B$_2$ (15)
Group V (administration of Chinese medicine)	V A (15)		V B (15)	

The Fourth Section Experimental Study

Group I: Control group with spleen. Firstly simulating spleen removal, after 7d transabdominal or percutaneous inoculation of Ehrlich ascites cancer cells 0.1ml, the number of cancer cells is 1×10^4 or 1×10^7 (table 2).

Table 2 Control group of simulating spleen removal (Group I)

Group I	Inoculated Cancer Cell Number	Inoculated Regions	Mice Number
I A$_1$	0.1×10^4	right armpit subcutaneousness	15
I A$_2$	0.1×10^4	abdominal cavity	15
I B$_1$	0.1×10^7	right armpit subcutaneousness	15
I B$_2$	0.1×10^7	abdominal cavity	15

Group II: Group of spleen removal before inoculation. Firstly spleen removal, after 7d percutaneous or transabdominal inoculation of Ehrlich ascites cancer cells 0.1ml, the number of cancer cells is 1×10^4 or 1×10^7 (table 3).

Table 3 Group of spleen removal before inoculation

Group II	Inoculated Cancer Cell Number	Inoculated Regions	Mice Number
II A$_1$	0.1×10^4	right armpit subcutaneousness	15
II A$_2$	0.1×10^4	abdominal cavity	15
II B$_1$	0.1×10^7	right armpit subcutaneousness	15
II B$_2$	0.1×10^7	abdominal cavity	15

Group III: Group without spleen, i.e. group of inoculation before spleen removal. Firstly inoculation of cancer cells, after 7d spleen removal. Both are right armpit subcutaneous inoculations. The number of cancer cells is 1×10^4ml or 1×10^7ml (table 4).

Table 4 Group of inoculation before spleen removal

Group III	Inoculated Cancer Cell Number	Inoculated Regions	Mice Number
III A	0.1×10^4	right armpit subcutaneousness	15
III B	0.1×10^7	right armpit subcutaneousness	15

Group IV: Group of spleen removal before inoculation, and further transabdominal transplantation of splenic cells or clear liquid of splenic tissue. Firstly remove spleen, after 7d inoculate cancer cells. In another 1d, transabdominal injection of living spleen cell suspension or supernatant liquid of splenic tissue (table 5).

Table 5 Group of spleen removal before transplantation of splenic cells or clear liquid of splenic tissue

Group IV	Inoculated Cancer Cell Number	Inoculated Regions	Processing Factor	Mice Number
IV A$_1$	0.1×10^4	trans-sub right armpit	injection of supernatant liquid of splenic tissue	15

IV A$_2$	0.1×10^4	transabdominal	injection of supernatant liquid of splenic tissue	15
IV B$_1$	0.1×10^7	right armpit subcutaneousness	transplantation of splenic cells of newborn mice	15
IV B$_2$	0.1×10^7	abdominal cavity	transplantation of splenic cells of adult mice	15

Group V: Group of taking Traditional Chinese Medicine (TCM) complex prescription with efficacy of strengthening the spleen and replenishing qi (table 6).

Table 6 Group of taking Traditional Chinese Medicine (TCM) complex prescription with efficacy of strengthening the spleen and replenishing qi

Group V	Inoculated Cancer Cell Number	Inoculated Regions	Processing Factor	Mice Number
V A	$10^7 \times 0.1$	right armpit subcutaneousness	firstly take TCM for 10d, after inoculation continue to take medication for 3 weeks	15
V B	$10^7 \times 0.1$	right armpit subcutaneousness	after inoculation take medication for 3 weeks	15

2. Instruments and Materials

(1) An animal sterile operating room and a set of sterile surgical instruments.

(2) Hank liquid, improved Hank liquid, calf serum, PRH, triple-distilled water, 0.9% sodium chloride solution for injection, ketamine, soluble phenobarbital, heparin sodium, trypan blue stain, Giemsa stain, Wright's stain, hydrochloric acid baking soda, L-glutamic acid, sensitization and non- sensitization zymosan.

(3) Centrifugal machine with 400 rounds per minute, glass homogenizer, medicine vibrator, filtering metal gauze (size 1000), funnel, thermostat, baker, low temperature water tank, microscope, relative sterile workbench.

(4) Animal feed are refined pellet feed. The drinking water is tap water. Rearing cage is plastic mouse cage.

3. Tumor Inoculation and Model Preparation

Ehrlich ascites tumor cell strain is introduced from Wuhan Biological Research Institute Cell Room. Ascites containing cancer cells are extracted from ascetic-type tumor animal abdominal cavity of mice Ehrlich ascites tumor. Firstly use improved Hank liquid to clean and centrifugate ascites for 3 times with 800 rounds per minute of centrifugal speed and five minutes. Remove supernatant liquid, and respectively combine deposited cancer cells with

Hank liquid to make up the cancer cell suspensions, containing 1×10^4 ml or 1×10^7 ml inoculated cells. The trypan blue dead cells exclusion test proves that the living cell rate is above 95%. Then inoculate cancer cells to experimental mice through right armpit subcutaneousness and abdominal cavity. Each mouse is inoculated with cancer cell suspension of 0.1ml, i.e. amounts of containing cancer cells are 1×10^4 ml or 1×10^7 ml.

4. Splenectomy Combine ketamine with soluble phenobarbital to execute intraperitoneal anesthesia. Dosages are 0.4mg/10g and 0.2mg/10g. After anesthesia, fix the mouse on surgery board. Shear the belly fur. Use iodine (2.5%) and ethanol (75%) to disinfect the belly. Bespread the sterile cloth on it. An incision is made into each layer of abdominal wall tissue through left lower abdomen. Then enter into abdominal cavity. Expose and dissociate the spleen. Use silk thread of size 0 to ligate the splenic stalk. Excise the spleen. Ensure the strict sterile operation, gentle action and thorough hemostases. During the operation, notice whether there is a splenulus. In case there is, excise it together. For simulating spleen removal of control group, only open the abdominal cavity; pull but do not excise the spleen. Antibiotics are not used in and after the operation. Infection of incisional wound is 1.0%. After operation, continue to feed the mouse with refined pellet feed.

5. Preparations of Splenic Cell Suspension and Supernatant Liquid of Splenic Tissue

(1) Preparation of splenic cell suspension: Execute newborn Kunming mice of 24~48h or adult mice. An incision is made into abdominal wall to take out the spleen. Cut off peripheral envelope and adipose tissue of spleen. Use Hank liquid to irrigate them in sterile glass culture dish for 3 times. Then put spleen into the glass homogenizer. Add in Hank liquid for 5ml. Grind up the splenic tissue. Filter it with stainless silk net of size 100. Centrifugate the filtering medium (1000 rounds per minute, 10 min). Remove supernatant liquid. Use Hank liquid to dilute deposited cells and make up the splenic cell suspensions of 5×10^7/ml. Suspensions are dyed by trypan blue stain and proved that the living cell rate is above 97%. Then transplant splenic cell suspensions into abdominal cavity of experimental mouse. Each mouse can only accept splenic cell suspensions of 2ml which belong to one receptor.

(2) Preparation of splenic cell homogenate: After excising the spleen, use quick freezing (-20 centi degree) and rapid rewarming to induce the cracking of dead splenic cells proved by trypan blue stain and microscopic examination. Then centrifugate the filtering medium (1000 rounds per minute, 10 min). Reserve

supernatant liquid and remove deposits. Inject supernatant liquid through abdomen into the experimental mouse.

6. Observation Item

(1) Observe success ratio of cancer cell inoculation, occurrence time of subcutaneous tumor nodi and speed of tumor enlargement.

(2) Every day use vernier caliper to measure diameter and size of subcutaneous tumor nodi; measure mouse' weight; observe metastasis condition and moving degree.

(3) Observe the quality of life, fur color, vitality, state of nutrition, breath, mental state of tumor-bearing mice and survival time of bearing tumor.

(4) Observe abdominal shape and prohection of ascetic-type tumor-bearing mice. Also according to prohection state, divide ascites content into 5 grades.

Grade 0: the abdomen is not of fullness, without ascites, note as (-).

Grade 1: slight prohection of abdomen, with a little ascites, note as (+).

Grade 2: prohection of abdomen, with medium content of ascites, note as (++).

Grade 3: obvious prohection of abdomen, with more ascites, note as (+++).

Grade 4: shape of frog abdomen, with plentiful ascites, note as (++++).

During necropsy, measure the content of ascites, microscopic examination of cancer cell shape, count living cell rate and content.

(5) Determine immunologic functional condition of red blood cells of tumor-bearing mice: test for measuring C_3b receptor garland with semi quantitative method.

(6) Necropsy and pathological section: dissect each dead experimental mouse. Observe tumor's size and weight, infiltrating and metastatic condition, morphological structure and involvement condition of visceral organs; measure the content of ascites; extract tumor tissue, liver, spleen, thymus gland, lung and other visceral organs to carry out the examination of pathological section.

[Experimental Result]

1. Resulting comparison and analysis on different groups with right armpit subcutaneous inoculation of small dose of 0.1×10^4 ml Ehrlich ascites tumor cells.

(1) Comparison on occurrence time of tumor nodi with different processing method (T test), see table 7.

Table 7 Comparison on occurrence time (d) of tumor nodi with different processing method (T test)

Group	Group I A$_1$ (Control group with spleen)	Group II A$_1$ (Group of spleen removal before inoculation)	Group IIIA (Group of inoculation before spleen removal)	Group IVA$_1$ (Spleen removal before inoculation+supernatant liquid of splenic tissue)
Occurrence time (d)	8	7*	9	9*

Note: ① *. Compared with Group I A$_1$, $P<0.05$ has remarkable significance; ② In Group I A$_1$ (control group with spleen), one experimental mouse (accounts for 7.6%) suffers no tumor nodi after inoculation of cancer cells. It survives for a long term (i.e. survival time is above 90d). No tumor is found during dissection. Treat it as inoculation failure. Not for statistical treatment; also in Group IVA (group with transabdominal injection of supernatant liquid of splenic tissue), 3 experimental mice (accounts for 25%) fail to be inoculated.

According to table 7, the earliest occurrence time of tumor nodi in above groups belongs to group of spleen removal before inoculation (Group II A$_1$). Control group and group with injection of supernatant liquid of splenic tissue have the later occurrence time.

(2) For different processing methods, maximum diameter comparison of each group's tumor nodi on the seventh, fourteenth and twentieth day, see table 8.

Table 8 Size comparison of each group's tumor nodi on the seventh, fourteenth and twentieth day after subcutaneous inoculation of 0.1×10^4 ml cancer cells (maximum diameter mm)

Group	Group I A$_1$ (Control group with spleen)	Group II A$_1$ (Group of spleen removal before inoculation)	Group III A (Group of inoculation before spleen removal)	Group IVA$_1$ (Spleen removal before inoculation+supernatant liquid of splenic tissue)	P
seventh	0	3.3±0.48	0	0	<0.01

fourteenth	11.43±5.99	14.4±6.2	11.8±7.45	8±4.33	<0.01
twentieth	18.92±9.98	21.12±8.28	19.7±5.98	13.89±7.63	<0.01

Note: Values P in the table are gained through analysis of diameter variance (F test).

From above results in the table, the tumor which belongs to group of spleen removal before inoculation (Group II A$_1$) appears first and grows fast. Before the fourteenth day, its tumor volume reaches biggest. On the twentieth day after inoculation, tumors' sizes of control group (Group I A$_1$), group II A$_1$ (group of spleen removal before inoculation), group of inoculation before spleen removal (Group III A) reach unanimity. While tumors which belong to group of injecting supernatant liquid of splenic tissue (Group IV A$_1$) have the smallest volume. That explains that during early growing stage of tumor (before the seventh day), spleen has tumor inhibitory action. But during medium and advanced stages (experimental group sets: medium stage is from eighth day to fourteenth day since the inoculation; since the fourteenth day, it is tumor advanced stage), the inhibitory action of spleen weakens or disappears. Furthermore, it can be observed that after cancer cells inoculation of spleen removal group, since the fourteenth day, tumor nodi often bear liquefaction, necrosis and ablation, which result in the shrinkage of tumor volume. Even some incisions have healed. Why does such phenomenon appear? That needs to have a further observation.

(3) Comparison of mean survival time (MST) for groups of subcutaneous inoculation with 0.1×10^4 ml cancer cells, see table 9.

Table 9 Comparison of each group's mean survival time (MST)

Group	Group I A$_1$ (Control group with spleen)	Group II A$_1$ (Group of spleen removal before inoculation)	Group III A (Group of inoculation before spleen removal)	Group IVA$_1$ (Spleen removal before inoculation+supernatant liquid of splenic tissue)	P
MST (d)	41.61±12.24	38.73±19.63	44.8±15.95	50±27.21	<0.05

Note: Values P in the table are gained through F test.

From table 9, mean survival times of groups I A$_1$, II A$_1$, III A are close to each other. T test shows there is no difference among these three groups, $P > 0.05$. While for injection of supernatant liquid of splenic tissue, mean survival time of this group is obviously longer than those of other groups, $P < 0.05$. The significant difference exists.

2. Resulting analysis of each group's transabdominal inoculation with 0.1×10^4 ml cancer cells After inoculation of cancer cells, experimental mice can survive above 90d without any ascite or tumor nodus. Also a dissection of corpse shows no tumor. The above results are treated as inoculation failures. It explains the fact that vaccinal cancer cells are rejected by the organism and no tumor forms.

(1) Comparison of inoculation failure rate for each group's transabdominal inoculation of 0.1×10^4 ml cancer cells without ascites, see table 10.

Table 10 Comparison of each group's inoculation failure rate (T test)

Group	Group I A$_2$ (Control group with spleen)	Group II A$_2$ (Group of spleen removal before inoculation)	Group II A$_2$ (Spleen removal before inoculation+supernatant liquid of splenic tissue)
failure rate	26%	0**	54%*

Note: **. indicates the comparison with control group, T test $P<0.01$, with high degree of significant difference; *. indicates $P<0.05$, with significant difference.

Results of table 10 show that all experimental mice in the group of spleen removal before inoculation form ascites, and failure rate is zero. The inoculation failure rates of control group with spleen and injection group of supernatant liquid of splenic tissue are 26% and 54% respectively. It process that tumor is easy to grow in the mouse without spleen after inoculation of tumor. That is, the removal of spleen promotes the growth of tumor. On the contrary, injection of supernatant liquid of splenic cells will suppress the growth of tumor.

(2) Comparison of survival time for each group's transabdominal inoculation of 0.1×10^4 ml cancer cells, see table 11.

Table 11 Comparison of each group's survival time (F test)

Group	Group I A$_2$ (Control group with spleen)	Group II A$_2$ (Group of spleen removal before inoculation)	Group IVA$_2$ (Spleen removal before inoculation+supernatant liquid of splenic tissue)	P
survival time (d)	51.46±29.35	35.6±18.93	57.6±14.85	<0.05

From table 11, the mean survival time of group with spleen removal before inoculation is 35.6±18.93 days. While mean survival times of control group with spleen and injection group of supernatant liquid of splenic tissue are 51.46±29.35 days and 57.6±14.85 days respectively, and P<0.05. Significant differences exist among these three groups. In three groups, group of spleen removal before inoculation has the shortest survival time. Group with spleen owns long survival time; while group without spleen owns short survival time. That shows the removal of spleen promotes the growth of tumor and shortens survival times of tumor-bearing mice. On the contrary, injection of supernatant liquid of splenic cells will suppress the growth of tumor and prolong survival times of tumor-bearing mice.

3. Results of each group's subcutaneous inoculation with 0.1×10^7 ml cancer cells

(1) Comparison on occurrence time of each group's subcutaneous tumor nodi, see table 12.

Table 12 Comparison on occurrence time of each group's subcutaneous tumor nodi

Group	Group I B$_1$ (Control group with spleen)	Group II B$_1$ (Group of spleen removal before inoculation)	Group III B (Group of inoculation before spleen removal)	Group IV B$_1$ (Spleen removal before inoculation+transplantation of fetal mouse's splenic cells)	P
Occurrence time (d)	5.5	5	7.5	9	<0.05

Mice of group IIIB are removed spleens on the seventh day after inoculations. So after seven days group IIIB and control group with spleen (Group I B$_1$) are in the same condition. The table shows that for the group with spleen removal first, occurrence times of subcutaneous tumor nodi are slightly earlier than these of other groups. While for group IVB$_1$ (transplantation of fetal mouse's splenic cells), occurrence times of tumor nodi are obviously later than these of other groups. It proves that the removal of spleen promotes the growth of tumor. While transplantation of splenic cells intensively suppresses the growth of tumor.

(2) Comparison of maximum diameter average on each group's subcutaneous tumor nodi on the seventh, fourteenth and twentieth day after inoculation, see table 13.

Table 13 Comparison of maximum diameter on each group's tumor nodi on the seventh, fourteenth and twentieth day (mm)

Group	Group I B₁ (Control group with spleen)	Group II B₁ (Group of spleen removal before inoculation)	Group III B (Group of inoculation before spleen removal)	Group IV B₁ (Spleen removal before inoculation+transplantation of fetal mouse's splenic cells)	P
seventh	5.07±1.847	10.88±5.278	2.83±1.948	3.0±1.56	<0.01
fourteenth	19.85±4.598	21.12±5.3	20.3±6.07	11±5.69	<0.01
twentieth	30.9±7.87	24±7.86	25.25±4.77	16±4.95	<0.01

Note: Values P in the table are gained through F test.

(3) Comparison of each group's mean survival time (MST), see table 14.

Table 14 Comparison of each group's mean survival time (subcutaneous inoculation of 0.1×10^7 ml cancer cells)

Group	Group I B₁ (Control group with spleen)	Group II B₁ (Group of spleen removal before inoculation)	Group III B	Group IV B₁ (Spleen removal before inoculation+transplantation of fetal mouse's splenic cells)	P
MST (d)	33.1±13.15	49.56±24.39	38.7±14.45	50.75±19.30	<0.01

From table 13 and 14, on the seventh day after inoculation, for the three groups-control group with spleen (Group IB₁), group of spleen removal before inoculation (Group IIB₁) and group of inoculation before spleen removal (Group IIIB), their maximum diameter averages of tumor nodi are $\bar{X}$ (IB₁) = (5.07±1.847) mm, $\bar{X}$ (IIB₁) = (10.88±5.278) mm, $\bar{X}$ (IIIB) = (2.83±1.948) mm respectively. $P<0.01$. Significant differences exist among these three groups. Tumors which belong to the group of spleen removal before inoculation (IIB₁) have the maximum volumes. Now on the seventh day, in fact groups IB₁ and IIIB have the spleen, which is in proliferative active phase. While group IIB₁ has no spleen. The tumor volume of group with spleen is smaller, and the tumor volume of group without spleen is larger. It indicates that the spleen can suppress tumor during early stage or the removal of spleen can promote the growth of tumor. While on the fourteenth day after inoculation, their average maximum diameters of tumor nodi are $\bar{X}$ (IB₁) = (19.85±4.598) mm, $\bar{X}$ (IIB₁) = (21.12±5.3) mm, $\bar{X}$ (IIIB) = (20.3±6.07) mm respectively. $P>0.05$. Significant differences disappear among these three groups. On the twentieth day after inoculation, the tumor volume of control group with spleen is larger than that of other groups. The maximum diameter $\bar{X}$ = (30.9±7.87) mm. At this time, the spleen of tumor-bearing mouse has extremely shrank, and lost the tumor inhibitory action. From the experiment, since the fourteenth day after inoculation, most mice tumors of group with spleen removal begin to bear liquefaction and necrosis. Some lumps ulcerate and ablate, whose volumes shrink. The reason that tumors in this period suffer from liquefaction, necrosis and ulceration is not clear at present. That needs to have a further observation.

Therefore, during the early stage of tumor, spleen can suppress the growth of tumor. For the group with spleen, the tumor growth rate is slower. Tumor volume is smaller. While on the advanced stage of tumor, the inhibitory action of spleen weakens or disappears. The tumor size of all groups reaches unanimity.

Furthermore, it can be seen from the stable that tumors of the group (IVB_1), which removes spleen before inoculation and transplants splenic cells of fetal mice, have obviously slower growth rate than that of other groups. The tumor volume is smaller. Its survival time is longer that that of other groups. These conditions prove that splenic cells of homogeneous variant fetus have obvious tumor-inhibitory action.

4. Results of each group's transabdominal inoculation with 0.1×10^7 ml cancer cells

(1) Comparison on occurrence time of ascites for each group, see table 15.

Table 15 Comparison on occurrence time of ascites for each group of transabdominal inoculation with 0.1×10^7 ml cancer cells

Group	Group I B_2 (Control group with spleen)	Group II B_2 (Group of spleen removal before inoculation)	Group IV B_2 (Spleen removal before inoculation+transplantation of splenic cells)
Occurrence time (median, d)	5	3*	4*

Note: **. indicates the comparison with control group, T test $P<0.05$, with significant difference.

(2) Occupying percentages of ascites content greater than (++) for groups on the fifth, seventh and fourteenth day after transabdominal inoculation of 0.1×10^7 ml cancer cells, see table 16.

Table 16 Comparison on ascites content of transabdominal inoculation with 0.1×10^7 ml cancer cells

Days after inoculation (d)	Group I B$_2$ (Control group with spleen)	Group II B$_2$ (Group of spleen removal before inoculation)	Group IV B$_2$ (Spleen removal before inoculation+transplantation of splenic cells)
2	0%	75% **	10% *
7	28%	100% **	70% *
14	100%	100%	100% *

Note: **. indicates the comparison with IB$_2$ (control group), T test $P<0.01$; *. indicates $P<0.05$; no *. indicates $P>0.05$.

(3) Comparison of survival time (d) for each group's transabdominal inoculation of 0.1×10^7 ml cancer cells, see table 17.

Table 17 Comparison of each group's survival time

Group	Group I B$_2$ (Control group with spleen)	Group II B$_2$ (Group of spleen removal before inoculation)	Group IV B$_2$ (Spleen removal before inoculation+transplantation of splenic cells)
survival time (d)	20.15±4.59	15.56±10.94*	16.67±8.34

Note: *. indicates the comparison with IB$_2$, $P<0.05$, with significant difference; no *. indicates the comparison with IB$_2$, $P>0.05$, without significant difference.

Integrating tables 15, 16 and 17, results show that for the group with spleen removal first (IIB$_2$), tumor growth rate is faster. Amounts of ascites are more. Survival time is shorter. Also visceral organs are easier to metastasize. Those explain that removal of spleen can promote the growth of tumor. Transabdominal transplantation of splenic cells of homogeneous variant adult mice can partially suppress the growth of tumor. But its inhibitory action is weaker than that of control group with spleen and group with transplantation of fetal mouse's splenic cells.

5. Results of necropsy and pathological examination Each mouse accepts the postmortem necropsy. Visually observe tumor shape, involved visceral organs and diffusion condition. And extract tissues for pathological section examination. The result shows that Ehrlich ascites tumor cell strain owns features of stable proliferation, strong invasiveness and so on. Subcutaneous inoculation is easy to induce the form of solid tumor. Necropsy proves that after inoculation tumors or ascites are easy to form in some regions, easily infiltrating to surrounding tissues. The metastases of

cancer cells rarely happen to mice with subcutaneous inoculation. While for mice with transabdominal inoculation, cancer cells easily metastasize to liver, kidney and lymph node in advanced stage. Only two of two hundred and seventy experimental mice suffer from splenic metastases, proving the weak affinity of spleen to cancer cells. This group of experiments has also found phenomena that for the group of spleen removal before transabdominal inoculation, multiple carcinomatous metastases appear in visceral organs of abdominal cavity. Metastatic ratio is up to 50%. These metastases invade liver, kidney, pancreas and mesenteric lymph nodes, always implicating more than two visceral organs. While for control group with spleen and group with transplantation of homogeneous variant splenic cells, carcinomatous metastases rarely occur. Metastatic ratios are 20% and 25%, which are obviously lower than those of the group without spleen. It shows that spleen can suppress the growth of tumor. While the group without spleens lose the inhibitory action, consequently leading to easy diffusion and metastasis of tumor.

Furthermore, dynamic observation of this group of experimental mice shows that thymus and spleen of tumor-bearing mice present a series of changes with the process of illness, which own certain regularity. About seven days after inoculation, the thymus presents acute and progressive atrophy. Its volume shrinks; the diameter of each normal lobule shortens from 5~8cm to about 1mm; the weight reduces from (70±10) mg to (20±5) mg. While soon after the inoculation of cancer cells, spleen becomes congested and tumid. The volume enlarges; weight increases; texture becomes fragile. Microscopic examination shows the increase of germinal centers and active cell proliferation. On the fourteenth day after inoculation, the spleen also quickly presents progressive atrophy. Its volume shrinks; the weight reduces from (140±15) mg to (50±10) mg. Germinal centers obviously decrease; cell proliferation is suffocated. The spleen also suffers from hyperplasia of fibrous tissues, fibrosis with gray color and rigid texture.

6. Testing results of erythrocytic immune function This group of experiments choose 100 mice to carry out the erythrocytic C_3b receptor garland test. The result shows that after the removal of spleen, bonding ratio of C_3b receptor garland of tumor-bearing mice is on a progressive declining tendency. That explains that after the removal of spleen, immunological adhesive competence of red blood cells drops to some extent.

[The analysis of the result]

1. As seen from experimental results, spleen can suppress the growth of tumor.

After the removal of spleen, compared with the control group, the growth rate is faster; the occurrence time and volume of subcutaneous tumor nodi is earlier and larger in the same period. For group with transabdominal inoculation of cancer cells and group with the removal of spleen, occurrence time of ascites is earlier; ascites content is greater; cells content is also higher. Survival time is shorter than that of control group. Necropsy finds that cancer metastatic rate of the group with the removal of spleen is 30% above that of control group (metastases to liver, kidney, pancreas and mesenteric lymph nodes). From table 13, group IIB_1 (spleen removal before inoculation) and group IIIB (inoculation before spleen removal) accept splenectomy in different time. On the seventh day after inoculation, maximum diameter averages of their subcutaneous tumor nodi are $\bar{X}(IIB_1) = (10.8 \pm 5.28)$ mm and $\bar{X}(IIIB) = (2.83 \pm 1.948)$ mm respectively. The former is obviously longer than the latter one. But on the fourteenth day after inoculation, the tumor of group IIIB quickly proliferates after the removal of spleen. The difference between them almost disappears. $\bar{X}(IIB_1) = (21.2 \pm 5.3)$ mm, $\bar{X}(IIIB) = (20.3 \pm 6.07)$, $P>0.05$, without significant difference. It prompts that the removal of spleen promotes the growth of tumor, i.e. spleen can suppress the growth of tumor.

In recent two decades, people find that spleen not only performs a great role in anti-infection, but also has the all-important influence on anti-tumor immunity. The active mechanism may be by producing Natural Killer cell, macrophage ($M\varphi$), Lympholine-Activated Killer cell, TH/Ti cell, B cell, Ts cell, etc. to realize the cellular immunity; and by secreting lymphokines of Tufisn factor, TNF factor, IL-2, interferon, addiment, antibody, etc. to kill tumor cells. Ge Yigong once used rat Lw56 pulmonary sarcoma model to the effect of removing spleen on tumor growth. Mr Ge holds that success ratio of tumor inoculation after the removal of spleen is higher than that of group with spleen. The metastatic ratio increases. Results are similar to this group of experimental results.

This group of experimental results also prompts that after the removal of spleen, bonding ratio of C_3b receptor garland of organism peripheral blood is 40% below that of healthy group with spleen. It explains that erythrocytic immune function of organism reduces after the removal of spleen.

2. Spleen's inhibiting action on tumor growth mainly occurs in the early stage of tumor course.

While in the advanced stage of tumor, spleen's inhibiting action on tumor growth weakens and disappears. As seen from tables 8 and 13, in the early stage of tumor (within 7d), the tumor of group without spleen has a faster tumor growth rate than that of control group with spleen. The volume of subcutaneous tumor nodi is large and ascites content is great. While in the advanced stage (after 14d) of tumor, tumor nodi of control group with spleen and group with the removal of spleen basically have the same volume. No significant comparability. No obvious difference between survival times. Necropsy and pathological examination of three hundred experimental mice find that spleen of tumor-bearing mice present a series of regular changes with the process of illness. In the early stage of tumor (within 7d after inoculation), due to the cytostimulation, the spleen becomes congested and tumid. The volume enlarges; cell proliferation accelerates; germinal centers increases. While in the advanced stage (since 14d after inoculation) of tumor, the spleen presents progressive atrophy. Its volume shrinks; germinal centers fall sharply. The spleen also suffers from hyperplasia of fibrous tissues. The fibrosis of spleen occurs; therefore, its anticancer immunization weakens or disappears. Even it can pass through the suppressor T cell. Macrophage and immune inhibiting factor can suppress the anticancer immunization of organism and promote the growth of tumor. That explains that spleen's effect on tumor immune state is bidirectional, has obvious time phase and is relevant to stadium. In early stage, the spleen owns the anti-tumor action. In advanced stage, the spleen owns immune inhibiting action. But the basic reason that leads to the immune inhibiting state of organism is the tumor itself. Spleen just plays a certain part in the forming process of this state.

3. Transabdominal injection of supernatant liquid of healthy splenic cells and transplantation of homogeneous variant splenic cells can suppress tumor growth.

For group of injection with supernatant liquid of splenic cells or transplantation of splenic cells (Group IV), comparative results with other groups show that the tumor growth rate is slower; the occurrence time of tumor nodi is later; the volume is smaller; ascites content is less. After the inoculation of small dose of 0.1×10^4 ml cancer cells, success ratio of inoculation for tumor-bearing mice is obviously lower than that of other groups. Moreover, after a little ascites or subcutaneous lesser tubercle firstly appearing in several mice, the tumor can disappear naturally. The survival time is above 90d (as long-term survivors). Especially splenic cells of homogeneous variant fetal mouse (group IVB_1) have obvious tumor-inhibitory action. The tumor inhibition rate is 54%. The survival time is 17d longer than that of control group. Pathological examinations of this group of tumor-bearing mice find that after transplantation of homogeneous variant fetal splenic cells, splenic islands grow on the abdominal cavity and (or) mesentery of seven mice (account for 50%). Pathological examination proves it as living splenic tissues. Fetal splenic cells have features of weak antigenicity, deficient quantity and strong cell proliferation, etc. After the transplantation of splenic cells of homogeneous variant mice, there is no sharp rejection. And moreover, it is not subject to blood group ABO. Do not need the cross test of different blood groups. Here in China some people use traumatic splenic cells to prepare LAK cells for treating advanced malignant tumors, which achieves better curative effects on inhibiting tumor growth and prolonging mouse's lifespan.

At present, adoptive immunotherapy of tumors with transplantation of fetal splenic cells has not yet been reported in the literature. This group of experiments needs to have a further observation.

4. Negative correlation between anti-tumor immunological action of the organism and the quantity of cancer cells

This group of experiments finds that anti-tumor immunological action of the organism is obviously affected by the quantity of inoculated cancer cells. The less the quantity of cancer cells, the stronger and more significant the anti-tumor effect; on the contrary, the weaker the anti-tumor effect. As for 0.1×10^7 ml inoculated cancer cells, immunological action of the organism is obviously suppressed. The tumor growth rates of group without spleen and group with spleen have bigger difference in the early stage. While after medium stage (after 7d), the difference will quickly disappear. There is also no significant difference in survival time. But for 0.1×10^4 ml inoculated cancer cells, anti-tumor action of the organism is relatively significant. The inoculated failure rate of group with spleen is obviously higher than that of group without spleen. The growth rate of tumor is slow; the volume of tumor nodi is small; and the survival time is long. Furthermore, after the transplantation of homogeneous variant splenic cells for small dose of inoculated cancer cells group, anti-tumor immunological action goes up remarkably. The growth rate of tumor decreases obviously. Some tumor nodi even can naturally disappear after its formation. Also the survival time is long. These results show the negative correlation between anti-tumor action of the organism and the quantity of inoculated cancer cells. While there is a positive correlation between cancer's immunological inhibiting action on the organism and the quantity of inoculated cancer cells. The spleen participates in tumor immunoregulation, which has double influences on immune state of tumor-bearing mice. In early stage, the spleen shows a certain anti-cancer action. As the development of tumor, the number of tumor cells is increasing. The spleen is shrinking gradually. Then the anti-cancer action is converted into immunological inhibiting action. But the basic reason of immune inhibiting state is the tumor itself. The progress of cancer, an increase in the number of cancer cells and the reinforcement of inhibiting action lead to the atrophia of spleen, thymus gland and other immune organs.

5. Experimental result prompts of this group

(1) The spleen has certain anti-tumor effects. In tumor's early stage, spleen can suppress the growth of tumor. While in advanced stage of the course of disease, the anti-tumor action of spleen weakens or disappears. The spleen even can promote the growth of spleen.

(2) Adoptive immunotherapy of tumors with transplantation of homogeneous variant splenic cells of fetal mice can reinforce anti-tumor immunological action of the organism, and suppress the growth of tumor.

(3) There is a negative correlation between anti-tumor action of the organism and the quantity of inoculated cancer cells. The more the quantity of cancer cells, the more easily the immunological action of the organism is suppressed or damaged. The faster the growth rate of tumor, the worse the prognosis.

3. The Experimental Observation of Effects on Thymus and Spleen from Tumor

It is usually considered that the immune functions of organisms affect the occurrence, development and prognosis, however at the same time tumors can inhibit the immune state of organisms. These two are mutually causal and intricate and complicated. When doing the animal experiments on the influences of spleen on the tumorous growth, the author have observed that the immune organs thymus, spleen of the cancer-bearing mice have changed a lot. It seems that this process presents a certain law. In order to study further on the relationship and laws between tumors and spleens or thymus, the following experiments are designed to observe dynamically the changes of conversion rates of thymus, spleen and lymphocyte of cancer-bearing mice in different phases and probe into the relationship between them. First, let's review the anatomy and physiology of the thymus.

1). Anatomy and physiology of thymus

1> Shape and position of the thymus

Thymus is cone-shaped and can be divided into left and right which are not symmetrical two leaves which is soft, elongated flat strip and is connected by connective tissue. The size of the thymus has a large difference in different age groups. Thymus grows fast in late period of embryonic development and neonatal, from birth to 2 years old, is the best period of development of the thymus, weighing 15 ~ 20g. With age, the thymus continues to develop to increase, but lower than during postnatal development is relatively slow to reach puberty 25 ~ 40g. After puberty, the thymus begins to shrink degradation. Adult thymus still maintain the original shape, but its structure has changed dramatically, a significant reduction in lymphocytes, thymus tissue is replaced by fat tissue more.

The adult thymus is behind sternum and on the front of mediastinum. Its rear is with the innominate vein and aortic arch adjacent to both sides of the adjacent mediastinal pleura and lung. Thymoma and thymic enlargement can compress the above organs, corresponding clinical symptoms.

Children thymus is larger, upper end extending root of the neck, some up to the lower edge of the thyroid gland, the lower end can be inserted into the anterior mediastinum, pericardial up front.

2>. Thymus structure

(1) Capsule or Coating: thymus tissue surface is coated with a film, a film composed of dense collagen fibers, elastic fiber and matrix and other substance. Coating of the connective tissue fibers extends into the substance of the thymus, the thymus is divided into many lobules. Leaflets are around the cortex, medulla is in the dark side, between the two there is a mesh stent composed of epithelial cells.

(2) Cortex: thymic cortex is located around the portion of the leaflets by dense lymphocytes and epithelial reticular cells. Lymphocytes near cortex is large which is original cell type. Middle lymphocytes were medium-sized, mostly small Lingpa is in the inner layer. Scattered macrophages is within the cortex. Hematopoietic stem cell proliferation and differentiation of T lymphocytes process is from shallow to deep.

(3) Medulla: thymic medulla is located deep leaflets by epithelial reticular cells and a small number of lymphocytes in the composition. Thymus bodies have scattered in the medulla. Small generally circular or oval, is made of several layers of epithelial reticular cells, arranged in concentric circles.

3>. Thymus function

A. **Secretion function**: Thymus function is more complex, the thymus is lymphoid organs and have endocrine functions. Some authors will be included in the endocrine system. Its main function is to develop and manufacture T lymphocytes and thymic hormone secretion. T cells within the thymus cultivate, need a suitable internal environment. Thymic epithelial reticular cells can secrete a variety of solidarity hormones: thymosin, thymus erythropoietin (thymopoietin), thymosin, thymic humoral factor(THF) and ubiquitin, etc. These hormones and macrophages within the thymus, Interdigitating cells together form a nurturing T cell microenvironment. Thymosin and thymopoietin can promote lymphoid stem cell differentiation to T cells, stimulation of T cell proliferation, the stimulation of the hypothalamus secrete ACTH and LH; thymopoietin can induce T cell differentiation; other hormones can promote early T cell division and have to promote synergy of T cell maturation.

Original lymph stem cells don't have immune function; have been further converted into T cells with immune function, then migrate to peripheral lymphoid organs, such as lymphoid tissue, lymph nodes, spleen, etc. by blood circulation to be involved in the immune response after antigen activation of proliferation. Although adult thymus atrophy and degradate, but there is still the ability to secrete thymic hormones. When the body's lymphoid tissue damage, T cells have a significant reduction. In thymic hormone action lymphoid stem cells in thymus can still be converted to T cells.

T lymphocyte

Two distinct types of thymocytes are produced in the thymus: CD4/CD8. All T cells originate from haematopoietic stem cells in the bone marrow. In the bone marrow haematopoietic stem cells become haematopoietic progenitors; on the way to thymus haematopoietic progenitors are expanded by cell division to generate a large population of immature thymocytes; in the thymus the earlist thymocytes are *double- negative* (CD4$^-$CD8$^-$) cells, later become *double-positive* thymocytes (CD4$^+$CD8$^+$); finally mature to *single-positive* (CD4$^+$CD8$^-$ or CD4$^-$CD8$^+$) thymocytes. About 98% of thymocytes die during the development processes in the thymus by failing either positive selection or negative selection, whereas 2% matured naïve T cells leave the thymus and begin to spread throughout the body, including the lymph nodes. As the thymus shrinks by about 3% a year throughout middle age, there is a corresponding fall in the thymic production of naive T cells, leaving peripheral T cell expansion to play a greater role in protecting older subjects. Lymphocytes differentiate and develop in Thymus.

T cell differentiation during development phenotypic change

Now known to induce T cell differentiation in the thymus, mature main factors include: ① thymic stromal cells (thymus stromalcell, TSC) interact directly with thymocytes by adhesion molecules on the cell surface; ② thymic stromal cells secrete a variety of cytokines (such as IL-1, IL-6, IL-7) and thymus hormone-induced thymocyte differentiation; ③ thymus cells themselves secrete a variety of cytokines (such as IL-2, IL-4) on thymocyte differentiation and maturation itself also It plays an important role. In addition, within thymic epithelial cells, macrophages and dendritic cells to thymocytes differentiation of self-tolerance, as well as the formation of MHC-restricted T cell subsets play a decisive role.

B. Thymus exocrine

Thymic hormone vitality can be detected by available bioassay method. The experiment proved the vitality of the thymus hormone decline with increasing age, with thymic atrophy and decreased removal of the thymus in an animal serum can not be measured, the thymus is the main origin of thymic hormone thymus hormone is a hormone secreted substance thymocytes, regulate immune function utility.

The thymus is the body's immune function important organization, secrete and generate thymosin (thymulin other hormones), and secrete intrinsic function and viability IL-1 and IL-2 and other interleukins ingredient to adjust the thymus; the same time regulated by the pituitary secretion of prolactin. Visibly, now the research of immunomodulatory thymus primarily provide evidence indicating that exogenous hormone (such as prolactin, growth hormone, thyroxine, etc.) can rejuvenate the thymus induced recession, maintain immunomodulatory force. Thymic involution can be reversed, it is common to study the development prospects of modern immunology and endocrinology.

C. Thymus immune function

From the beginning it is believed that it was independent to other physiological systems controlled single regulatory system, the development so far is that the thymus and the neuroendocrine system is interconnected functional network system harmonization. Since the late 1970s, Besedovsky (1977) proposed neuroendocrine immune network theory (NIM), has been recognized as the thymus and immune function to guide the core idea. Thymus and central nervous system and peripheral immune response functions form the system's three-point line connection. Central cerebral cortex, hypothalamus, pituitary regulation center is higher; peripheral lymphoid organs and tissues, cells and cytokines to regulate and implementation units subordinate immune network; intermediate hub of the thymus, can be called NIM middle line. NIM path can be divided into three: ① down line that reached down from the central median line and off the assembly line each unit; ② uplink from each cytokine offline feedback information to the central site; ③ middle line access to thymus for the spindle,

25

combined with the spleen and other lymphoid tissue and bone marrow progenitor cell nucleus. Recent studies have shown that the thymus plays an important role in the NIM activities. For example, Fabres (1983) put forward - the concept of "thymic neuroendocrine network", Goldstein AL (1983) that "neuroendocrine - thymus axis" of thought, expression can be described as the thymus special significance in the NIM network.

Thymus starts to degrade after sexual maturity, secreted thymosin and other hormones are also reduced, so that blocked T lymphocyte differentiation, decreased immune function. The main reason for human and mammalian aging degeneration has the close relation to atrophy of the thymus.

While Increasing age, thymic atrophy naturally and life is gradually aging, the thymus is an important factor affecting the level of the body's immunity. Experiments show that adult rats (2 months) removal of the thymus can accelerate its own immune dysfunction and aging. Rats (2 months) after surgery six months to the thymus, the spleen lymphocyte immune activity decreased, only of 51.6% in the same age did not remove the thymus.

The Body's immune function, especially cellular immune, T lymphocyte function decreases with age, the structure and function of thymus gradually degenerate in adulthood. Thymus is a central organ of immune system and the base of T lymphocyte differentiation and maturation. Thymic epithelial cells produce and release Thymosin which plays an important role in differentiating T lymphocyte precursors into mature T cell immune activity. Thymus is the first organ of the body degradation, and then began a decline after sexual maturity, the ability to produce and secrete thymosin also gradually decreased with age.

Thymus research began in the early 1960s, it was found that closely related to immune function. Miller et al (1960) found that the thymus to animals (neonatal mice) immune function hypoplasia, the number of circulating T cells was significantly reduced. Since 50 years thymus has been recognized as the center of the organ animal immune system, is the first body's organs mature, the structure and function of the thymus reach a peak while sexual maturity, and thereafter with age gradually shrinking and degradation, which immune function in adult animals is gradually being replaced by the spleen and other lymphoid tissues. The thymus is the core of tissue T lymphocyte development, but it is also the base of producing a variety of immune factors (lymphokines, cytokines), thymosin is the main secretion of immune modulators, now has a variety of thymosin (peptide) products for the Clinical and Experimental Research. Foreign specialized periodicals have been called "thymus" (thymus), regularly publishes reports on the thymus research and clinical treatment.

2). The experimental study on tumor bearing mice

[Material and Methods]

A. Experimental animal and grouping

Use 40 Kunming mice and divide into four groups at random with the age of 40~50days and the weight of 15~18g, ignoring the sexes.

Group I: Control group of healthy mice which are not inoculated with cancer cells. After executing them, take away their thymus, spleens and circumferential blood to do the experiment.

Group II: Inoculate the mice with 0.1×10^7 ehrlich ascites carcinoma through abdominal cavity, execute them after 3 days and observe.

Group III: Inoculate the mice with cancer cells (as the above) execute them after 7 days and observe.

Group IV: Inoculate the mice with cancer cells, execute them after 14 days and observe.

Use the results of anatomizing 100 cancer-bearing mice after natural death as the alterant results of thymus and spleen in terminal period. In this period the average diameter of thymus of cancer-bearing mice is 1.2 ± 0.3mm, average weight is 20 ± 5 mg with a bit hard texture. While spleens are extremely easy to atrophy, whose average weight is 60 ± 12mm, texture is hard, and its color is gray, with the germinal center reducing and fibrosing.

B. Experimental methods

Execute the mice of each group by digging out their eyes and blooding them at the preconcerted time. Reserve the whole blood of each mouse (using heparin for anti-coagulation) to do the experiment of lymphocyte conversion and then anatomize them immediately; observe the range of soakage, volume of ascites and the situation of all viscera; emphasize on observing the anatomical shape of thymus, spleens and lymph nodes and take out the thymus and spleen integrally, then measure their volume with a vernier caliper; weigh them respectively using analytical balance and send them to the department of defection.

C. Measuring the conversion rate of peripheral blood lymphocytes of mice in each group

Measure by digging out their eyes and blood with heparin for anti-coagulation.

D. Making tumor model

As same as the experimental part 1.

【Experimental Result】

1. Thymic weights of mice in each group after inoculated with cancer cells in different phases (see table 1)

Do analysis of variance with the statistical data in table 1, see table 2. Using a curve to present the results of table 1 and table 2, draw the curve of change in the thymic weights (chart 1); the thymic weights of the 25th day and 30th day in the chart are quoted from the results of the experimental part 1.

Table 1 Comparison of thymic weights of mice in each group (mg)

Group	Group I healthy	Group II on the 3rd after inoculated	Group III on the 7th after inoculated		Group IV on the 14th after inoculated
	72.8	78.2	90.0		40.0
	50.0	83.4	66.0		32.2
	56.4	89	85.4		39.8
	96.4	68	106.5		23.5
	77.4	74.8	51.7		38.0
X_i	100.7	95.4	77.8		36.0
	87.5	115.0	73.0		46.0
	76.8	56.4	60.0		20.0
	112.7	43.0	49.4		55
	51.0				20
ΣX	781.87	703.2	736.3	350.5	ΣX 2 571.7
N_i	10	9	10	10	N 39
$\bar{X}_i$	78.17	78.13	73.63	35.05	$\bar{X}$ 65.94
$\Sigma_i X^2$	6 6261.79	58 566.66	57 033.75	18 467.25	ΣX^2 191 324.75

Table 2 Analysis of variance of table 1

Resources of variation	SS	V	MS	F	P
Between groups	12967.10	3	4322.36	12.85	<0.01
Within groups	11777.12	35	336.48		

28

It can be noticed that thymuses of the cancer-bearing mice present the regular change from

Table 1, table 2 and chart 1. Within 7 days after inoculation, thymuses have no obvious change observed by eyes; however their weights begin to lose weight. After 7 days, they present acute progressive atrophy; in the later period, the diameter of the thymuses reduce from the normal level 5~8 mm to about 1mm and the weights decrease from 76.1mg to 20mg with the texture becoming hard and the functions declining even lost, which indicates that the cellular immune functions are operated and inhibited increasingly with the development of tumors, and the immune functions are declined to a lower level with tumors growing more and more rapidly.

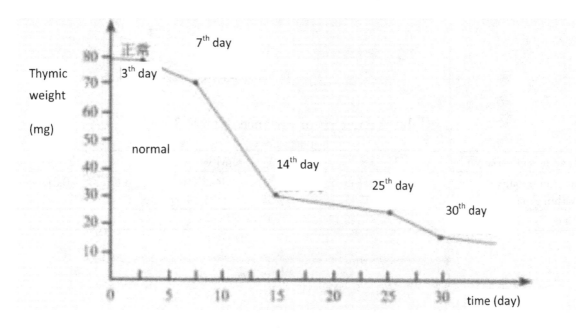

Chart 1 the curve of variation on the thymic weights

2. Splenic weights of mice in each group after inoculated with cancer cells in different phases (see table 3 and 4)

Table 3 splenic weights of cancer-bearing mice in each group in different phases

Group	Group I healthy	Group II on the 3rd after inoculated	Group III on the 7thafter inoculated		Group VI on the 14th after inoculated
组别	I 组正常组	II 组接种后第 3 天	III 组第 7 天		IV 组第 14 天
	98.4	103.0	152.8		120.7
	86.0	110.3	175.8		96.9
	139.0	153.2	154.5		103.0
	126.0	96.7	154.0		102.0
	194.4	206.0	290.4		91.0
X_i	130	137.0	156.0		122.3
	107.4	174.0	184.0		88.6
	82.8	143.0	232.0		109.0
	86.0	160	86.3		102.4
	82.0				119.0
ΣX	1 256.4	1 209.0	1 720.9	1 021	ΣX 5 210.2
N_i	10	9	9	10	N 38
$\bar{X}_i$	125.84	134.43	172.09	102.1	$\bar{X}$ 133.59
ΣX^2	169 020.88	175 088.97	322 834.65	106.41	ΣX^2 773.385

Table 4 Analysis of variance of table 3

Resources of variation	SS	V	MS	F	P
Between groups	25345.12	3	8448	5.68	<0.01
Within groups	51983	35	1485.24		
Total	77328.12	38			

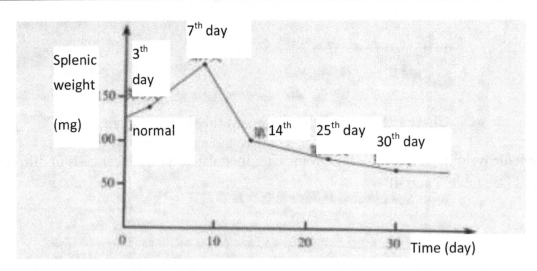

Chart 2 the curve of variation on the splenic weights

Inspect the 100 corpses in the experimental group in part 1 and get the average splenic weight is 60+12 mg. Use a curve to describe the change in splenic weights (chart 2).

From the statistical data in table 3, 4 and chart 2, it can be found that spleens of cancer- bearing mice in the early stage the volume is enlarging gradually and the weight is increasing, while in the later stage, the spleens present progressive atrophy. The above indicates that in the early period, cellular proliferation is active and the effects of immune response are reinforced as well as the inhibition on tumors due to the tumor simulation so as to react on inhibiting the growth of tumors; while in the latter period, as the number has enlarged plentifully, a great of inhibitory factors are produced to inhibit cells and immunity to stop the proliferation of splenic immune cells and consume effector cells, which results in atrophy and fabric tissue hyperplasia, the inhibition on tumors is weakened even promote the growth of tumors.

3. Comparison of experimental results of peripheral blood lymphocytes of the cancer-bearing mice conversion at different time (see table 5 and 6)

Table 5 Comparison of the conversion rate of peripheral blood lymphocytes in each group at different time (%)

Group I healthy	Group II on the 3rd after inoculated	Group III on the 7th after inoculated	Group VI on the 14th after inoculated		
45	53	43	31		
40	62	32	28		
51	48	26	19		
42	43	45	21		
60	52	30	22		
39	51	32	23		
	50				
ΣX 277	359	208	144	ΣX	988
N, 6	7	6	6	N	25
X̄ 46.17	51.29	24		X̄	39.52
ΣX² 13 111	18 611	7 498	3 560	ΣX²	12 780

Table 6 Analysis of variance of table 5

Resources of variation	SS	V	MS	F	P
Between groups	2820.64	3	940.21	21.614	<0.01
Within groups	913.59	21	43.51		
Total	3734.23	24			

Using a curve to present the results of table 5 and table 6, draw the curve of lymphocyte conversion rate of the cancer-bearing mice at different time (chart 3).

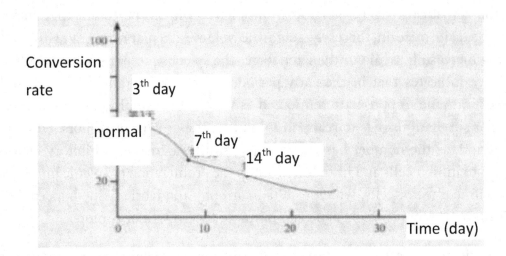

Chart 23-3 curve of lymphocyte conversion rate

From table 5, 6 and chart 3, it can be seen that the change in lymphocyte conversion rate of the cancer-bearing mice presents certain regularity: after inoculation the conversion rate increase slightly and then presents an acute progressive decrease. Until 14th day (later period), it declines to normal level about 50% and continue declining after that, which indicates that in the whole course of diseases, tumors produce inhibitory effect on the cellular immunity; what's more, with the course of diseased this effect becomes more intensive and the immune functions are damaged.

From chart 1, 2 and 3 it can be known that the changes in thymic volume and weight are extremely similar to the curve of lymphocyte conversion rate presented as synchronism. By contrast, the changes in splenic volume and weight are different from them with increase in the early period and the decrease, which indicates that during the middle and later period, both the organismal humoral immunity and cellular immunity are damaged and inhibited.

4. Changes of thymic and splenic pathology

(1) Thymus presents progressive atrophy during the whole course of disease; on the 3rd day after inoculated with cancer cells, thymus shrinks slightly and the color is gray; on the 7th day, thymic volume shrinks obviously and the cellular proliferation is stopped with reduced mature cells; during the later period of tumors, thymus shrinks extremely and its volume is as big as a sesame with the diameter of 1 mm and hard texture.

(2) Spleen is congested and tumefied; the volume is augmenting with being black red and crisp. The number of germinal centers increase and mature decrease; while from the 14th day after inoculation, spleen also presents progressive atrophy.

Discussion

1. The effect of tumor on the structure and function of the spleen

The experimental results show that the tumor affects the immune function of the body, the spleen of tumor-bearing mice will have a regular change. In the early stage it is splenomegaly, active cell proliferation, germinal centers increased, mature cells increased, the inhibition of tumor growth, The late spleen showed progressive atrophy, cell proliferation is limited, the germinal center decreased, accompanied by fibrous tissue proliferation and fibrosis, hard texture, loss of anti-tumor immunity. Why does spleen have such a change? The mechanism is unclear, which need to be further explored, presumably as follows: on the one hand tumor cells stimulate the host immune system through the tumor-specific antigen, to stimulate the immune effect to kill tumor cells, to get the protective effect on the body. On the other hand, tumor cells can induce inhibition of immune cells T suppressor cells and macrophages) and the production of inhibitory factors, together with tumor cells secrete many immunosuppressive factors, thereby inhibiting the body's immune anticancer effect, to escape the immune killer effect, then to survive and develop. The spleen is the body's largest peripheral Lymphoid organs, can produce immune lymphocytes and antibodies, and can produce anti-tumor effect of body fluid molecules Tuftisin. When cancer cells invade the body early, spleen is stimulated and gets response, cell proliferation is active, and the function is strong and it produces more immune effector cells and lymphokines which can inhibit the growth of the tumor. In the late stage, due to tumor progression, it results in a large number of immunosuppressive factors, leading to spleen atrophy; its function is limited or injury, and thus lost the positive role of anti-tumor immunity.

2. The effect of tumor on Thymus

The results of the tumor on the thymus showed that after inoculation of tumor cells, thymus is inhibited immediately, and the whole progressive atrophy, thymus thus immediately lost the anti-tumor immune response.

Observed in experiments: shortly after inoculation of tumor cells the morphological change of thymus occurs, and the whole course was progressive atrophy. To advanced cancer, thymus by weight of 78.13 ± 13.2mg decreased to 20 ± 5mg, the volume is reduced by the diameter of 5 ~ 8mm to 1mm. Cell proliferation was blocked.

Since the thymus atrophy, cell proliferation is blocked, reduced or mature cell depleted, the index declined, weakening the metabolism, decreased cell viability, with thymic hormone secretion also decreased and cellular immune function is inevitably damage, the defense capability in mice is low, namely a large number of cancer cells transplanted grew and reproduced. Similar reports by Zhang Tong Wen et al. was that mice thymus atrophy, it is also accompanied by the proliferation of bone marrow cells is blocked, nucleated cell activity decreased, and believe there is a close relationship between the two. Thus, inhibition of tumor or injury of host immune function is multifaceted, affecting the body's entire immune system. The group of lymphocyte transformation rate tests showed that after inoculation of cancer cells, the lymphocyte transformation rate decreased progressively, until late fall more than 50 percent, also shows that immune effector cells is inhibited. As for why the thymus of mice was inhibited atrophy requires further experimental research and observation.

Thymus also produces a variety of hormones, to promote the differentiation of immune lymphoid stem cell maturation. Although thymus is lymphoid organs, but due to the presence of blood thymus barrier, thymus doesn't contact with the antigens directly to play a role in the effect. Therefore there are not tumor-specific antigen stimulation and proliferation of enlargement. The tumors secrete immunosuppressive factors able to act on the thymus, so that thymus is atrophy, dysfunction.

Immunotherapy cancer, many doctors committed to developing great interest in this area.

Since the 1980s, due to the rapid development of immunology and biotechnology, provided an opportunity for tumor underwent immunotherapy, biological response modifiers proposed theory, established in addition to surgery, radiotherapy, chemotherapy fourth treatment program, That tumor biological therapy (BRM). Use of biological modulators to treat cancer, the tumor may have hoped to promote the development of effective new therapies for immune therapy.

In short, the host and the tumor is a contradiction in the whole process of tumor incidence, there has been a development. In a healthy immune system function, the body can respond to tumor through their cell immune and humoral immune in order to limit and eliminate tumors. On the other hand, the growth of the tumor produces a lot of influence on the body's immune system which suppresses immune function and promotes tumor development.

Chapter 2 The Experimental Study of Improving immune and curbing tumor progression

1. EXPERIMENTAL STUDY ON TREATMENT OF MALIGNANT TUMOR BY ADOPTIVE IMMUNOLOGIC RECONSTITUTION THROUGH COMBINED TRANSPLANTATION OF FETAL CELLS

1). Experiment on Adoptive Immunologic Reconstitution of Fetal Liver, Spleen and Thymus Cells through Combined Transplantation

The author introduces the experiment on the systematic adoptive immunologic reconstitution with the mice bearing Ehrlich ascites cancer (EAC) subcutaneous solid tumor through combined transplantation using the same kind of fetal liver, spleen and thymus cells. In this experiment, set up groups of monomial transplantations of fetal liver, spleen and thymus respectively; the groups of bigeminal transplantation of fetal liver and spleen cells, fetal liver and thymus cells as well as fetal spleen and thymus cells, and then observe the time of the growth, regression and survival, index of cellular immunity as well as all items of pathological examination in each group respectively; compare the curative effects of each groups. The research results show that the curative effect of trigeminal group is better than that of the bigeminal group which is better than the individual groups in turn. For the experimental group of trigeminal cell transplantation, the complete regression rates of the tumor in near and forward future are 40% (n=15) and 46.67% (n=15) respectively, and the partial regression rates (the percentage of the tumor regression is more than 50%) are 26.67% and 13.33% respectively. Those whose tumors regress completely can survive for a long time and the lifetimes of those whose tumors regress partially are prolonged for more than a month on average, and their immune index improves obviously and the immune organs are of hypertrophy. The sections of immune organ tissue reveal the active cell proliferation. Moreover, the pathological sections of tumor tissue show that a large amount of lymphocytes soak around the tumor tissue and in stroma, and then form parcel; flaky concretion, liquefaction necrosis, karyorrhexis and other pathologic phenomena emerge in the central tumor tissue. For the experimental groups of bigeminal cell transplantation, except a few cases of partial regression, there is no complete one. All

35

the improvement of the immune indexes, the prolonged lifetime, and the soakage of lymphocytes in tumor tissue are less obvious than those of the experimental trigeminal group. As to monomial groups of cell transplantation, the results of regression, lifetime and immune indexes as well as the pathological examination results are less apparent than the former two groups, but better than the control group of the tumor-bearing mice. It can be implied that compared with partial reconstitution, systematic adoptive immunologic reconstitution can develop the anti-carcinomatous immunologic function and improve the curative effects though overall systematic synergism.

Thanks to the theory of biological response modifier (BRM), treatment of tumor has been experiencing a profound reform. The fourth generation of the modality of tumor therapy, biological treatment of tumor has become the focus in the field of tumor therapy after surgeons, chemotherapy and radiotherapy. According to a large number of clinical and experimental researches, it can be found that the organismal immune state exhibits progressive inhibition with the evolution of the stadium. Therefore, how to restore and reconstitute the anti-carcinomatous immunologic function is the core of the research of tumor biological treatment. The adoptive immunotherapy developed by Rosenberg who is the representative has got outstanding achievement in this field. Except transferring the active factors amplified in vitro and various kinds of artificial immunologic factors, fetal immune organs and cell transplantation are promising researches. Although the technique of biotherapy is expensive, it possesses several advantages like economy, convenient technique and easy popularization in that the sources of embryo are broad in China, which is worthy of thorough research and exploration. In recent years, many scholars at home have developed the research on transplantation of fetal liver, spleen and thymus from the level of cells to tissue and then to the level of organs for curing advanced malignant tumors and they have achieved some curative effects. The thorough researches can explain the source, proliferation, differentiation and the function of lymphocytes as well as the function and effects of reconstituting immune organs and peripheral immune organs clearly. Currently, in many cases of adoptive immunologic treatment with transplanting fetal immune organs, only single fetal organs is utilized, cell transplantation of fetal liver, spleen and thymus cells as well as tissue transplantation, etc. there is no similar literature or reports on the question that it is possible to carry out adoptive reconstitution systematically and integrally. The combined transplantation of fetal liver, spleen and thymus cells, in which the transplantation of fetal liver cells has analogous function of marrow transplantation and is combined with the transplantation of fetal thymus and spleen cells, can make the adoptive reconstitution approach to the systematical and integral level. But it is worthy of researches and exploration that whether it can bring synergism into play and improve curative effects.

【Material and Methods】

1. Animals and tumor model

(1) Experimental animals: 200 cross bred Kunming mice in closed flock, 5 to 6 weeks old, 18±2.1g in weight, no gender limitation.

(2) Facilities for model of planting tumors: prepare mice of ascitic type after the anabiosis of the root of Ehrlich ascites tumor ; when the ascites are formed, draw out the ascites of the cancer cells and centrifuge washing with Hank for three times(800r/min), five minutes for one time; remove the supernatant liquid, then dilute the liquid with the precipitated cancer cells to the concentration of 10^7/ml; use eosin exclusion teat to verify that the percentage of living cells is above 95%; inoculate the experimental mice under the skin of the right hollow viscera, 1ml for each mouse; after a week, all the mice have tumor nodes with the diameter of 9.5±1.5mm in the point of inoculation to make the subcutaneous solid tumor model bearing Ehrlich Ascites tumor.

2. Grouping

Group the experimental animals with random into control group bearing tumors (Group B, n=9), observation group for combined transplantation of fetal liver, spleen and thymus cells in forward future (Group CI, n=15), observation group in near future (Group CII, n=15, carry on combined transplantation to this group once a week for successive 5 weeks and then execute the mice), treatment group with transplantation of fetal liver cells (Group F), treatment group with transplantation of fetal spleen cells (Group G), treatment group with transplantation of fetal thymus cells (Group H), treatment group with combined transplantation of fetal liver and spleen cells (Group I), treatment group with combined transplantation of fetal liver and thymus cells (Group K), $n_F=n_G=n_H=n_I=n_J=n_K=$ 12. When the model is prepared, carry out correspondent cell transplantation once a week for each group respectively for five times in a row. As to the control group, use Hank as comparison.

3. Preparing of the suspension of fetal liver, spleen and thymus

Use the female mice that copulate naturally by stages and have been pregnant for 15 to 18 days; paunch them aseptically to take out the fetal mouse, liver, spleen and thymus; rinse them through the Hank individually under 4°C, then individually mix them with aseptic homogenate to the full; dilute the mixture with Hank under 4°C and filter them to collect the suspension with adequate cells; Sample the suspension and do bacterial culture and pyrogen experiment; if the experimental results are negative, divide them and package as standby.

4. The approach and method for cell transplantation

(1) Transplantation of fetal liver cells: use the prepared suspension of fetal liver cells for caudal vein injection, 0.2ml for each mouse at a time.

(2) Transplantation of fetal spleen cells: use the prepared suspension of fetal spleen cells for intraperitoneal injection, 0.2ml for each mouse at a time.

(3) Transplantation of fetal thymus cells: use the prepared suspension of fetal thymus cells for intramuscular injection in the back leg, 0.2ml for each mouse at a time.

The treatments for the experimental mice mentioned above begin after a week from cancer cell inoculation, once a week for successive five weeks. As to the control group, use the same amount of Hank as comparison.

5. Observation item

(1) General items: after cancer cell inoculation, observe the time when tumor emerges; measure the size of the tumor nude with a vernier caliper every two days (the average vertical diameter, mm), the quality of life, the situation of the tumors and the lifetime (d).

(2) Dynamic observation on T cells in peripheral blood: in this experiment, use Alpha Naphthyl Acetate Esterase (ANAE) staining method to take count of the T cells in peripheral blood. Prepare six pairs of nitrogen magenta solution and 2% ANAE solution respectively, store them in the shade under 4°C; before using the prepared solution, add 89ml, 1/15mol/L, pH=7.6 phosphate buffer into the 6ml nitrogen magenta solution gradually and mix up fully, then add 2.5ml, 2% ANAE solution gradually, then mix up to the full. The final sample is amber with pH being 6.4 as solution for incubation. Put this into the water bath of 37°C for warm-up. Cut the tip of the mouse's tail, and get the section. After the section has dried by natural wind, soak it into the solution for incubation for 1 to 3 hours, then wash it clear by tap water and air it. Use 1% methyl green to dye for 1 to 3 minutes, wash with tap water. After airing, observe the section under microscope. There are black red granules, namely ANAE positive cells in different size and quantity (the amount generally is 2 to 5). Count 200 lymphocytes and then calculate the percentage of T lymphocytes. Observe the

percentage dynamically after a week from having built the model and from treatment respectively and measure it every two weeks.

(3) Dynamic observation on the conversion rate of lymphocytes: Measure the conversion rate with the morphologic method of microdose whole blood culture in vitro. Prepare RPMI 1640 complete medium (1640 is the product of Japanese Juchheim, containing 10.4g dry powder in each bag), which consists of 1ml, 20%, 30.0g/L L- glutamine of killed calf blood serum, 3ml 60.0g/L aseptic $NaHCO_3$, 10000U penicillin and 10000μg streptomycin. Sanitize the tail strictly and cut the tip for 0.2mm; collect blood aseptically for 0.1ml with heparinization microdose sampler; add 1.8ml complete medium and then o, 1ml PHA; cultivate the sample in the water-jacket incubator under constant temperature of 37°C for 72 hours and stir it once a day. After the cultivation, draw most of the supernatant liquid out and add 4ml 8.5g/L NH_4Cl to mix up; place the mixture in the water-bath of 37°C for 10 minutes, then centrifugalize it in 2500r/min, discard the supernatant liquid; Add 5ml fixation fluid (9 units of methanol and an unit of glacialaceticacid; place the sample under ambient temperature for 10 minutes and centrifugalize it in 1500r/min for 5 minutes, discard the supernatant liquid and reserve the precipitate. Add Hank to the precipitate to the volume of 0.2ml, mix the precipitate and Hank and drop on a clean glass to stretch uniformly. After natural airing, dye it with Giemsa for 5 minutes, then wash with tap water. After drying, observe 200 lymphocytes under the microscope and calculate the percentage of the conversion rate of the metrocyte. As same as T cells, observe the percentage dynamically after a week from having built the model and from treatment respectively and measure it every two weeks.

(4) Measuring the green weights of immune organs: do comprehensive autopsy in detail for each dead or the executed mouse, cut the thymus and spleen and observe their sizes, then weight them with a torsion balance; calculate the ratio of the green weight of the immune organs to the body weight for each mouse.

(5) Pathological examination: do systematic pathological autopsy to each dead and the executed mouse, observe the tumor soakage and tumor metastasis; reserve tumor tissue, thymus, spleen, lung, liver, kidney, etc. for tissue pathological section ant attach importance to observe the lymphocyte soakage in tumor tissue and the pathologic changes in the immune organs.

【Experimental Results】

1. Comparison of the average lifetime of the mouse in each group (geometrical average) and the persistence in different ages of tumors

According to Table 1, the lifetimes of all treatment groups are prolonged obviously compared with the control group with P being less than 0.05. Especially, the effect of the treatment group of trigeminal cell transplantation is most obvious, with P being less than 0.01. Other treatment groups have significant difference compared with the trigeminal treatment group with P being less than 0.5. In Group CI, the tumors in 7 cases regress completely, which gain a long- term survival and no tumor relapse. The rate of tumor regression in 2 cases is more than 50%, in which the two mice survive for 2 months and die of tumor relapse. Regarding the persistence in different ages of tumor, in the third week after bearing tumor, all treatment groups have significant differences compared with the control group. With the extent of the stadium and observation period, compared with the control group, Group CI shows notable differential all along, but other treatment groups lose the difference from the control group gradually and show the significant difference from that of Group CI.

Table 1 comparison of the average lifetime of the mouse in each group and the persistence in different ages of tumors

Group	N	Lifetime(d) $\bar{X}$+S	The persistence in different ages of tumor							
			1week	2week	3week	4week	5week	6week	2weeks	3months
GroupB	9	13.3±1.2	100	55.6	11.1	11.1	0	0	0	0
GroupF	12	22.5±1.6△*	100	83.3	58.3*	50	33.3	33.3	0△	0△
GroupG	12	21.4±1.9△*	100	75	75*	50	33.3	16.7△	0△	0△
GroupH	12	26.2±1.4△*	100	100	100*	58.3*	41.7	33.3	0△	0△
GroupI	12	27.4±1.7△*	100	91.7	91.7*	50	33.3	33.3	8.3△	0△
GroupJ	12	28.3±1.8△*	100	83.3	83.3*	66.7*	41.7	41.7	16.7	0△
GroupK	12	23.5±1.5△*	100	100	100*	58.3*	33.3	25	16.7	0△
Group CI	15	47.2±2.0**	100	93.3	93.3*	73.3*	66.7*	60*	46.7*	46.7*

Note: ①in Table 1, Group B is the control one bearing cancer; Group F is the treatment group with fetal liver cells; Group G is the treatment group with fetal spleen cells; Group H is the treatment group with fetal thymus cells; Group I is the group of combined treatment of fetal liver and spleen cells; Group J is the group of combined treatment of fetal liver and thymus cells; Group K is the group of combined treatment of fetal spleen and thymus cells; Group CI is the group of combined treatment of fetal liver, spleen and thymus cells; ②*means that comparing the each treatment groups with the control group, P <0.05; **means P <0.01; △ means comparing the treatment groups with Group CI, P <0.01.

2. The curative effect and the analysis on the effect

Table 2 the analysis on the curative effect

Group	N	Curative rate	The rate of apparent effect	Effective rate	Rate of inefficiency	Total effective rate
GroupB	9	0△△	0	0	100	0
GroupF	12	0△△	0	34.4(4)	66.4(8)	33.4(4) △△
GroupG	12	0△△	0	25(3)	75(9)	25(3) △△
GroupH	12	0△△	8.3(1)	33.4(4)	58.3(7)	41.7(5)△*
GroupI	12	0△△	8.3(1)	33.4(4)	58.3(7)	41.7(5)△*
GroupJ	12	0△△	26.67(2)	41.7(5)	41.7(5)	58.3(7)*
GroupK	12	0△△	26.67(2)	33.4(4)	50(6)	50(6)*
GroupCI	15	46.7**	13.3(2)	20(3)	20(3)	80(12)**

Note: *means P <0.05 compared with the control group, ** means P <0.01 compared with the control group; △ means P <0.05 compared with Group CI, △△ means P <0.01 compared with Group CI

The standards of curative effects:

① Cure: The tumors regress completely, the suffers regain long-term survival without relapse;

② Apparent effects: The tumors regress partially (the regression rate is more than 50%), and the survival time is more than 2 months;

③ Being effective: The lifetime is prolonged for more than one time without obvious tumor regression.

④ Inefficiency: The tumors grow progressively leading to death in short term (3 to 4 weeks).

According to Table 2, the curative effect of Group CI reaches 46.67%, and is obviously different from other groups with P <0.01. There is no obvious difference among each group as to the rates of apparent effect and being effective respectively. The comparison of the total effective rate shows that except the treatment groups of unitary fetal liver or spleen cells, the total effective rate of all other treatment groups have visible distinction from the control group, with their curative effects being in the rank that the trigeminal is better than the bigeminal which is above the monomial. Moreover, in the groups of monomial cell transplantation, the curative effect of TH cells treatment group is the best, and in the groups of bigeminal cell transplantation, the curative effect of the group containing TH cells is better than that of the groups without TH cells, which indicates that thymus cells play an important role in the course of treatment, but sole liver or spleen cell transplantation have little effects. However, if two of liver, spleen or thymus cells are combined, the curative effect can be improved. And the combination of the three can improve the curative effect significantly.

3. Observing and comparing the growth rate of tumors, the regression and prognosis

In this experiment, the mimic clinical method is used to file case history for all the experimental mice in each groups to record their growth rate of tumors, regression and the prognosis. Measure the average vertical diameter every two days. For the cases of death, all the terminal measured values are regarded as effective sample parameter in the following measures within the same group. After a week from the establishment of the model, tumors grow rapidly with the average vertical diameter being 9.5±1.5mm. After a week from beginning the treatment, tumors continue to grow. Until the second week, the results of each group become differential that the mice bearing tumors have progressive exhaustion with the tumors growing rapidly in the control group; within four weeks, all mice are dead. In the group of sole cell transplantation, the life quality of the experimental mice are improved apparently with their tumors growing slowly, but all the mice bearing cancer die within two months. In the groups of bigeminal cell transplantation, the growths of the tumors are inhibited obviously. Five cases have partial regression but all the mice die with three months. In the group of trigeminal cell transplantation, there are nine cases with apparent tumor putrescence, fall off and ulcer, then scab. In other seven cases, the tumors regress completely, and then canker, scab. In two cases, the regression rate of tumors is more than 50%. As to other cases, except the mice in two cases die in the second and the third week respectively, tumors in the residual cases are in dead state until the death from exhaustion. The sufferers whose tumors regress completely regain long-term survival without relapse for more than six months, and they have normal capacities to become pregnant and give birth. From the above observation, it can be found that the sole or bigeminal cell transplantation is able to inhibit the growth of tumors, improve the life quality and prolong the lifetime; the trigeminal cell transplantation can not only inhibit the growth of tumors, but also result in apparent complete or partial regression and prolong the lifetime.

4. Dynamic observation on the number of T lymphocytes in peripheral blood and the conversion rate of lymphocytes

From table 3 and 4, after a week from the establishment of the model, the cellular immune indexes of the experimental groups decline obviously with the average decrease being more than 50% compared with that of the control group (the number of T cells in the normal group X is 62.5±1.7 and that of lymphocyte transformed X is 66.8±4.8), indicating that the development of tumors does inhibit immune function. After a week from beginning treatment, all immune indexes are improved (P<0.05) and there are no apparent differential among all treatment groups from the comparison between the treatment groups and the control group as well as the comparison of the indexes before and after the treatment. Seen from the growth of tumors, the immune indexes are improves, but the inhibition of tumors is not apparent. The continuous dynamic observation shows in the groups of sole and bigeminal cell transplantation, the inhibition of tumors and the improvement of immune indexes last for a certain period (3 to 4 weeks), after that period the immune indexes tent to decline, so that the state of the mice bearing cancer deteriorates, which is consistent with the reports on the clinical monitor of immunologic functionand the prognosis. In the group of trigeminal cell transplantation, the immune indexes have persistent improvement, especially the tumors regress obviously. For those who regain long-term survival, the above indexes measured two months later are still close to the indexes of normal mouse. By contrast, for those suffering deterioration, the indexes measured before their deaths have declined below the level before treatment. The above indicates that the cellular immune indexes do reflect the curative effects and can be regarded as a good prove for prognosis; at the same time it can indirectly prove that immunocyte transplantation is able to achieve the aim of immunologic reconstitution for cancer-bearing organisms.

Table 3 dynamic observation on the number of T lymphocytes in peripheral blood (ANAE)

Group	N	\multicolumn{8}{c}{The number of T lymphocytes ($\bar{X}\pm S$)}
		n	1 week	n	2 weeks	n	4 weeks	n	6 weeks
GroupB	9	9	3.42±4.8	5	29.1±2.9	1	32	0	
GroupF	12	12	31.4±3.6	10	54.6±5.12△*	6	48.7±2.2△	4	36.7±4.9
GroupG	12	12	35.5±3.9	9	52.5±4.7△*	6	46.6±3.3*	2	33.4±5.1
GroupH	12	12	32.6±4.1	12	56.6±4.1△*	7	50.9±2.1△	4	40.7±3.8△
GroupI	12	12	36.2±2.7	11	53.4±3.5△*	6	55.3±3.6△	4	39.3±4.2△
GroupJ	12	12	30.8±4.3	10	55.8±3.8△*	8	56.4±1.9△	5	42.6±2.7△
GroupK	12	12	33.7±3.4	12	57.3±4.4△*	7	55.8±2.8△	3	41.3±4.5△
GroupCI	15	15	31.8±3.1	14	59.6±2.6△*	11	62.5±1.7△	9	67.8±3.4△

Note: * means P<0.05 compared with the control group; △ means P<0.05 in the comparison before and after the treatment

Table 4 the dynamic observation of the conversion rate of the lymphocytes in peripheral blood

Group	N	The conversion rate of lymphocytes ($\bar{X} \pm S$)							
		n	1 week	n	2 weeks	n	4 weeks	n	6 weeks
GroupB	9	9	3.25±5.4	5	25.51±3.6	1	28	0	
GroupF	12	12	31.6±3.7	10	51.2±2.7$_\triangle$*	6	54.2±6.1$^\triangle$	4	36.1±5.4
GroupG	12	12	29.8±4.3	9	48.4±4.6$_\triangle$*	6	52.8±1.8*	2	33.5±2.5
GroupH	12	12	34.1±4.1	12	56.5±2.1$_\triangle$*	7	52.4±3.7$^\triangle$	4	40.7±1.9$^\triangle$
GroupI	12	12	28.5±5.1	11	53.4±3.5$_\triangle$*	6	50.5±2.9$^\triangle$	4	37.3±3.2$^\triangle$
GroupJ	12	12	29.4±2.9	10	58.1±3.5$_\triangle$*	8	60.6±3.4$^\triangle$	5	46.5±4.5$^\triangle$
GroupK	12	12	30.7±1.8	12	54.9±5.2$_\triangle$*	7	57.5±4.3$^\triangle$	3	45.8±3.9$^\triangle$
GroupCI	15	15	31.5±3.2	14	55.8±2.8$_\triangle$*	11	63.9±3.2$^\triangle$	9	66.8±4.8$^\triangle$

Note: * means P<0.05 compared with the control group; △ means P<0.05 in the comparison before and after the treatment

5. Anatomic observation of immune organ and comparative analysis of immune organ's green weight

The observation results are seen in table 5 and table 6. In this experiment, in order to see the changes in immune organs of cancer-bearing organisms and the relevance to the curative effects, another near-future observation group of trigeminal cell transplantation is set up (Group CII, n=15, the tumors in six cases regress completely and the regression rates in four cases are more than 50%). After building the model, give the treatment to the mice in Group CII for five times and then execute them. At the same time, set a normal group for comparison, using Hank to simulate the model and execute the mice in the sixth week. Anatomize the mice and observe the changes in their immune organs; measure the green weight of the immune organs and calculate the ratio of immune organs to the body weight; compare the values in Group CII with those of the other groups. From the results, it can be found that in all the cases that in all experimental groups, the tumors develop progressively and lead to death, the thymus shrink apparently and the degree of atrophy is relevant positively to the tumor development. The atrophied thymus is dull-colored and of crisp texture. As to spleen, its change is not as obvious as that of the thymus. In most cases, the spleens are congested and swelling. Only in a few cases the spleens are atrophied. However, in Group CII in all the cases that the tumors regress completely and partially, the thymus and spleens are hypertrophied, so as the indexes of thymus and spleen increase.

Through statistical disposition, these indexes are not only differential apparently from the death cases in each group (or the cases without tumor regression), but also different from the normal control group.

Table 5 the comparison of the green weight of the immune organs between the death cases and the normal control group.

Group	N	Thymus(mg)/body weight(g) $\bar{X}\pm S$	spleen(mg)/body weight(g) $\bar{X}\pm S$
Normal	10	2.97±0.38	3.80±0.23
Group B	9	1.02±0.32**	4.01±1.32
Group F	8	1.21±0.41**	4.213±0.87
Group G	10	1.18±0.46**	4.45±1.63
Group H	8	1.28±0.25**	4.47±1.24
Group I	8	1.34±0.43**	4.67±0.48
Group J	7	1.47±0.28**	4.56±0.62
Group J	9	1.43±0.35**	4.89±1.47
Group CII	5	1.96±0.37**	5.12±1.56

Note: * means P<0.05 compared with the control group; ** means P<0.01 compared with the normal control group

Table 6 the comparison of the green weight between the cases of complete or partial tumor regression and the cases without apparent regression in Group CII

Immune organ(mg/g)	Normal group (N=10, $\bar{X}\pm S$)	Group with tumor regression (N=10, $\bar{X}\pm S$)	Group without tumor regression (N=10, $\bar{X}\pm S$)
thymus	2.79±0.38	4.65±2.21 $_{\triangle\triangle}$ **	1.96±0.37
spleen	3.80±0.23	10.15±2.29 $_{\triangle\triangle}$ **	5.12±1.56

Note: ** means P<0.01 compared with the normal control group; △△means P<0.01 in the comparison between the group with tumor regression and the group without tumor regression.

6. The comparison of pathological examination

In this experiment, anatomize the mice in each group and observe the pathologic section. Observe the tumor soakage and metastasis as well as the changes in immune organs like thymus, spleen, etc. Reserve the viscera like tumor tissue, lung, kidney, thymus and spleen as tissue pathological section for observation. The results show that with the course developing, the range of local tumor soakage expends and the tumor becomes hypertrophied without apparent remote organ metastasis. The thymus shrinks obviously, which has positive relevance to the evolution of the tumor. As to the spleen, it is congested and swelling. In the near-future observation group of trigeminal cell transplantation, the thymus, spleen and liver in the cases of complete or apparent partial regression do not become hypertrophied obviously, which exhibits significant differences from the normal group. When the mice in the cases of complete regression are anatomized, no residual cancer cells can be found in the part of tumor inoculation with both naked eyes and microscope. At the 3rd or 4th week when the tumor putrescence is the most apparent, reserve the tumor tissue as pathological section for observation. It can be found that there are large amount of lymphocytes soakage around the tumor tissue and in the stroma which wrap the tumor tissue resulting a wide range of tumor cells are liquefied and solidified to be dead. The sections of immune organs show that the thickness of the thymus cortical area and the denseness of lymphocytes as well as the increase in epithelial reticular cell, phagocytotic phenomenon and thymus corpuscles. In the spleen, the white pulp area enlarges and the lymph nodes increases, also the lymphocytes become dense. In the control group, the sections of tumor tissue show that the tumor cells soak into the deep-layered muscular tissue and there are cancer embolus formed by tumor cell transplantation in the blood vessels but no lymphocytes soakage. As to the thymus, the cortex atrophy and the cells are sparse, the blood vessels are congested. In the spleen, the amount of lymphocytes decreases significantly and the cells are sparse. In other treatment groups, the tumor sections show that the boundary of the tumor are clear with a little lymphocyte soakage and the changes in thymus and spleen is between the group of trigeminal cell transplantation and the control group. Moreover, the arrangement of the cells is dense with light atrophy.

【Discussion】

1. Therapeutic evaluation

It can be found from the results of the above experiment that the adoptive immunological therapy through transplantation of immunocyte with the origin of embryo can inhibit the growth of tumor and improve the life quality in different extend and force the tumor to regress completely or partially, and then improve the immune indexes apparently and prolong the lifetime, which indicates that immunocyte transplantation with the origin of embryo can reconstitute the anti- carcinomatous immunologic functionfor cancer-bearing organisms. The combined reconstitution of central immunity and the peripheral immunity at the same time is the best and better than the partial reconstitution of bigeminal and monomial cell transplantation.

2. Possible mechanism

The possible mechanisms to take effect are mainly the following: ①After the cancer-bearing organisms accept the same kind of xenogenous embryo cell transplantation, the immune system of the organism gets non-specific simulation to produce immune hyperplasia so as to improve the immunologic function to resist tumors. ②Cell transplantation belongs to organ transplantation, which can keep active for a certain period of time in the acceptor. By immunocyte transplantation with the origin of embryo, fetal liver cells can provide stem lymphocytes, which is combined with thymus and spleen cell transplantation so as to achieve the combined reconstitution of central immunity and peripheral immunity and enable the organism to gain adoptive immunity. A large number of researches home and abroad on the proliferation, differentiation and function of fetal immune organs and histiocytes show that when fetal immune organs are in their 16 weeks, they put up obvious proliferation to the original simulation of division, which becomes more intensive in the 24th week. In the 8th week of pregnancy, lymph tissue begins to emerge in the fetal thymus and lymph nodes as well as the cells with secretion in the 20th week. All these researches indicate that fetal immunocytes are able to bring immunoreaction into play. ③Some researches show that both the supernatant liquid from fetal thymus tissue cultivated outside the body and thymus extractive have the ability to promote the formation rate of the acceptor's E- wreath and the transformation of lymphocytes obviously. Therefore, fetal immunocyte transplantation can strengthen the cellular immunity of the cancer-bearing organism for cancer-bearing organism. ④ low immunogen of the fetal organs and the homology between the transplanted fetal organs and the acceptor's immune organs are in favor of forming immunologic tolerance to the transplanted for the acceptor, which can not only avoid rejection or have light rejection, but also simulate each other to achieve synergetic effects so as to reconstitute immunity. Moreover, as the curative effects of the trigeminal cell transplantation group are much better than those of the other groups, it is be believed that the effects result from the relatively complete reconstitution of central immunity and peripheral immunity at the same time which lead to the synergetic effects. In a word, the mechanism is much more complex than the above mentioned. It will be useful to step further to make the mechanism clear if the level of the immune factors that are closely relevant to anti-tumor immunity like IL-2, TNF, INF, etc. and the activity of the immunocytes that relate directly to anti-tumor immunity like NK, LAK, TIL, etc. in peripheral blood can be detected and the transplanted cells can be marked to make clear their distribution and survival inside the acceptor.

3. Problems about the barrier of transplantation

Although fetal organs have low immunogen, it is still impossible to avoid rejection, just in different degree. Therefore, the problem about the barrier of transplantation exists and directly relate to the success of transplantation and that whether the transplant can continue to act inside the acceptor. In this experiment, the animals used belong to the hybrid species in closed flock, which ensures largely that the mice in each experimental group have relatively close genetic background. It is probably the important reason for the success of transplantation with tissue matching except the low immunogen of embryonic tissue. Apart from those, it is possible that the mismatch of histocompatibility leads to the cases with inconspicuous curative effects in Group CI and Group CII. Thus, the key of improving curative effects may lie in studying and solving the barrier of transplantation.

4. The choice of the approach and method of transplantation

The transplantations of fetal immune organs from the level of cells, to tissue, then to the level of entire organ belong to adoptive immunity. In terms of the current repots, for fetal liver and spleen, blood cell transplantation is the best; for thymus, spleen and tissue, omentum embedding is the best. Although the technique of cell transplantation is simple and easy to be successful, it can only last for a short time. Therefore, the best approach of transplantation needs further observation and research.

2). The Study on Treatment of Tumor by Adoptive Immunity through Transplantation of Immunocyte with the Origin of Embryo

According to a large amount of clinical and experimental researches, the immunity of the tumor-bearing organisms tent to be in progressive inhibition with the course the disease. So how to reconstitute the anti-tumor immunity is the core of the research on immunological therapy. In 1980s, the fourth generation of tumor treatment mode, namely biological treatment of tumor, brought tumor therapeutics into a new era, when the adoptive immunotherapy was the most outstanding achievement. For those whose tumors were in the advanced stage, several kinds of the conventional therapies were of no effects. However, adoptive immunotherapy of LAK, TIL and gene-modified TIL, which is represented by Rosenberg gained prominent curative effects, attracting the attention all over the world. In this technique, it is needed to gain a great amount of artificial synthesized IL-2 with high purity by biotechnology and plentiful immune competent cells through cultivate and proliferation in vitro in a long term to reach the aim, so the cost was very expensive. Currently, this project is still in depth research.

As only a few institutes at home have developed the research in this area, there is no doubt that the above mentioned therapy is an extremely prominent research direction in treatment of tumor, however it is some difficult to become popularized in China. Besides, treatment of tumor by adoptive immunity through transplantation of immune cells, tissue and organs with the origin of embryo is another prominent research in the treatment of tumor by adoptive immunity, which is featured by simple technique, low cost and popularity. In recent years, some researchers have used embryonic liver, spleen and thymus to do transplantation from the level of cellular tissue to organs with vessel pedicles, which has been applied in the treatment of advanced malignant tumor gaining some curative effects, and paid much attention gradually.

i. Research status of fetal liver cell transplantation (FLT)

In 1958, Uphoff was the first one to fetal liver cells into the mice who died from ray of fatal dose with the remarkable effects of regaining hematopiesis. From then on, that fetal cell transplantation can be applied in curing the diseases in hemopoietic system and in the therapy of regaining hematopiesis after chemotherapy and radiotherapy for those with malignant tumors is researched extensively. In the following researches it has been found that FLT can not only reconstitute hematopiesis, but also reconstitute immunity. Wu Zuze and other researchers have found that FLT is able to reconstitute T and B lmphyocytes. They have also found that founder cells in fetal liver and spleen nodes are possessed with the basic features of several kinds of hematopoietic stem cells or lymph myeloid stem cells through the comparative research on the proliferation and differentiation between fetal liver cells and myeloid hematopoietic stem cell. Fetal liver cells contain a small amount of macrophages and lymphocytes. After 5 months from being pregnant, the amount of T lymphocytes begins to increase gradually, which is thought to be the substantial foundation of applying FLT to cure hematopoietic disorders immunologic deficiency disease to reconstitute hematopiesis and immunity. These features of fetal liver cells, especially the ability to reconstitute immunity make FLT play an important role in improving immunity. In recent years, there have been more and more researches on applying FLT to treatment of tumor.

ii. Research status of treatment of tumor through fetal spleen cell transplantation

1. Research on the relationship between spleen and the growth of tumor

It has been thirty years since Old and others began to study the influence of spleen to the growth of tumor. During this period, many scholars have done a large number of experiments and clinical researches on the effect of spleen in anti-tumor immunity, but they can not get a consistent conclusion as they hold that spleen has both positive and negative effects on anti-tumor immunity. With more deep researches on splenic surgery and its function, most scholars tent to confirm the anti-tumor immune function. As spleen is the biggest immune organ in bodies, it is the place where Th and Ts cells become mature. The antibodies, Fibronetin, Tufftsinr-1NF and IL-2, etc. immune factors secreted by Th and Ts cells as well as killer cells like LAK and NK, etc. play an crucial role in anti-tumor immunity. Ge Yigong, etc. have found when researching the effect of ablating spleen to the growth of W256 rat's sarcoma that in the group of spleen ablation, the survival rate of the tumor inoculation and the diameter of tumor are higher apparently than those of the control group. Meanwhile, in the former group, the postoperative changes of T cell subgroup in peripheral blood are manifested by the reduction in T and Th cells and slight increase in Ts cells which is on the low level continuously after inoculation and have remarkable differential from the group without tumor and the tumor-bearing control group(P<0.001). That is consistent with the research on the effects of spleen to the growth of tumor that was done before. They have also found that after ablating spleen, there was positive correlation between the decline in the ratio of Th/Ts in T cell subgroup and the diffuse and metastasis of tumor. Lersch has reported that lymphocytes inside the spleen of tumor-bearing mice decline progressively with the growth of tumor, which is consistent with the experimental results mentioned above. All these researches can indicate that spleen plays an important role in anti-tumor immunity.

2. Researches on treatment of tumor through fetal spleen cell transplantation

Based on the understanding of the action of spleen in anti-tumor immunity, many scholars have begun to develop the experimental and clinical researches on treatment of tumor through fetal spleen cell or tissue transplantation. Ma Xuxian, etc. report that fetal spleen cell transplantation has been used in nine cases of advanced malignant tumor. All sufferers in these cases feel better after the treatment. The author also has found that fetal spleen cell transplantation can inhibit the growth of tumor apparently when studying the effects of spleen to the growth of tumor. What's more, some scholar has studied the feature and approach of fetal spleen transplantation and found that transplantation through vein is the best, intramuscular injection and celiac injection follow. For tissue transplantation, omentum embedding is the best; both HVGR and GVHR are few. The mechanism of spleen cell transplantation is still in research.

iii. Research status of treatment of tumor through fetal thymus transplantation

Among immune organs, thymus has the closest relation to anti-tumor immunity and the researches on thymus are the most profound. Thymus plays a decisive role in cellular immunity and even the entire immunoregulation as thymus is the central immune organ where T cells develop and grow up.

1. Research on the relationship between thymus and the growth of tumor

The function of thymus has close connection with the occurrence of tumor that can lead to thymus atrophy, low level of thymosin or lack of analogous thymic factor. For those experimental animals, that the thymus are ablated or irradiated by dead dose ray can promote the tumor metastasis. Therefore, fetal thymus transplantation or thymic epithelial cell transplantation as well as injection of thymosin can put off thymus atrophy and reconstitute immune function. The above researches indicate that thymus plays an extremely important role in anti-tumor immunity.

2. The application of fetal thymus transplantation in treatment of tumor

Many scholars have done plentiful researches on treatment of tumor through fetal thymus transplantation. Zhou Shifu, etc. have performed the treatment of tumor through fetal thymus transplantation for 14 tumor cases. After 46 hours, the immune indexes have been improved and the conditions of the sufferers have been remitted and improved. Song Ruze, etc. have used the treatment of advanced malignant tumor through fetal thymus tissue omentum transplantation and gained the same curative effects. Liu Dungui, etc. have used cell transplantation, tissue transplantation and transplantation of thymus with vessel pedicle to treat advanced liver cancer resulting in that tumors in some cases shrunk significantly and the lifetime was prolonged for six months. All these can indicate that fetal thymus transplantation is an effective approach of immunotherapy of tumor.

Moreover, some scholars have studied on the features of the immune organs in different ages with the origin of embryo like the activity and the saving time, etc. They have found that the activity of fetal organs after five months' pregnancy is best. The researches on the approach of transplantation show that fetal liver and spleen cell transplantation through vein is the best, and omentum embedding is best for spleen and thymus tissue transplantation.

All these researches provide precious theoretic and experimental basis for treatment of tumor by adoptive immunity through immune organ transplantation with the origin of embryo and contribute to further studies.

2. TG'S INHIBITION ON ANGIOGENESIS OF TRANSPLANTATION TUMOR OF MICE

Since Folkman presented the concept that the growth of tumor depends on vascularization in 1971, the following researches further confirm that angiogenesis is a key factor for the growth of tumor. Thereafter researchers have brought forth the concept of anti-angiogenic therapy, that is, by preventing neovascularization and (or) spread of new-born rete vasculosum and (or) destroying new-born blood vessels to stop the production or establishment of small solid tumor, and finally to prevent the growth, evolution and metastasis of tumor. At present, foreign experts have done a lot of studies in this respect and made gratifying progress. Therefore anti-angiogenic therapy is expected to be an effective means to cure tumor. But domestic relative studies start fairly late; and very few reports are given to it except some counts about capillary density of tumor tissues.

Along with the deepening research of Common Threewingnut Root, its new pharmacological actions are constantly to be found, such as anti-tumor action and two-way regulating action on immune system. Especially the recently discovered Common Threewingnut Root, which inhibits in vitro the formation of lumen that induced by the migration, proliferation and differentiation of vascular endothelium cells, has a better inhibiting action on neovascularization. In order to further explore the inhibiting action of Common Threewingnut Root on new-born blood vessels of tumor in vivo, the writer adopts transplantation tumor model of mouse's abdominal muscles. Based on the observation of formation characteristics of tumor blood vessel and its relation with tumor, researchers' new findings in recent years and the writer's experimental results both prove that Common Threewingnut Root has the two-way regulating action with dose dependent on immune system. Choose adequate doses of TG with no effect on the body's immune function to carry out the experimental study of TG's inhibiting action on new-born blood vessels of transplantation tumor of mouse's abdominal muscles. The study is to know about TG's inhibiting capability on tumor angiogenesis, which can provide experimental references for further anti-tumor study in terms of blood vessels.

1). Experimental Study on Observation of Angiogenesis of Transplantation Tumor at Mouse's Abdominal Muscle

This experiment depends on the anatomical position and structural features of mouse's abdominal muscle, adopts EAC transplantation tumor model of abdominal muscle, fixes and displays blood vessels with transparent specimen, which are all for finding out the formation characteristics of tumor blood vessel and its relation with tumor.

[Material and Method]

1. Materials

   (1) Animals: 20 Kunming mice, 18~22g, a 50:50 proportion of male and female.

   (2) Cancer-bearing mouse: Kunming mouse with the intraperitoneal inoculation of EAC cells.

   (3) Instrument and apparatus: mouse retaining plate, 1ml injector, test tube and heparin tube, glass slide, ophthalmic scissors, microsurgery scissors and surgical clamps, small cutting needle, 1-0 silk thread, ophthalmic needle holder, glass petri dish, light microscope, Olympus Japanese microscopic observation and photographic system of type BH-2.

   (4) Reagent: Wright stain, 0.2% physiological saline of trypan blue, Hank solution, depilatory, 1% pentobarbitale sodium solution, 10% formaldehyde solution, tertiary butyl alcohol solution of 70%, 80%, 90%, 95% and 100%, methyl salicylate.

2. Method

   (1) Prepare EAC cell suspension (6.0×10^7/ml): Aseptically draw ascites of cancer-bearing mouse with the inoculation for 7~9d; put ascites in a sterile tube; draw another little ascites in a heparin tube for cell count; store tubes in ice blocks. Drop remaining ascites in the empty needle on a glass slide, cover with another slide and stain the specimen with Wright stain, finally use it for differential counting of cells, the proportion of cancer cells $\geqq 95\%$ (if insufficient, choose another cancer-bearing mouse). Dilute ascites in the heparin tube with physiological saline to 10 times and 100 times; respectively take 0.95ml blending with 0.1ml trypan blue physiological saline of 0.2%; use the counting method of white blood cells to count the total number of tumor cells and dead tumor cells, calculate the survival rate, which should be $\geqq 95\%$ (if insufficient, choose another cancer-bearing mouse). Finally dilute ascites in the tube with sterile pre-cooling Hank solution to 6.0×10^7/ml and use it for the inoculation.

   (2) Inoculation in the area of peritoneum: Use depilatory in advance to clean a mouse's ventral seta two days ago; anaesthetize it injecting with 1% pentobarbitale

sodium (0.3mg/10g weight) into the abdominal cavity; lie on its back and fix it on mouse retaining plate; sterilize the abdominal skin; cut open the skin about 1.2cm long from the middlemost place about 1cm below the processus xiphoideus; conduct the blunt separation to one side gently and carefully, then find an area on this side with few blood vessels in the abdominal muscle; inoculate 0.04ml EAC cell suspension with the concentration of 6.0×10^7/ml, then present a full small "swelling" without any collapse, which explains the correct inoculation location without penetrating the peritoneum. Finally stitch the skin and isolate this mouse for protection until it regains consciousness safely.

Note: During the process of inoculation, always store the test tube with cancer cell suspension in ice blocks so as to ensure the constant survival rate. And also require a fast and stable manipulation.

(3) Group and make transparent specimen: 20 inoculated mice, randomly divide into 10 groups with 2 mice of each group. Since the first day after the inoculation, pull off the cervical vertebra to execute one group each day for making transparent specimen. The specific making procedures are as follows.

Submerge and fix the execute mice in formaldehyde solution with the concentration of 10% for 24h. Take out the mice, cut open their skin, peel off the whole abdominal muscle membrane, rinse it with distilled water for 1 min, and submerge it orderly in the tertiary butyl alcohol with different concentration (70%, 80%, 90%, 95% and 100%) to dehydrate for 6~8h. Finally submerge it directly into the methyl salicylate until the tissue is completely transparent.

(4) Observe and shoot tumor vessels: Use Olympus microscope of type BH-2 to observe the transparent specimen in the small petri dish with methyl salicylate. Note the shape, quantity and distribution of new born capillary around tumor tissues and in the tumor. Then take microscopic photos and use Olympus microcirculation microscopic photographic system to observe the flow rate of new born capillaries.

[Experimental Result]

On the first day after the inoculation, there is no new born vessel in the inoculation area, around which the original host's capillaries slightly exude. On the second day, tumor cell mass swells. It is clear that original host's capillaries put forth slim but crooked new vessels, which invade into the tumor. There is no continued vessel segment. On the third and fourth day, the tumor tissue has a further growth. The density of new vessels outside the tumor increases; the caliber is irregular; vessels array in disorder. In the tumor, incontinuous and imperfect new vessels with maldistribution and various thicknesses are obviously in the direction of muscle fiber. Some vessels are comma-shaped or bud-shaped, and irregular bud-shaped vessels connect each vessel. On the fifth and sixth day, the tumor presents the progressive growth. Capillaries outside the tumor twist or distend or cluster to distribute with various thicknesses; vessels in the tumor start to interlace with each other or show irregular sinusoid dilatation. On the seventh and eighth day, the color in the tumor becomes red. Capillaries outside the tumor distend, twist and come in different shape and size; in the tumor only a few incontinuous and short vessels present an irregular distribution, most vessels have no any figure and fuse in the shape of flake or mass. On the ninth and tenth day, there is only a red mass-shaped zone in the tumor, which is fused by vessels. Brown area of hemorrhage and necrosis appears in the centre of the tumor. Vessels with extreme dilatation and distortional appearance can be made out in some areas.

Transplantation tumor model of mouse's abdominal muscles helps to have a more intuitional observation, from inflammation changes of stimulating the angiogenesis since the first day after inoculation to tumor vessels that gradually appear later. It reflects the formation characteristics of tumor's new-born capillaries and their relations with the tumor. That is, new-born capillaries generally register as the abnormal route, irregular arrangement, irregular diameter, the lack of continuity and integrity, and even comma-shaped or bud-shaped immature differentiation and growth. The relation between capillaries and tumor is the continued proliferation and enlargement of tumor cell cluster along with the formation and growth of new-born capillaries in the inoculation area. Simultaneously, the tumor mass characterized by progressive growth causes the blood vessels in the central part to bear the rise in blood pressure, dilatation, and necrosis, which appear as a red fused mass.

2). Experimental Study on Effects of TG with Different Dosages on Immunologic Function of Mice

In recent years, reports about Common Threewingnut Root having the two-way regulating action with dose dependent on immune system have continued to arise. TG is a refined product that separated and abstracted repeatedly from the crude drug—Common Threewingnut Root. In order to have a better understanding of the two-way regulating action, this experiment chooses three different doses of TG to act on the phagocytic function of mice celiac macrophages (Mφ) and immune organs. Their drug reactions can basically reflect TG's effect on the immune function of mice.

i. TG's effect on the phagocytic function of mice celiac macrophages (Mφ)

[Material and Method]

1. Materials

   (1) Animals: 40 Kunming mice, 18~22g, a 50:50 proportion of male and female.

   (2) Drugs and reagents: ① TG turbid liquor: Pulverize TG tablets; use 0.5% Carboxythmethyl Cellulose (CMC) to respectively prepare turbid liquors of three different concentrations, TG_1 10mg/10ml, TG_2 10mg/20ml and TG_3 40mg/10ml; ② 0.5% CMC solution; ③ 2% chicken red blood cell (CRBC) suspension: Sterile venous sampling of 2ml under the chicken wing; put the blood sample in a heparin tube; clean it for three times with physiological saline; after centrifugation, abandon the supernatant fluid and white blood cell layer at the interface; when the specific volume of blood cells keeps stable, use physiological saline to prepare 2% (V/V) red cell suspension; ④ Sterile calf serum; ⑤ 1:1 acetone- methanol solution; ⑥ 4% (V/V) Giemsa-phosphate buffer.

   (3) Instrument and apparatus: Gastric lavage needle, thermotank, and for the rest, please sees "Experimental Study on Observation of Angiogenesis of Transplantation Tumor at Mouse's Abdominal Muscle".

2. Method

   (1) Grouping: 40 mice are randomly divided into 4 groups with 10 mice of each group, group TG_1, TG_2, TG_3 and control group.

   (2) Gastric lavage: According to the proportion of 0.2ml/10g (weight), respectively inject TG suspension into the stomach with corresponding concentrations (group TG_1 20mg/kg, TG_2 40mg/kg and TG_3 80mg/kg) and 0.5% CMC solution for 12 days.

   (3) Induction and functional examination of celiac Mφ: On the tenth day after gastric lavage, sterile injection of 0.5ml calf serum into each mouse's abdominal cavity. On the thirteenth day, inject 1ml CRBC suspension with the concentration of 2% into each mouse's abdominal cavity. 30min later pull off the cervical vertebra

to execute the mouse. Cut open the abdominal wall skin from the middlemost place. Inject 2ml physiological saline into the abdominal cavity and turn the mouse's body. Aspirate 1ml celiac lotion, averagely drop it on two glass slides and put slides into an enamel box with wet paper cloth. 30 min after moving the box into 37°C thermotank for warm cultivation, rinse the two glass slides with celiac lotion in physiological saline, dry by airing, fix in 1:1 acetone- methanol solution, dye them with 4% Giemsa-phosphate buffer, rinse with distilled water and dry by airing. Finally conduct the count of Mφ (200 Mφ on each slide) under the oil immersion lens of microscope. See the following mathematical equation to calculate the phagocytose percentage.

$$\text{Phagocytose Percentage} = \frac{\text{Amounts of M}\varphi \text{ that phagocytizes CRBC}}{200 \, \text{M}\phi} \times 100\%$$

(4) Statistical treatment: The data is represented by average ± standard error ($\bar{X} \pm S$), and analyzed by t test.

[Experimental Result]

Determination result about TG's effect on the phagocytic function of mice celiac Mφ can be seen in table 2-1.

Table 2-1 TG's effect on the phagocytic function of mice celiac Mφ ($\bar{X} \pm S$)

Group	Dosage(mg/kg)	Case load	Amounts of Mϕ that phagocytizes CRBC (%)
Control group	-	10	44.83±0.41
TG$_1$	20	10	47.20±0.35*
TG$_2$	40	10	45.72±0.25
TG$_3$	80	10	44.40±0.45*

Note: Compare to the control group, *P<0.05

As seen from the table 2-1, in low doses of 20mg/kg, TG can obviously activate the phagocytic function of Mφ (P<0.05); in median doses of 40mg/kg, TG has no obvious effect on the phagocytic function of Mφ (P>0.05); in high doses of 80mg/kg, TG will inhibit the phagocytic function of Mφ (P<0.05). The above results indicate that TG can affect the phagocytic function of mice celiac Mφ and have the obvious characteristic of dose dependent, that is along with the gradual increase of TG dosage, the phagocytic function of mice celiac Mφ can respectively present three different effects of being activated, no obvious effect and inhibition.

ii. TG's effect on immune organs of young mice

[Material and Method]

1. Materials

(1) Animals: 40 three-aged Kunming mice, 10~12g, a 50:50 proportion of male and female.

(2) Drugs and reagents: TG suspension and 0.5% CMC solution: Preparation is same as stated before.

(3) Instrument and apparatus: Analytical balance and for the rest, please sees "Experimental Study on Observation of Angiogenesis of Transplantation Tumor at Mouse's Abdominal Muscle".

2. Method

(1) Grouping and gastric lavage: see "Experimental Study on Observation of Angiogenesis of Transplantation Tumor at Mouse's Abdominal Muscle".

(2) Weighing of thymus gland and spleen: On the thirteenth day after the experiment, pull off the cervical vertebra to execute the young mouse. Cut open its skin, chest cavity and abdominal cavity. Excise the whole thymus gland and spleen. Use filter papers to suck dry the blood and finally weigh thymus gland and spleen on an analytical balance.

(3) Statistical treatment: The data is represented by average ± standard error ($\bar{X}\pm S$), and analyzed by t test.

[Experimental Result]

Weighing results of thymus gland and spleen can be seen in table 2-2. As seen from the table 2-2, TG at different dosages has different effect on immune organs of young mice. In low doses of 20mg/kg, TG can stimulate the weight gain of young mouse's thymus gland ($P<0.05$); in median doses of 40mg/kg, though there is a trend in weight loss, no obvious difference exists when compared with control group ($P>0.05$); in high doses of 80mg/kg, thymus gland appears as obvious atrophia compared with control group ($P<0.01$). Only in high doses, TG can inhibit the growth of young mouse's spleen ($P<0.05$); while in median and low doses, there is no obvious effect ($P>0.05$).

Table 2-2 TG's effect on immune organs of young mice ($\bar{X} \pm S$)

Group	Dosage(mg/kg)	Case load	Thymic weight (mg/10g weight)	Spleen weight (mg/10g weight)
Control group	-	10	26.38±1.22	70.43±0.76
TG$_1$	20	10	30.20±0.74*	72.65±0.83
TG$_2$	40	10	23.48±0.88	69.88±0.56
TG$_3$	80	10	21.12±0.76**	68.44±0.42*

Note: Compare to the control group, *$P<0.05$, ** $P<0.01$

Experiments about TG's effect on the phagocytic function of mice celiac Mφ and weight of young mice's immune organs can basically reflect TG's two-way regulating action with dose dependent on mice's immune function. That is, along with the gradual increase of TG dosage, there are three different immune effects of enhancement, no obvious effect and inhibition. It prompts that the application range of TG can be expanded by different effects of choosing different dosages of TG on immune system.

3). Experimental Study on Inhibition of TG of Different Dosages on Angiogenesis of Transplantation Tumor at Mouse's Abdominal Muscle

i. Observation on new-born capillaries of transplantation tumor at mouse's abdominal muscle

Researches in recent years have found that Common Threewingnut Root has the characteristic of inhibiting migration and proliferation of endothelial cell to suppress angiogenesis. In order to have a further exploration of its inhibiting action on tumor angiogenesis, this experiment bases on the previous experiment and chooses adequate doses of TG (40mg/kg) that have no effect on mice's immune function. Through observation in vivo by microcirculation microscope, experts can carry out an experimental study on angiogenesis of transplantation tumor at mouse's abdominal muscle.

[Material and Method]

1. Materials

(1) Animals: 40 Kunming mice, 18~22g, a 50:50 proportion of male and female.

(2) 6.0×10^7/ml EAC cell suspension; see [Experiment 1] for preparation.

(3) 20mg/10mg TG suspension and 0.5% CMC solution; see [Experiment 2] for preparation.

(4) HH-1 microcirculation detection system (microcirculation microscope, photomicrography system and display system, video light mark blood flow meter, etc.), other required reagents and instruments are same as those mentioned in the previous experiment.

2. Method

(1) Inoculation: see this chapter "Experimental Study on Observation of Angiogenesis of Transplantation Tumor at Mouse's Abdominal Muscle".

(2) Grouping: 40 inoculated tumor-bearing mice are randomly divided into medication administration group and control group with 20 mice of each group. Then each group is also randomly divided into four groups with 5mice of each group, which is the third day, sixth day, ninth day and twelfth day.

(3) Gastric lavage: Since the first day after inoculation, medication administration group and control group begin to undergo the gastric lavage of 20mg/ml TG suspension and 0.5% CMC solution according as the proportion of 0.2ml/10g (weight).

(4) Observation of new-born tumor capillaries: Respectively on the third day, sixth day, ninth day and twelfth day, observe new-born capillaries of tumor at mouse's abdominal muscle among the proper group of medication administration group and control group (groups of the third day, sixth day, ninth day and twelfth day). Specific method and procedure are as follows: ① Carry out the anesthesia with the injection of 1% sodium pentobarbital (0.3mg/10g weight) in abdominal cavity before operation, carefully cut open the skin below the processus xiphoideus to the lower abdomen, conduct blunt separation of skin to the middle axillary line of one side, and then cut open the abdominal muscle along the white line. This operation should be careful and gentle. If there is a little oozing of blood, use small gauze dipped in tepid physiological saline to stanch the bleeding. ② Make the mouse lie on side on the self-made observation platform, overturn the abdominal muscle that is detached from one side of the skin, and fix incision edge on the outer margin of the window of observation platform, which lets the half-side abdominal muscle cover the whole window and makes the tumor mass be located in the middle of the window. ③ Put the observation platform with mouse on the microscope carrier that is in a thermotank (Refer to the

preparation of Tian Niu and make an improvement), and drop 37°C Ringer-Locke liquor in the overturned abdominal muscle to moisten it. ④ Start the cold light source and bring into focus for observation.

(5) Observation project: Use HH-1 microcirculation detection system to observe the shape and quantity of new-born capillaries in and around the tumor, and take microscopic photos. Measure the density of new-born capillaries which enter and leave the tumor, as well as the average diameter and flow rate of tumor arterioles and venules. Use a vernier caliper to measure the maximum diameter and transverse diameter of tumor, and calculate its maximum transverse section.

(6) Statistical treatment: The data is represented by average ± standard error ($\bar{X} \pm S$), and analyzed by t test.

[Experimental Result]

1. Changes in the shape and quantity of new-born capillaries in and around the tumor. See table 3-1.

2. The density of new-born capillaries which enter and leave the tumor (the number of new-born capillaries around tumor cell cluster/mm²). See table 2-4.

The above results indicate that the density of new-born tumor capillaries of group TG is obviously lower than that of control group ($P<0.05$), which shows that TG has an inhibiting action on tumor vascularization. Especially on the third and sixth day, this manifestation is more apparent ($P<0.05$). The angiogenesis speed of control group is faster during the previous six days, but then it gradually slows down. While the angiogenesis speed of group TG during the previous six days is slower than that during the next six days and capillaries are obviously smaller that those of control group, indicating that TG significantly slows down angiogenesis speed during the previous six days and suppresses the angiogenesis. During the next six days, the angiogenesis speed of group TG gradually increases to that of control group on the tenth day to twelfth day. It shows that during the next six days TG's inhibiting action on tumor vascularization begins to remit. But as seen from table 3-1, on the twelfth day the density of new-born tumor capillaries of group TG is still obviously below that of control group, indicating that the comprehensive effect of drugs still appears as the inhibition of tumor vascularization up to now.

Table 3-1 TG's effect on the shape and quantity of new-born capillaries in and around the tumor

Observation Date	Control Group	Medication Administration Group of TG
The Third Day	Obvious, unbalanced and new-born capillaries in the tumor; unbalanced and crooked capillaries around the tumor; capillaries unevenly enter and leave the tumor. The whole tumor body is light red.	No crooked new-born capillaries enter and leave the tumor; capillaries around the tumor grow straight in the original direction; no obvious, unbalanced and new-born capillaries in the tumor. The whole tumor body is milky white.
The Sixth Day	Abundant capillaries with various thicknesses around the tumor branch from minute blood vessels of the host, twist into the tumor and form a nodular capillary network, which make the whole tumor body become light red.	Slender earthworm-shaped capillaries grow around the tumor; there are new-born capillaries without dilatation and distortion in the tumor. The whole tumor body is light red.
The Ninth Day	Abundant twisty and spreading capillaries grow around the tumor; abundant unbalanced and new-born capillaries appear in the tumor and intertwine with each other to form the shape of fasciculation and twist. There are new-born vascular buds resembling a pointed cone or cyst. The whole tumor is flesh-colored.	A small quantity of new-born circuitous capillaries start to grow around the tumor; capillaries in tumor grow in number and begin the irregular dilatation. The whole tumor body is light red.
The Twelfth Day	Abundant capillaries around the tumor look like a string of beads, or intertwine with each other to cause an irregular arrangement, or penetrate the tumor and form into concentrated clumps; capillaries in the tumor extremely distend and fuse into the shape of mass or anal sinus, which form a vast light-tight area of hemorrhage and necrosis in the centre of the tumor. The whole tumor body is maroon.	New-born slender capillaries around the tumor grow in number without interlaced phenomenon. Capillaries in the tumor distend and fuse, but there is no the area of hemorrhage and necrosis. The whole tumor is flesh-colored.

Table 3-2 TG's effect on the density (the amount of capillaries/mm^2) of new-born tumor capillaries ($\bar{X} \pm S$)

Group	Case load	The Third Day	The Sixth Day	The Ninth Day	The Twelfth Day
Control Group	5	3.40±0.14	8.34±1.05	11.26±1.28	13.1±0.90
TG Group	5	1.84±0.12**	3.64±0.64**	6.58±1.20*	9.90±0.92

Note: Compare to the control group, *$P<0.05$, ** $P<0.01$

3. The average diameter and flow rate of tumor arterioles and venules

Results can be seen in the table 3-3, 3-4, 3-5 and 3-6.

Table 3-3 TG's effect on the diameter (μm) of tumor arterioles ($\bar{X} \pm S$)

Group	Case load	The Third Day	The Sixth Day	The Ninth Day	The Twelfth Day
Control Group	5	15.0±0.71	18.8±1.07	20.8±0.84	21.4±0.75
TG Group	5	14.2±0.97	19.0±1.14	18.0±0.71*	19.2±0.58*

Table 3-4 TG's effect on the diameter (μm) of tumor venules ($\bar{X} \pm S$)

Group	Case load	The Third Day	The Sixth Day	The Ninth Day	The Twelfth Day
Control Group	5	22.6±0.68	24.0±0.71	25.6±0.51	26.8±0.58
TG Group	5	22.4±0.93	23.2±0.86	23.4±0.75*	19.2±0.68*

Table 3-5 TG's effect on the flow rate (mm/s) of tumor arterioles ($\bar{X} \pm S$)

Group	Case load	The Third Day	The Sixth Day	The Ninth Day	The Twelfth Day
Control Group	5	0.42±0.014	0.45±0.022	0.39±0.011	0.36±0.015
TG Group	5	0.43±0.018	0.47±0.013	0.42±0.012	0.41±0.013*

Table 3-6 TG's effect on the flow rate (mm/s) of tumor venules ($\bar{X} \pm S$)

Group	Case load	The Third Day	The Sixth Day	The Ninth Day	The Twelfth Day
Control Group	5	0.35±0.016	0.32±0.014	0.28±0.014	0.23±0.016
TG Group	5	0.34±0.014	0.35±0.013	0.32±0.012	0.29±0.015*

Note: Compare to the control group, *$P<0.05$

As seen from the above tables, on the ninth and twelfth day, diameters of tumor arterioles and venules of TG group are obviously thinner than those of the control group ($P<0.05$); on the third and sixth day, there is no significant difference between the two groups ($P>0.05$). On the twelfth day, flow rates of tumor arterioles and venules of TG group are faster than those of the control group ($P<0.05$); on the third, sixth and ninth day, there is no significant difference between the two groups ($P>0.05$). It indicates that TG also has an influence on minute blood vessels (feeding the tumor) of the original host. Especially during an advanced stage, narrowing the diameter and quickening the flow rate can affect the amount of tumor blood supply.

4. The maximum cross section of tumor

Results can be seen in the table 3-7.

Table 3-7 TG's effect on the tumor size ($\overline{X} \pm S$, mm)

Group	Case load	The Third Day	The Sixth Day	The Ninth Day	The Twelfth Day
Control Group	5	9.46±0.65	21.78±1.90	34.11±1.62	65.99±2.21
TG Group	5	4.91±0.76**	14.01±1.27**	27.09±2.16*	62.64±2.45

Note: Compare to the control group, *$P<0.05$, ** $P<0.01$

The above results indicate that in the previous nine days TG inhibits the growth of tumor ($P<0.05$); especially in the previous six days, this effect is more obvious ($P<0.06$). On the twelfth day, there is no significant difference between the tumor size of TG group and that of control group ($P>0.05$). It prompts that TG can obviously inhibit the growth of tumor in an early stage. While in the middle-late stage, this effect decreases. Finally in the advance stage, there is no significant inhibiting action.

ii. Determination of plasma endothelin (ET) in mice with transplantation tumor at abdominal muscle

ET is a kind of biologically active peptide synthesized by epidermic cells with extensive biological effects. Recently, increasing researches indicate that ET has an intimate relation with the growth and development of tumor, and also can participate in and promote the vascularization. In order to have a further understanding of tumor, ET and TG's effect on ET of tumor mice, experts carry out the following experiments.

[Material and Method]

1. Materials

(1) Animals: 60 Kunming mice, 18~22g, a 50:50 proportion of male and female.

(2) EAC cell suspension of 6.0×10^7/ml, 20mg/10ml TG suspension and 0.5% CMC solution: Preparation is same as stated before.

(3) Endothelin radioimmunoassay kit.

(4) The gamma (γ) radioimmunoassay counter of SN-682.

Other required reagents are same as those mentioned in the previous experiment.

2. Method

(1) Grouping and gastric lavage according to the table 3-8.

Table 3-8 Grouping and gastric lavage of experimental mice

Animals (mice)	Grouping	Gastric lavage (0.2ml/10g)
20 uninoculated mice	Normal group ① 10 mice	physiological saline×6d
	Normal group ② 10 mice	physiological saline×12d
40 inoculated mice	Control group ① 10 mice	0.5% CMC×6d
	Control group ② 10 mice	0.5% CMC×12d
	Administration group ① 10 mice	20mg/10ml TG×6d
	Administration group ② 10 mice	20mg/10ml TG×12d

*. The inoculation method refers to "Experimental Study on Observation of Angiogenesis of Transplantation Tumor at Mouse's Abdominal Muscle".

(2) ET determination: Six days after gastric lavage, collect specimens of blood from the eye socket of mice with 2ml of each mouse in normal group ①, administration group ① and control group ①. Put the blood sample in the tube with 10% EDTA · Na 230μl and 40μl aprotinin. Lightly shake the mixture well. Centrifuge for 10min with 3000 revolutions per minute at 4°C. Separate plasma and store it at -20°C for determination. Twelve days after gastric lavage, for the mice of remaining groups to adopt the same method to collect specimens of blood, separate plasma. Use the specific radioimmunoassay and gamma (γ) radioimmunoassay counter of SN-682 to measure both the present and previous plasma. Operating procedures should be seriously carried out according to instructions of radioimmunoassay kit.

(3) Statistical treatment: The data is represented by average ± standard error ($\bar{X}\pm S$), and adopt analysis of variance — F test to carry out the comparison among groups.

[Experimental Result]

Determination results of plasma endothelin (ET) in mice can be seen in the table 3-9.

Table 3-9 TG's effect on the plasma endothelin (ET) in mice with transplantation tumor at abdominal muscle ($\bar{X}$±S, pg/ml)

Group	Case load	The Sixth Day	The Twelfth Day
Normal group	10	93.6±4.72	93.4±4.83
Control group	10	126.4±3.87**	132.8±4.02**
Administration group	10	106.4±4.49*ΔΔ	114.6±5.41*Δ

Note: Compare to the normal group, *P<0.05, ** P<0.01; while compare to the control group, Δ P<0.05, ΔΔ P<0.01

The above results indicate that ET of administration group and control group is obviously higher than that of normal group (P<0.05), which shows that the tumor can increase the plasma endothelin (ET) of mice. While ET of administration group is apparently lower than that of control group, and this phenomenon is significant during the previous six days (P<0.01), which shows that TG can reduce the increase of plasma endothelin (ET) caused by the tumor and effects in the early stage are stronger.

Results of observation on new-born capillaries of transplantation tumor at mouse's abdominal muscle with microcirculation detection system indicate that TG can inhibit the growth of new-born capillaries in and around the tumor, reduce the density of new-born capillaries which enter and leave the tumor and suppress the growth of tumor. Furthermore, those effects of TG are significant in the early stage, and TG can change the diameter and flow rate of tumor arterioles and venules in the advanced stage to narrow the diameter and quicken the flow rate. Determination results of plasma endothelin (ET) show that the tumor can increase the plasma endothelin (ET) of mice. But TG can reduce the increase of plasma endothelin (ET) caused by the tumor with stronger effects in the early stage.

[Discussion]

1. Analysis and evaluation on the observation method of new-born capillaries by building the transplantation tumor model of mouse's abdominal muscles

At present, the methodology of tumor capillaries research is still in the process of constant exploration and improvement. Generally choose the rabbit cornea, chorioallantoic membrane (CAM) and yolk sac of chick embryo, and hamster cheek pouch for in vivo techniques; and also insert manual apparatus into rabbit ear chamber and subcutaneous air pouch of rat's back, which are called "sandwich" observation room, as the location of transplantation tumor for viviperception. In recent years, corrosion casting and immunohistochemistry are also used to display and identify vascular composition. Each of the above methods has its merits and drawbacks. At present, experts are still exploring to find a kind of simple, economical model and method with high quantitative feature and repeatability for the angiogenesis research. Therefore, combining concrete conditions of this laboratory, the writer has studied and designed the transplantation tumor model of mouse's abdominal muscles, applying improved microcirculation observation techniques to observe new-born capillaries of tumor. This method is easy, convenient and intuitional, and finally becomes a new approach for the tumor capillaries research on the methodology.

(1) Model evaluation: The approach of transplanting tumor at mouse's abdominal muscles is adopted to study and observe the relation between tumor and capillaries, as well as the drug effect on tumor capillaries, which has the reliable theoretical and practical basis.

The abdominal muscle layer of mouse is thinner. A thin layer of aponeurosis lies between the exterior of abdominal muscle layer and skin. The interior of abdominal muscle layer links closely with the abdominal membrane. The Hunter's line divides the abdominal muscle layer along the centre position into right and left halves, which are provided blood circulation by inferior epigastric arteries and veins. The right and left halves diverge one more into tiny branches (arterioles and venules) and capillary branches, which form rich anastomoses around the abdominal muscle of each side. The center position has fewer vascular branches and ramus anastomoticus and becomes an area with rare vessels, where is convenient for the observation of new-born capillaries.

When EAC cell suspension is injected into the abdominal muscle layer, tumor cells will quickly begin the infiltrative growth and expand along the flat surface of abdominal muscle without any adhesion of skin and organs in the abdomen. When the tumor grows up to a certain extent, it will gradually break through the abdominal muscle layer, penetrate inward through the abdominal membrane, move into organs in the abdominal cavity through implantation metastasis and finally produce ascites.

Consequently, the better choice is to inoculate in the area with rare vessels and observe tumor capillaries during the period of the tumor not yet penetrating through the abdominal membrane, which can both make a clearer observation of the emergence and change of new-born capillaries and avoid many factors' combined effects on new-born capillaries, such as ascites and tumor diffusion caused by the tumor's penetration through the abdominal membrane.

Combined with this experiment content, in order to have a better reflection and observation of the transplanted tumor in abdominal muscle and the whole growing and developing process of new-born capillaries, the writer has carried out repeated trials and finally chosen EAC cell suspension with the concentration of 6.0×10^7/ml for inoculation. According to the growth status of tumor, the writer arranges 10 days' observation and 12 days' treatment. Divide four time spans of the third day, sixth day, ninth day and twelfth day to reflect the tumor's reaction to drugs in the early, intermediate and advanced stages.

The transplantation tumor model of mouse's abdominal muscles can intuitively and clearly reflect the formation and change of new-born tumor capillaries, and it also provides new idea and method for studying new-born tumor capillaries' selection of transplantable parts and preparation of animal model. There are a few points that should be remembered when preparing the model: ① Inoculation site should be chosen in the abdominal muscle with rare vessels, not penetrating the peritoneum. The mark is a full small "swelling" without any collapse on the inoculation site. ② The experimental operation should be gentle and careful. Try to keep away from the tiny venous tributary (generally only 1~2 vessels) that links skin and abdominal muscle, so that no local hemorrhage is caused. Then the inoculation effect and the growth of new-born tumor capillaries after inoculation will be unaffected. ③ Appropriately increase the number of experimental mice to reduce errors of different location of rare vessels of abdominal muscle caused by individual difference.

(2) Evaluation of observation method

① Observation of transparent specimen: The tissue of abdominal muscle membrane is thinner. After transparent treatment, other sites are all transparent except vessels are red. Naked eyes can clearly see vessels' routes. Microscope observation can show the shape, distribution and interrelation of capillaries. The transparent specimen is not only convenient and intuitive but also preserves the natural form of vessels and associative perception. When preparing the transparent specimen, do not inject with Chinese ink or other pigments, but directly display vessels through natural color of blood, which prevent particle size, dispersion degree and viscosity of perfusate from affecting the specimen quality and changing the shape of vessels due to improper injection pressure. The transparent specimen must completely reflect the condition in vivo so as to make displayed vessels be closer to the reality.

The transparent specimen of abdominal muscle- membrane can clearly display various vessels in the abdominal muscle, involving the route, shape and distribution of capillaries around and in the tumor as well as localized congestion, oozing of blood and bleeding, which make it more convenient for observing new-born capillaries inside and outside of the tumor. The transparent specimen can only show the change of capillary form after animals have died, but it cannot reflect their blood flow state. Therefore, combined with the dynamic state of vital blood flow and functional parameters to have observation, it will be more favorable to have a complete understanding of new-born tumor capillaries' features.

② In vivo observation with microcirculation microscope: The mouse's abdominal muscle membrane is thinner with the shape of film and is easy to transmit light, whose vascular form and fluid state can be clearly seen through the microcirculation microscope. Inoculated tumor cells begin the infiltrative spreading growth in the abdominal muscle. In the early stage, the abdominal muscle membrane still can transmit light and display the vascular form in tumor tissue due to unobvious increase in thickness. In the advanced stage, the tumor tissue grows and thickens; the pressure of central part increases; necrosis and hemorrhage arise, which appear as a light-tight solid mass; vessels in this part cannot be seen, but the form of vessels in other transparent parts of tumor can be seen at present. The microcirculation microscope is used to observe new-born capillaries inside and outside of transplantation tumor at abdominal muscle and those which enter and leave the tumor as well as tumor arterioles and venules, which can completely reflect the relation between tumor and vessels as well as drugs' effect on new-born tumor capillaries in the respect of vascular form and fluid state.

The above two observation methods can complement each other with joint application. Observation of transparent specimen can cover the shortage of not observing vessels in a light-tight part of tumor in vivo; while in vivo observation makes up for the observation of dynamic state of blood flow. The above methods can only make one-off observation and cannot have a continuing dynamic monitoring in a long term, so they also remain inadequate. In order to have a more accurate and deeper research, the methodology needs the further improvement and completeness.

2. Evaluation of experimental drugs Common Threewingnut Root generally refers to the plant belonging to Tripterygium of Celastraceae. There are three varieties in China, which are Common Threewingnut Root, Tripterygium Hypoglaucum and Common Threewingnut Root of North-East (Tripterygium regelii Sprague et Take). This kind of drug has an acrid-bitter flavor and medicinal properties of

cold and hot. The drug passes through main channels of liver and spleen as well as twelve regular channels, which has efficacies of clearing away heat and toxic material, expelling wind and removing dampness, relaxing the muscles, stimulating the blood circulation and removing obstruction in channels, reducing swelling and alleviating pain, destroying parasites and relieving itching. This drug, which contains about 70 components, is recorded in *Sheng Nong's herbal classic* at the earliest. Since the 1970s, it has been used in treating rheumatoid arthritis, which results in certain curative effect. In recent twenty years, it has been widely used in treating chronic nephritis, hepatitis, purpura haemorrhagica and all kinds of skin diseases. At the same time, the research of pharmacological action also becomes deeper, widely covering adrenal gland, immunity, generation, micturition, central nerve and blood system. Experts all agree that this drug can enhance adrenal cortex function, relieve inflammation and alleviate pain, resist fertility and prevent tumor activity. Only as to its effect on immune system, experts each sticks to their own viewpoint. There were many controversies and inferences. In an early period, experts embarked on the research of its effect on immune system because of its unique effect on treating rheumatoid arthritis. The earliest result indicates that this drug can suppress immunity. As more and more researches are done deeply, most researchers gradually tend to the viewpoint of "two-way regulation". They hold that Common Threewingnut Root has the two-way regulating action with dose dependent on immune system. For instance, Zheng jiarun, Yan Biyu, Luo Dan, Lei Yi and Fan Yongyi respectively report that Common Threewingnut Root has the two-way regulating action on mouse's thymic weight, human thymocyte hyperplasia, NK activity of mouse's spleen cells, T and B cell function of mouse's spleen and proliferation of T cells in vitro. Through the experiment of the effect of TG with different dosages on Mφ function of mice abdominal cavity and immune organs by the writer, it reflects that Common Threewingnut Root has the two-way regulating action on immune system. The above results indicate that Common Threewingnut Root does not have the only effect of immunological suppression. Many experiments have proved that a small dosage of Common Threewingnut Root can enhance the immunization to some extent. While within a certain limits, there will be a reversible manifestation between enhancement and inhibition. It can also show nearly no appreciable effect on immunologic function. When further increasing the dosage, this drug will show the complete inhibiting action on immunization. The inhibiting action of Common Threewingnut Root is obviously related to its dosage.

Given the above conclusions, the writer chooses the dosage of TG, which has no appreciable effect on immunologic function, to carry out the experiment. It can avoid drugs' influence on immunologic function, which may complicate the research of TG's inhibiting action on tumor capillaries. At the same time, it can provide experimental considerations and exploring foundations for experiments and clinical researches of TG's anti-tumor action on the premise that Common Threewingnut Root will not damage the body's immunological function.

The drug of this experimental research is a kind of prepared product after repeated separation and abstraction. The amount of active principle is higher and the untoward effect is less. In order to have a further exploration of angiogenesis inhibition of active principle in this drug, various chemical compositions and monomers after the second separation and purification still need further study.

3. Features of tumor angiogenesis Under normal conditions, the angiogenesis only limits in embryonic development, repair in trauma and endometrial regeneration. Furthermore, the host can strictly control its growth with various mechanisms. But in the recent twenty years, experts haven't found any mechanism which can suppress tumor angiogenesis. It indicates that tumor angiogenesis has its own features.

Through the observation on new-born capillaries of transplantation tumor at mouse's abdominal muscle, it is easy to find that as the formation and growth of capillaries in the inoculation area, tumor cell cluster constantly proliferates and its volume continually expands. It starts with the exudation of original host's capillaries, and then slender and crooked new-born capillaries gradually come out with the characteristics of disorganized arrangement, uneven distribution and irregular diameter. Especially these capillaries, which enter into the tumor, have incontinuous routes, lack completeness and present the shape of comma or bud. The above signs indicate that those capillaries are not fully mature and cannot form complete and continuous basilar membrane. Furthermore, they are not blocked and packed by well-differentiated vascular walls with multilayered structure, which make vessels expand irregularly in the shape of nodositas or sinus. Along with the progressive growth of tumor, dust-color area of hemorrhage and necrosis appears in the centre of the tumor. Capillaries in adjacent sites are hard to be seen because of extreme dilatation, which may be due to the constantly rising pressure within tumor caused by the continuous proliferation of tumor cells. The pressure of central part in tumor is relatively highest, and the central part is far away from new-born capillaries that penetrate from the outside of tumor, so the central part is easy to suffer from necrosis because of ischemia, involving the necrosis and hemorrhage of vessels. But there still are different-shaped tumor capillaries with active proliferation at the margin of tumor, which can ensure the required nutrition for the further infiltrative growth. This phenomenon also indicates that the tumor grows indefinitely and cannot be adjusted and controlled.

At present, experts have been adopting various methods to study tumor vessels. The existing achievements have proved that the formation of tumor vessels is different from the angiogenesis in a normal physiological state. It has its own special uniqueness, such as infantile differentiation, incomplete vascular wall and out of the body's control, etc. While the whole process and regulatory mechanism of tumor angiogenesis remains obscure and are still in further exploration. This experiment just superficially reflects the relation between tumor and vessels, as well as some features of tumor vessels. The deeper study also needs the breakthrough of methodology, and the continued clarification of biological characteristics of tumor vessels in terms of the physiology and pathology of angiogenesis, biochemistry and molecular biology.

4. Exploration of TG's inhibiting action on new-born tumor capillaries Since Common Threewingnut Root is explored and applied, domestic and foreign medicine circles have been starting to pay great interest and attention to it and carrying out multi-disciplinary study and exploration one by one for broadening the application range. The recent researches show that Common Threewingnut Root can inhibit the migration and proliferation of vascular endothelial cells (EC). Zhu Jinbo and another two Japanese scholars utilize self-made F-2 and F-2C of EC strain to study the effect of Common Threewingnut Root on the process of angiogenesis. The result shows that Common Threewingnut Root can directly act on EC and inhibit its migration, proliferation, differentiation and the formation of lumen, which prompts that Common Threewingnut Root has a better inhibiting action on angiogenesis. The experimental study of TG's inhibiting action on new-born capillaries of transplantation tumor at mouse's abdominal muscle finds that TG can suppress tumor angiogenesis with stronger effects in the early stage. Presumably TG's active mechanisms may include the following respects.

(1) Directly act on new-born tumor capillaries: The experimental results indicate that TG can obviously suppress the growth of capillaries in and around the tumor and reduce the density of new-born capillaries which enter and leave the tumor. Thus it can be inferred that TG may directly act on endothelial cells of tumor vessels, suppress the migration and proliferation of cells and reduce the formation, differentiation and growth rate of tumor vessels.

(2) Directly act on tumor cells: TG's direct damaging effect on tumor cells has been proved in an early period. It is generally acknowledged that TG comes into the effect of cell toxicant by directly interfering with DNA replication of tumor cells and suppressing RNA and protein synthesis. During the process of angiogenesis, the tumor cell itself can produce multiple angiogenesis factors, such as fibrocyte

growth factor (FGF), angiogenine, transfer growth factor (TGF) and tumor necrosis factor (TNF-2), etc. Furthermore, the tumor cell can release some chemical mediators to induce the angiogenesis of host and tumor. The above substances that are released by tumor cells and can induce angiogenesis are collectively called "tumor angiogenesis factor (TAF)" by Folkman. TG can reduce the production of TAF by directly killing tumor cells, which indirectly inhibits the angiogenesis.

(3) Change of tumor blood flow: Determination result of the average diameter and flow rate of host's tumor arterioles and venules shows that TG can change the blood flow in the tumor and affect the growth and change of tumor and its new-born capillaries by acting on the blood supply of tumor.

(4) Reduction of plasma ET content: The recent researches indicate that ET has the effect of growth factor on promoting cell proliferation, which can stimulate the growth of endothelial cell and the proliferation of vascular smooth muscle cells. ET has an intimate relation with the tumor, which can promote the transcription and expression of proto-oncogene and the growth and differentiation of tumor, increase the blood flow of tumor tissue and stimulate the angiogenesis. The determination result of mouse's plasma ET indicates that ET of inoculated group is obviously higher than that of normal group. It proves that ET has an intimate relation with tumor and the tumor can increase mouse's plasma ET content. While ET of TG group is apparently lower that that of control group, which indicates that TG can obviously lower mouse's plasma ET content and reduce the growth effect on promoting tumor and angiogenesis caused by ET.

Furthermore, TG has a feature in this experiment that its inhibiting action on tumor angiogenesis in the advanced stage is weaker than that in the early stage. In addition to TG's pharmacological characteristic of suppressing angiogenesis, its inhibiting power is also related to drugs' accumulative action. It is conjectured that TG accumulates in vivo and plays an extensive pharmacological effect with prolongation of medication time, and thus affects its inhibiting action on tumor angiogenesis.

This research result indicates that TG can suppress tumor growth by inhibiting tumor angiogenesis with no significant effect on the immune system, and moreover, TG's effect in the early stage is significant. This study provides references for the further multi-field and multi-angle TG researches, and also new ideas for the research of TG anti-tumor mechanisms. Without doubt, this conclusion still needs extensive repeated experiments to be verified. At the same time, drug purification and methodology improvement are necessary for the further deeper study.

Inhibiting the formation of new-born tumor capillaries to suppress the tumor growth is a new idea on oncology that emerges in recent years.

This topic is on the basis study of formation features of new-born capillaries of transplantation tumor at mouse's abdominal muscle as well as capillaries' relation with tumor and TG's two-way regulating action with dose dependent on the immune system of mouse, and thus by choosing the TG dosage (40mg/kg weight) of no obvious effect on mouse's immune function to carry out experiments of TG's effect on the shape and quantity of new-born capillaries of transplantation tumor at mouse's abdominal muscle, the density of new-born capillaries which enter and leave the tumor, the average diameter and flow rate of tumor arterioles and venules, tumor size and plasma ET. The above experiments find that TG can inhibit tumor angiogenesis through various mechanisms of direct action on new-born tumor capillaries as well as tumor cells, the change of tumor blood flow and the reduction of plasma ET content, and moreover, TG's effect in the early stage is significant. This research result shows that the anti-tumor study of TG from the angle of vessels has certain significance and needs the further study confirmation and deepening.

4). The Significance of Inhibition of Angiogenesis in Treatment

Tumorigensis is a complicated process and is affected by many factors, involving the foundation of tumor vascular net. Many researches have proved that tumor growth must depend on angiogenesis. By inhibiting certain steps or the whole process of tumor angiogenesis to control tumor growth is of great importance to tumor therapy and prevention of tumor's distant metastasis.

i. The relation between tumor angiogenesis and the generation and growth of tumor

At present, the question about tumor generation mainly focuses on the study of oncogene; nevertheless, malignant change of tissues, tumor formation and tumor gene activity are just necessary conditions instead of the whole. Folkman Judah and other scholars in Children's Hospital of Harvard Medical School do a series of studies about the generation of pancreatic islet B cell tumor of mutant mice. The study result finds that tumor gene activity is related to the proliferation of B cells, and moreover, angiogenesis plays an important role during the generation of B cell tumor. The generation of tumor is caused by getting angiogenic ability of hyperplastic tissue. The research proves that one of evident characteristics of most precancerous lesions is the lack of obvious neovascularization. Compared with the tumor with abundant new-born vessels, the transition from precancerous condition and lesion to blood vessel phase may be the "switch" for tumor generation. It indicates that the induction of angiogenesis and the consequent neovascularization are both ahead of the tumor generation. Once the tumor is found, its further growth must depend on the continuous generation of vessels. This concept has been put forward by Folkman in 1971. He holds that tumor cells and vessels combine into a highly integrated ecological system. If there is no angiogenesis, the tumor will not swell. Many experimental research evidences in recent years further support the above views.

The growing period of solid tumor cells can be divided into invading prophase without vessels and invading growth phase of vascularization. During the invading prophase, the growth of tumor cells mainly depends on diffusion to gain nutrition. When the diameter of solid tumor exceeds 1~3cm and cell number is up to about 10^7, tumor's central part and its continued growth must be provided with oxygen and nutrient substance by vessels. ① Observe the black tumor cell cluster of mouse that is cultured in agar. When the cluster grows to 1mm³, the proliferation of its peripheral cells and the necrosis of central cells are equivalent. When the tumor body continues to swell, the proliferation and necrosis achieve a dynamic equilibrium. If the tumor grows in the organism, then this phase can also be called the blood vessel phase of tumor growth. Breaking this state needs the growth of new and functional capillaries so as to provide adequate oxygen and nutrient substance. ② Observe the growth rate of transplantable tumor in the subcutaneous transparent cavity of mouse. The tumor shows a slow linear growth before angiogenesis. While after angiogenesis, the tumor shows a rapid exponential rise. ③ Implant tumor tissue masses into the rabbit cornea. The tumor stands back from the host's vascular bed. The new-born capillaries around the cornea are found to gather toward the tumor. The growth rate averages 0.2mm/d. After new-born capillaries grow into the tumor, the tumor mass begins to grow rapidly and exceeds 1cm³. ④ The tumor grows in the isolated perfused organ of mouse. Because there is no vascular proliferation, the tumor limits in 1mm³. If this tumor is transplanted into the mouse, it will rapidly grow to 1~2cm³ after angiogenesis. ⑤ Suspend tumor cells in the aqueous humor of anterior chamber of rabbit eyes. Because there is no vessel, the tumor size is less than 1mm³. If this tumor is transplanted into iris vessels, it will grow rapidly with 1.6 times of its original volume in two weeks. ⑥ When the human retina blastoma is transplanted into the vitreous body or anterior chamber, the growth of this tumor will be limited due to the lack of vessels. ⑦ Use ³H- thymine to label tumor cells of fixed cancer. The label index of tumor cells reduces with the increase of distance between the nearest open capillaries and tumor cells. The mean value of label index of tumor cells is the function of label index of tumor vascular endothelial cells. ⑧ Transplanted tumor in CAM. During the avascular period (≥72h), the growth of tumor is restricted. A set of experiments show that the tumor diameter is no more than (0.93±0.29) mm. In 24 hours after the vascularization, the tumor starts growing rapidly. On the seventh day, the average diameter of tumor is (8.0±2.5) mm. ⑨ Oophoroma metastasizes to the abdominal membrane. Before the vascularization, this tumor grows slowly and its size seldom exceeds 1mm³. ⑩ If the tumor diameter is less than 1mm, there will be no vascularization in the metastatic cancer of rabbit cornea. All other metastatic cancers, whose diameter is greater than 1mm, have the formation of vessels.

All these above can indirectly or directly prove that tumor growth must depend on vascularization and the vascularization is a key factor for tumor development.

ii. The anti-tumor action of angiogenesis inhibitors

In the early 1970s, along with the presentation and research of the concept that tumor growth depends on vascularization, researchers also bring forth the relevant concept of anti-angiogenic therapy. That is to say, by preventing neovascularization and (or) the expansion of new-born vascular net and (or) destroying new-born vessels to stop the generation or establishment of small solid tumor and also arrest the growth, development and metastasis of tumor. Ways of adopting anti-angiogenic therapy: ① Suppress tumor to release tumor angiogenic factors (TAF); ② Neutralize the tumor angiogenic factors (TAF) that have already been released; ③ Inhibit the reaction of vascular endothelial cells (EC) on angiogenic factors; ④ Disturb the synthesis of basilar membrane; ⑤ Destroy the formed new-born tumor vessels, etc. In conclusion, ideal tumor angiogenesis inhibitors must be able to suppress one or more procedures or the whole process of tumor angiogenesis.

At present, people have done a lot of researches in this respect. Experimental results indicate that angiogenesis inhibitors (AI) can inhibit the growth of tumor. ① According to more domestic reports, the combination of heparin and hydrocortisone is acknowledged as an effective angiogenesis inhibitor. Experiments prove that their combined application can suppress the angiogenesis in CAM, promote tumor regression, prevent metastasis and inhibit the neovascularization of rabbit cornea that caused by tumor. That this kind of inhibitor is used to cure some mice tumors can bring about a striking effect. For instance, after the oral administration of heparin (200U/ml) and subcutaneous injection of hydrocortisone (250mg), 100% reticulum cell sarcoma, 100%

Leuis lung cancer and 80% B16 melanoma can have a complete regression. What's more, 80% tumors will not suffer from the relapse after regression. ② Fumagillin is a kind of antibiotic which is naturally secreted by aspergillin. For the in vitro experiment, Fumagillin can inhibit the proliferation of endothelial cells. For the in vivo experiment, Fumagillin can inhibit the angiogenesis caused by tumor and also suppress the tumor growth of mice. For example, 30mg/kg of Fumagillin can inhibit the growth of Lewis lung cancer and B16 melanoma. ③ 1µg/ml TNP-470 (a kind of Fumagillin synthetic analogue) can inhibit the growth of cultural endothelial cells of human umbilical vein. 3~10mg/kg TNP-470 can suppress the growth of nude mice's transplanted tumor of human oophoroma. ④ Platelet factor 4 (PF_4) is a kind of 28kDa protein that is released by the dense body when blood platelets aggregate together. There is a great affinity between PF_4 and heparin. Taylor and other scholars have found that PF_4 can effectively inhibit the growth of CAM vessels. Recently Maione and others have discovered that recombination of human PF_4 ($rHuPF_4$) can suppress the reproduction and migration of human endothelial cells, and also produce an avascular area in chick embryo CAM. Sharpe has carried out the research about mice melanoma and human colon cancer, which proves that human PF_4 ($rHuPF_4$) has an inhibiting action on the growth of solid tumor. ⑤ α-Difluoromethylornithine (DFMO) is a kind of nonreversible ornithine decarboxylase inhibitor. It can inhibit the angiogenesis caused by melanoma in chick embryo CAM, and then inhibit the tumor growth in CAM. ⑥ The latest approved angiogenesis inhibitor - Angio stain is a kind of 38kDa protein, which can inhibit the generation of endothelial cells and angiogenesis in the Lewis mice tumor. When Folkman injects Angio stain into the mouse with transplanted tumor, this new type of inhibitor can keep this transplanted tumor in a state of dormancy, that is to say, the multiplication rate of tumor is equal to the death rate of cells. In addition, Angio stain can suppress the growth of human tumor.

At present, people have realized that the anti-tumor effects of many anti-tumor methods directly or indirectly act on the structure or function of tumor vessels, such as anti-tumor angiogenesis, the change of tumor blood flow and its regulation, etc. That by inhibiting the angiogenesis of malignant tumor to suppress the growth and metastasis of tumor is a new way to fight against cancer, and meanwhile adopting angiogenesis inhibitors to cure tumors will open up a new and promising therapeutic area clinically. For instance, cooperating operation, chemotherapy, radiotherapy and immunological therapy will certainly improve the overall tumor treatment level.

Tumor cells produce multiple tumor angiogenesis factors (TAF), such as basic fibroblast growth factor (bFGF), acid fibroblast growth factor (aFGF), endothelial cell growth factor (ECGF), vascular endothelial cell growth factor (VEGF), platelet derivation endothelial cell growth factor (PDECGF), epidermal cell growth factor (EGF), transforming growth factor (TGFα, TGFβ), tumor necrosis factor (TGF-α), granulocyte colony stimulating factor (G-CSF) and granulocyte macrophage colony stimulating factor (GM-CSF), etc. TAF has the promotional effects on tumor generation, development and metastasis. Exploring the generative mechanism of tumor capillaries and the inhibition of capillaries' formation and growth is one of the effective measures to prevent and cure tumors, and may also become a new promising anti-cancer therapy after the surgical treatment, radiotherapy, chemotherapy and biological therapy.

Chapter 3 The Experimental Study on Anti - cancer Effect of Traditional Chinese Medication

1. Overview

1). The source and background of the research topics

In April 1991 the author applied for the "85" critical research and technology projects from China scientific department, which this project was named as "further develop the preventing the cancer and anticancer Chinese herbs which can treat the stomach cancer an liver cancer and the precancer of the stomach with the combination of the Chinese medicine and western medicine in the basic and the clinical research". In June the xxx in Hubei organized three persons who is responsible for these projects to report to Hygience and health department in Beijing. After two months the providence xxx with these three persons went to Beijing to further report these projects and accepted these important projects. After two months, these projects were approved as << 85 Chin national important scientific and technology projects>>, however the author suddenly had the heart attack which he had acute myocardiac infarct in the anterior walls and lateral walls. After the therapy of hospitalization half years, he was discharged and his health was recovered gradually. However this critical project was stopped since then.

In 1993 the author started to conduct these projects again after his healthy condition was getting better so that he followed up his patient who had the cancer surgery done. The results showed that the recurrence and metastasis after the surgery is the key toaffect the treat the long-term treatment and must be researched to prevent the recurrence and metastasis for the basic and clinical concept and the effective method. He set up his mind to do good research on these topics and started to raise money for this research. In 1993 his wife was retired and opened her own private practice, which she used these income to help with these research projects. He also applied the support from the university such as sharing the small animals and other instruments for these projects. In brief, these projects started soon after the author got small amount funding, later he built the animal experimental laboratory which is a building with two floors and six rooms. In 1996 the author was already 63 year old and retired from the university, however he continued to do the research and clinical research under the low income. After 10 years of the hard work, he almost finished these national projects and gathered all of the experimental and clinical research material and data together and summarize them, consistencely published two books which are : 1. << the new concepts and ways of treatment of the cancer>>, Xu Ze, Jan, 2001, published in book press by Hubei Science and technology company. 2. << the new concepts and ways of treatment of the cancer>>, Xu Ze, published by People's military medical press.

2). Scientific study route and methods

Our oncology clinical research work principle is: "following the scientific development concept, based on known science, facing future medicine"; "seek truth from facts, speak out with the experimental data and clinical efficacy, The basic methods is described below:

1>> To discover the questions--- to post the experimental research projects--- to seek for the methods of solving the questions

Through following up most of the patients, it was found that the keys of effects on the longterm curative effects are the reccurence and metastasis after the surgery.

Suggest that research and solve the recurrence and metasatasis problems can improve the long term curative effects which set up the targets or aims of how to antimetasatasis.

Set up the research center and do some research to investigate the mechanism of the metastasis and antirecurrence reasons and to look for the new drugs such as 48 chinese herbs of 200 chinese herbs were selected as anticancer and antimetastasis medications.

Conduct the clinical research to investigate the rules of the tumor metastasis and to find the new anticancer therapy models and upto the automatic new theory and new anticancer therapy models.

2>> This research is from the clinical to the experiments to the clinics to the experiments to the clinic again, to solve the clinical problems

3>>Combined the theory and the practice : these research started from the clinics, searched the questions and the clinical breakthrough. After experimental research and clinical research, then applied into the clinics again to solve the clinical practical questions.

4>> This research took the combination of the Chinese medicine and the western medicine

to macroscopic combination to molecular level combination, and use the new theory of the modern tumor molecular transferring mechanism and eight steps, three stages to search and to select the new anticancers from 200 oldest herbs to protect the immune organs and activate the cell factors and immune factors and make the old medication into the modern medicine and to merge them into the international levels and combined the modern medicine with the older Chinese herbs in the molecular level and BRM level.

5>> Obey the medicine rules and keep the truth and scientific facts. To prove the facts by the evident and get the experimental research and the clinical verified.

6>>The curative therapy evulation standard and the long term curative effects: living longer and observed in the clinics 3-5 years, even 8-10 years so as to evaluate the long term curative therapy.

Obeying the all the research ways:

1. Combined scientific study with clinics, first serve the patients, the incomes from the private outpatient service were used as a research fee.

2. Built the outpatient medical records and kept them and follow the patients up: many years of the following up and called them to aske the questions and educated the diet habits and other important things to pay attention to be healthy. Kept the following tables and chemotherapy tables and the medication tables.

3. Built up the associate of the research group and the projects associate and did the research according to the research plans such as the research tables.

4. Built the detail medical records such as the patients' epidemiology and deeply analyze the successful experience and failure of the experience and specific medical condition for each cases such as analysis of the medical records.

5. Wrote the summary of analyzing the cases after following up more six months to one year. After three year of the follow-up the cases had the written summary of the analysis of the curative experience and lessons such as the medical summary.

6. Build the big tables and statistic one by one such as on the wall put the big tables includeing all of the epidemiology information, the tumor metastasis rules and information and the curative therapy experience and lessons.

7. Sharing the instruments and the materials and sharing the research awards and we didn't buy the big instruments which we used them in the university.

8. Didn't apply for money from the province, however we reported our research results and scientific evaluation to Province and the city.

3). Pay attention to the accumulation and management of scientific research experimental data

(A) In medical research, why should it attaches great importance to the accumulation of raw data

The purpose of medical research is to study the disease, to understand the disease, to seek new methods and new technologies and new theory, to improve the level of medicine and disease prevention, health services for the people, and to contribute to national construction. However, outstanding medical research is characterized by its research object which is the human body itself, and the results of its research and application is to the human body so that its results must be **strict scientific, accurate and reliable, harmless to the human body**. An outcome of the scientific nature, reliability, correct, the analysis of which the argument is logical is based on the original data from the statistical data processing, analysis, synthesis, induction. If you ignore the complete and accurate raw data, it is difficult to analyze and the inductive argument is more difficult to draw the right conclusion. **People are the most valuable,** many experiments and observations are not allowed to direct the test in the human body by the researcher, should be taken to simulate the method, the establishment of animal models for the experimental study. After being fully aware of the human body harmless, and then it can be applied to the human body. This will increase the experimental procedures to extend the work cycle, especially the national research topics, most of which are the disease pathogenesis of basic theoretical research, these issues need to be completed in a few years, complex technology, difficult, involving in many disciplines, if there is not accumaltion of all of the information without central management for a long time, it is impossible to do analysis, synthesis, induction and summary or summary stage. T herefore, each medical research, each medical research topics (such as the amount of the original data) should have responsible person who must pay the heavy and strict attention to accumulat the original data and data managerment for scientific research. The author personally participated in experimental work to obtain first-hand information.

2. How to Accumulate Original Data of Medical Research

Accumulation of scientific information should be carried out in three steps:

(1). data collection and analysis. (2). experimental design, experimental observation, the collection of experimental or observation data (3). data processing, analysis and argument, presenting the conclusions

1>>Developing a plan

There are clear objectives to be drawn up for the project, research methods and procedures to be studied, and the necessary physical equipment, in addition to the overall plan, a phased plan should be developed. In the process the actual situation should be changed at any time to make the appropriate adjustments, such adjustments in the exploratory research process, is often encountered, so the plan must be left room for the idea of topic selection, subject design guidance, and the implementation plan and procedure; the instrument design principle, the drawing, the raw material, the mold, the cooperation plan, the contract signed by several parties, all original data, need to save and schedule inspection plan for execution and agreement or contract execution.

In order to understand the experience and achievements of the predecessors and others, it is necessary to find out what the work has been done on the subject, what are the achievements, what differences exist, what issues have not yet been resolved. It is necessary to access the literature, read the title of the relevant literature and the establishment of literature data cards and classified archive.

The relevant domestic and international profiles, project plans, design drawings, scientific research cooperation contracts are the original data. Accumulate and management should be categorized. Strategic management needs to be hand-derived and the assistants should help make this work and become the good assistant for the main charge person.

2. The experimental observation

After the preparation is done, observations should be recorded one by one, observe the specimen should be consistent. Observation should be objective, practical and realistic, research process found that special changes in the research process should be carefully observed and the results of the study should be carried out in accordance with the plan. Even if it is fully inconsistent with the original assumption, it should also pay attention to and detailed records. Observing the record must be correct response to the objective facts seen in the study. The inspection report must be reliable, inspection methods and results to determine the criteria should be determined, The information should be reviewed regularly. Team leader should personally participate in specific work. If you do not personally participate in specific research work, the experience is not deep, it is difficult to detect problems in time to solve the problem.

All the raw materials (records, laboratory tests, special examinations, specimens, photographs, real objects, etc.) obtained during the whole research, experiment and observation shall be collected in full. The research materials shall be the important property of the subject, and be the confidentiality and proper custody of the original material. As a lot of very complex, not systematic, involving a wide range of storage time is long, there must have an assistant to assist the project leader to help with managing these original data, structuring well.

3. Analysis and Arrangement

When the research work reaches a certain stage, the original data should be analyzed and collated so as to carry out a comprehensive review of the whole research work and to make the necessary modifications and additions to the research plan in time, which will depend on the original data for analysis, (The equivalent of secretarial work) should be provided in a timely manner to the custody of the information in the analysis and make any judgments should be on the research methods, the reliability of the original data and whether it can be analyzed Such as the special test by whom, how reliable? Do not rush to make conclusions. This requires the integrity of the original data, system, reliable and no omission.

In the course of analyzing and sorting out the original data, we must be good at finding out the law of things, and analyze, synthesize, summarize and ascend into the theory from the obtained data, carry on the logical analysis and argumentation, and compare with the predecessors. Whether the new knowledge, new theory, new technology, what value has not been found by the predecessors.

Throughout the process, if the findings are in doubt, doubt, you must review the original audit information in order to correct errors, or modify the plan, or further add research information.

The work of the above stages requires the project leader to seize the accumulation of the original data and all the staff of the research group attach importance to the accumulation and management of the original data.

(C) It should take the serious attitude towards the accumulation of medical research of raw data

The quality and level of the results depends on the level of design and the quality of the original data, and if the quality of the original data is not the same as the quality of the original data, Research design is a strategic measure, the collection of raw data is a tactical measure is the key to success.

The original data records must pay attention to scientific, advanced, innovative, (try not to repeat the low level) Seek truth from facts, is one to one, is the second on the success of the record should be truthful, the failure to truthfully record Truthful records, to be faithful to objective information.

All the objective data of the whole process including the topic, the plan, the field observation, and the summary process, and even the work log are included in the original data record of scientific research, which contain the contents of the experimental part of the topic, and should be kept confidential. Cabinet lock), no one is allowed to take out of the house or hospital, the end of the subject with the identification of materials with the archive.

For the primitive material accumulation, it must have the strict style and the strict request and it should seek truth from facts, respect the primitive data, be faithful to the original data (if the method is really reliable) and have the real work style; the subject person in charge must be new to participate in the practice without the slightest empiricism and preconceived; the person should be the main thing; the successful experience is important, but the lessons of failure is equally important; it should respect every objective observation of the experimental data; whether you think it is important or not, all of them should be collected. No matter what you think of at that time the main topic is not successful, all of them should be collected. Simetimes you the main topics were not successful, but accidentally get other results or discover; in the world some new theories, new technologies and new discoveries are from those results and there are many cases as the samples, so we must attach importance to the first-hand the original data which are valuable wealth. In our laboratory all the original plans, drafts, work contact notes, etc. about the scientific research are saved and had good summary in the end of the subject. These raw materials may sometimes trigger our new ideas, research is not based on unthinkable thought of inspiration, but it is in the repeated thinking on the basis of practice to stimulate a sudden awakening to open a crux.

It is necessary for the research chief to have a strict style, a serious attitude and a real management way; for the research chief to have the spirit of hard work and tell the truth and serious attitudes. The research members should conscientiously implement and seriously implement the plan, meticulous and meticulous. The assistants should be organized and sorted according to the order of the project, and collect and store the original data, and comply with the corresponding secret class, at any time to provide information required for the project leader to facilitate the consolidation, induction, analysis, summary or Summarized as a paper.

2. The experimental research and clinical observation of immune regulation anti-cancer medications

In order to look for the traditional herb medicine with actually curative effect and without toxication and adverse reaction, this surgical tumor research institute has screened 200 kinds of Chinese herbal medicines with so-called anticancer reaction recorded on Chinese herbal medicine books for tumor-inhibition reaction on the solid carcinoma in the tumor-bearing animal models one by one in the past 4 years. Through long-term in-vivo tumor-inhibiting animal experiments, we have screened 48 kinds of Chinese herbal medicines with relatively good tumor-proliferation inhibition rate. Through the better combination, and then tested in the experiments on the animal models such as liver cancer, lung cancer and stomach caner, etc, formed Z-C 1-10 particles, Z-C1 significantly inhibits cancer cells without affecting the normal cells; Z-C4 can protect thymus and increase the immune function; Z-C8 can protect bone morrow. Z-C immune regulation medications can prolong the patients survival time, improve the life quality in advanced patients and increase the immune function and increase the patients appetite and strengthen the body.

I. Experimental Study on Animal

1. Materials and Method

(1) Experimental animal: 260 Kunming clon white rats, half of male and female respectively, weight:21±2g, 8~10 weeks.

(2) Cell strains and inoculation: hepatic carcinoma H_{22} cell strains, the fresh tumor bodies from the rats with tumor were prepared into the single cell suspended

liquid, after dyeing and counting of the cancer cells (1×10^6/ml), 0.2ml normal saline of cancer cell was subject to subcutaneous vaccination at the front axilla at the right side of each rat.

(3) Drugs and experimental group: the traditional herb medicines $Z-C_1$ and $Z-C_4$ were entirely developed and prepared by Hubei Branch of China Anti-cancer Research Cooperation of Chinese Traditional Medicine and Western Medicine, the former was a compound and the latter was a medicinal powder. The chemotherapy control medicine used by the chemotherapy group was cyclophosphane (CTX).

Experimental group: the animals with H_{22} cancer cell transplanted were divided into four groups randomly: ① traditional herb medicine $Z-C_1$ group (90 rats). The rats were subject to gastriclavage once every day after 24h of transplantation of cancer cells, 0.8ml per rat every time, equivalent to 1.4mg of the dried medicinal herbs. ②Traditional herb medicine $Z-C_4$ group (90 rats), as to the dose and gastriclavage method, ditto. ③Chemotherapy group (50 rats), from the next day after transplantation of cancer cells, they were subject to gastriclavage with CTX50mg/kg weight every other day. ④Control group (30 rats), they were subject to gastriclavage with normal saline every day from the next day after transplantation of the cancer cells, 0.8ml/rat.

(4) Observation of indexes: measure the weight of the rats every 3d, measure the diameter of the tumor with vernier caliper, measure the immunologic function and blood picture. Half of each group as Group A, subject to tumor-bearing experiment, regular killing of the rats in batches, separation of tumor and weighing of the tumor and then calculation of tumor-inhabiting rate. The tumor was subject to the pathological section and a few of the specimens were subject to the observation of ultra-structural organization. The rest half of each group as Group B. The tumor-bearing experimental rats were drenched for a long time until they met with natural death. Then the tumor was separated and weighed, the long-term inhibition rate and life elongation rate of the tumor was calculated.

2. Experimental result

(1) The tumor-inhibition effect of Z-C Medicine on Rats bearing hepatic carcinoma H_{22}: in the second week after administration of $Z-C_1$, the tumor-inhibition rate was 40% and the one in the fourth week was 45% and 58% in the sixth week. The tumor-inhibition rate after administration of $Z-C_4$ was 55%, 68% in the

fourth week and 70% in the sixth week. (P<0.01) the tumor-inhibiting rate after administration of CTX was 45% in the second week, 45% in the fourth week and 49% in the sixth week (See Fig. 1 and 2).

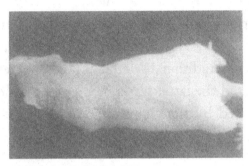

Fig. 1 Z-C$_1$ and Z-C$_4$ therapy group
30d after inoculation of hepatic carcinoma H$_{22}$

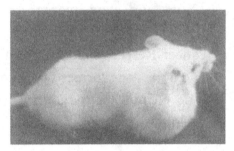

Fig. 2 Control group
30d after inoculation of hepatic carcinoma H$_{22}$

(2) The effect of Z-C medicine on the survival time of the rats bearing hepatic carcinoma H$_{22}$: the average survival time of Z-C$_1$, Z-C$_4$ and CTX was longer than the one of the normal saline control group (P<0.01); Z-C medicine played a role in obviously prolonging the survival time. Through comparison with the control group, the life elongation rate of Z-C$_1$ group was 85%, the one of Z-C$_4$ group was 200% and the one of CTX group was 9.8%. The rats in Z-C$_1$ and CTX in Group B met with death in 75d. 6 rats bearing carcinoma in Z-C$_4$ survived after seven months.

(3) Both Z-C$_1$ and Z-C$_4$ medicine improved the immunologic function and Z-C$_4$ obviously improved the immunologic function, increased the white blood cells and red blood cells, without any effect on the hepatic function and kidney function and without damage to the hepatic and kidney section. CTX decreased the white blood cells and reduced the immunologic function with the renal damage to the kidney section. The thymus in the control group was obviously atrophic (Fig. 1-4) while the one of Z-C$_1$ and Z-C$_2$ therapy group was not atrophic but a little hypertrophic (Fig.1-3).

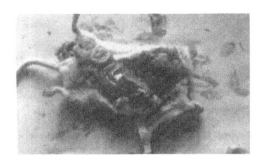

Fig. 3 Z-C4 therapy group

The thymus was obviously hypertrophic in 30 days after inoculation of hepatic carcinoma H_{22}

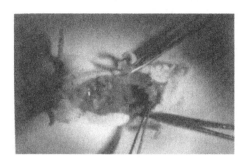

Fig. 4 Control group

The thymus was obviously atrophic in 30 days after inoculation of hepatic carcinoma

H_{22}

Pathological section of thymus in the control group: the cortex of the thymus was atrophic, the cells were discrete and the blood vessel met with sludge (Fig. 1-5). The pathological section of the thymus in Z-C_4 therapy group displayed that the cortical area of the thymus built up, the lymphocyte was dense, the epithelium reticulocyte increased and the thymus corpuscles increased (Fig. 1-6).

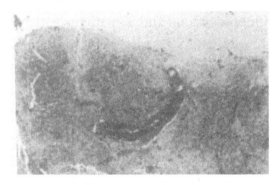

Fig. 5 Pathological section of the thymus in tumor-bearing control group

HE x 100 cortex atrophia   lymphocyte obviously decreased, cortical area formed an empty band of lymphocyte and the sludge appeared in the blood vessel.

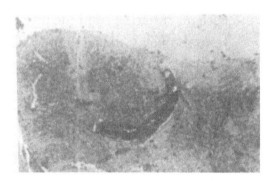

Fig. 6 Thymus of Z-C_4 control group

HE x 100 the cortex and medulla of the thymus built up and the lymphocyte was highly dense

II. Observation on Clinic Application

1. Clinical information

(1) Hubei Branch of China Anti-cancer Research Cooperation of Chinese Traditional Medicine and Western Medicine, Anti Carcinoma Metastasis and Recurrence Research Office and Shuguang Tumor Specialized Outpatient Department had treated 4, 698 carcinoma patients in Stage III and IV or in metastasis and recurrence with Z-C medicine combined with western medicine from 1994 to Nov. 2002, among which there were 3, 051 men patients and 1,647 women patients. The youngest one was 11 years old and the oldest one was 86 years old, the high invasion age was 40~69 years. All groups of the patients were entirely subject to the diagnosis of pathological histology or definitive diagnosis with ultrasonic B, CT and MRI iconography. According to the staging standard of UICC, all the cases were entirely the patients in medium and advanced stage over Stage III. In this group, there were 1,021 hepatic carcinoma patients, among which there were 694 primary lesion hepatic carcinoma patients and 327 metastatic hepatic carcinoma patients; there were 752 patients suffering from carcinoma of lung, among which there were 699 patients suffering from the primary carcinoma of lung and 53 patients suffering from the metastatic carcinoma of lung; there were 668 gastric carcinoma patients, 624 patients suffering from esophagus cardia carcinoma, 328 patients suffering from rectum carcinoma of anal canal, 442 patients suffering from carcinoma of colon, 368 patients suffering from breast carcinoma, 74 patients suffering from adenocarcinoma of pancreas, 30 patients suffering from carcinoma of bile duct, 43 patients suffering from retroperitoneal tumor, 38 patients suffering from oophoroma, 9 patients suffering from cervical carcinoma, 11 patients suffering from cerebroma, 34 patients suffering from thyroid carcinoma, 38 patients suffering from nasopharyngeal carcinoma, 9 patients suffering from melanoma, 27 patients suffering from kidney carcinoma, 48 patients suffering from carcinoma of urinary bladder, 13 patients suffering from leukemia, 47 patients suffering from metastasis of supraclavicular lymph nodes, 35 patients suffering various fleshy tumors and 39 patients suffering from other malignancies.

(2) Medicine and medication: the treatment aims to support healthy energy to eliminate evils, soften and resolve the hard mass and supplement qi and blood. $Z-C_1$ is the compound, 150ml to be taken on the daily basis, $Z-C_4$ is powder, 10g to be taken on the daily basis. According to the analysis and differentiation of the diseases, anti-cancer powder shall be taken orally and the

anti-cancer apocatastasis paste shall be applied externally for the solid tumor or the metastatic tumor. In case of being in pain, anti-cancer aponic paste shall be applied externally. Icterus removal soup or dropsy removal soup shall be taken orally for the patients suffering from icterrus and the ascites.

(3) Therapeutic evaluation: it pays attention to the short-term curative effect and iconography indexes as well as the survival time of long-term curative effect, quality of life and immunologic indexes. Attention shall be paid to the changes in subjective signs in administration of drugs. It will be effective when the subjective signs are improved and last over one month; otherwise, it will be ineffective. As to the quality of life (Karnofsky Performance Status), it will be effective when it is improved and lasts over one month, otherwise, it will be ineffective. As to the evaluation standard of the curative effect of solid tumor, it can be divided into four levels according to the changes in size of tumor: Level I: disappearance of tumor; Level II: tumor reduces 1/2; Level III: softening of tumor; Level IV: no change or enlargement of level tumor.

2. Curative results

(1) The symptom was improved, the quality of life was improved, the survival time was prolonged: among the 4,277 carcinoma patients in medium and advanced stage who took Z-C medicine with the return visit over 3 months, the case history had the specific observation record of the curative effect. It improved the quality of life of the patients in an all-round way, see Table 1-2.

Table 1-1 Observation of curative effect on 4 277 patients: fully improving the quality of life of the carcinoma patients in medium and advanced stage

Improvement	Vigor	Appetite	Reinforcement of physical force	Improvement in generalized case	Increase of body weight	Improvement of sleep	The restriction of improvement activity and capability released activity	self servicing normal walking	Resumption of work Engaged in light work
No. of cases	4071	3986	2450	479	2938	1005	1038	3220	479
(%)	95.2	93.2	57.3	11.2	68.7	23.5	24.3	75.3	11.2

In this group, all of them were the patients in medium and advanced stage. After taking the medicine, their symptoms were improved to different extents with the effective rate of 93.2%. With respect to the improvement of the quality of life (as per Karnofsky Performance Status), it rose to 80 scores on average after administration from 50 on average before administration; the patients in this group met with the different metastasis and dysfunction of the organs about Stage III. It was reported by the previous statistic information that the mesoposition survival time of this kind of patients was about 6 months. The longest time among this group of the cases reached up to 11 years; another patient suffering from hepatic carcinoma had taken Z-C medicine for ten years and a half; two patients suffering from hepatic carcinoma met with frequency encountered carcinomatous lesion in the left and right liver and it entirely subsided through secondary CT reexamination after the patient took Z-C medicine for half a year and the state of the disease had been stable over half a year. One patient suffering from double-kidney carcinoma met with the widespread metastasis of abdominal cavity after removal of one kidney, after taking Z-C medicine, he was entirely recovered and began to work again. 3 patients suffering from carcinoma of lung, with the lung not removed through explaraton, had taken Z-C medicine over three years and a half. 2 patients suffering from gastric remnant carcinoma had taken Z-C medicine for 8 years. 3 patients suffering from reoccurrence of rectal carcinoma had taken Z-C medicine for 3 years. 1 patient suffering from metastatic liver and rib of the mastocarcinoma had taken Z-C medicine for 8 years. 1 patient suffering from the recurrent bladder carcinoma after operation of renal carcinoma had not met with the carcinoma for 9 years and a half after taking Z-C medicine. All of these patients were the ones in the medium and advanced stage that could not be operated once more or treated with radiotherapy or chemotherapy. They only took Z-C medicine without other medicines for treatment. Up to today, they are reexamined and get the medicine at the out-patient department every month. Through taking the medicine for a long time, the state of the disease is controlled in the stable state to make the organism and the tumor in balanced state for a relatively long time and get a relatively good survival with tumor, in this way, the symptoms of the patients are improved, the quality of life is improved and the survival time is prolonged.

(2) As to 84 patients suffering from solid tumor and 56 patients suffering from enlargement of upper lymph node of metastatic compact bone, after taking Z-C series medicines orally and applying Z-C3 anti-cancer apocatastasis paste, they met with good curative effects, see table 1-3.

Table 1-2 Changes of 84 patients suffering from solid tumor and 56 patients suffering from metastatic mode after applying Z-C paste externally

Solid tumor				Enlargement of upper lymph node of metastatic compact bone			
Disappearance	Shrinkage 1/2	Softening	No change	Disappearance	Shrinkage 1/2	Softening	No change

No. of cases (%)	12 14.2	28 33.3	32 38.0	12 14.2	12 21.4	22 39.2	14 25.0	8 14.2
Total effective rate (%)		85.7				85.7		

(3) 298 patients suffering from carcinoma pain obtained the obvious pain alleviation effects after taking Z-C medicine orally and applying Z-C anti-cancer apocatastasis paste externally, see Table 1-3.

Clinical menifetation	Pain			
	Light alleviation	Obvious alleviation	Disappearance	Avoidance
No of cases	52	139	93	14
(%)	17.3	46.8	31.2	4.7
Total effective rate (%)			95.3	

3. Discussion on Anti - cancer Pharmacological Action of Traditional Chinese Medicine

1). The Pharmacology of XZ-C Immune regulation medication:

Compared with Western medication immunity pharmacology, traditional Chinese medication pharmacology has own characteristics and advantages which long-term clinical experience Chinese medicine has accumulated a large number of prescriptions regulating body's immune function, especially beneficial traditional Chinese medicines generally have dynamic regulation of the immune benefits.

Whether single herb medicine or prescription will have a variety of active ingredients, and unlike Western medicine (synthetic drugs) is a matter of a single structure. The role of traditional Chinese medication are many aspects, in addition to the regulation of immune function, which has a certain role on the whole system function.

The main role of XZ-C medicine immunomodulator in regulating cellular immunity (cellular immunity) regulate various immune cell-mediated disease-free response, including cytokines (cytokines) or (lymphoknes), XZ-C medicine immune function has major role on stem cells immunity, such as the thymus, gonads and lymphatic systems and T, B cells and various cytokines.

China has the concept which righteousness ancient medicine had not imaginary, evil does not go into, constitute an integral part of traditional Chinese medicine theory. Its essence is to maintain the balance of the overall function, enhance resistance to disease. Its main role is to enhance immune function, in fact, is to avoid disease tonics based pharmacology. Immunity pharmacology is an emerging interdisciplinary, serves as a bridge contact between pharmacology and immunology. XZ-C immunomodulatory medication has obvious immune function, as an effective immune enhancers, this area should be vigorously developed, to be made according to a new type of immune accelerator, making the treatment of patients with reliable, efficient and safe drugs. XZ-C4 in various Chinese herbs have substantially immune enhancers effect. In animal experiments have proven to significantly promote the thymus function. The main role of medicine immunomodulator in regulating cellular immunity, regulate various immune cell-mediated immune response, including cytokines or lymphokines.

2). XZ-C Study of immune regulation of Chinese medication

1. To sum anticancer pharmacology and experimental cancer-bearing animal solid tumors in vivo anti-tumor experiments, xz-c drugs have significant anti-tumor effect. Antitumor activity xz-c1 the first six weeks inhibition rate xz-c medicine for liver cancer H22 bearing mice 58%, xz-c4 first six weeks inhibition rate was 70%, cyclophosphamide amine (CTX) first 6 weeks inhibition rate was 49%. XZ-C1 life span was 9.8% indicates xz-c drug has a good anti-cancer effect.

2. XZ-C drug have synergistic effect of attenuated toxicity from chemotherapy drugs, said anti-cancer pharmacology 3,6 xz-c4 has been shown to have better function to reduce the toxicity from anticancer drugs of chemotherapy.

3. XZ-C anti-cancer medicine protective immune regulation hematopoietic system function. In MMC or cyclophosphamide amine (CTX) in cancer-bearing mice, chemotherapy drugs cause bone marrow hematopoietic system suppression, and then served xz-c4 for 4 weeks Hb, WBC, PLT were improved significantly.

4. XZ-C immunomodulatory anticancer medicine has a role in protecting the immune organs and improvement human immune function.

Above H22 cancer-bearing mice with cyclophosphamide (CTX)has leukopenia, reduced immune function, kidney damage sliced, ; dried xz-c4 can significantly improve immune function and can make white blood cells, red blood cells increase, not thymic atrophy but a little hypertrophy, lymphocytes intensive, increased epithelial reticular cells in xz-c treatment group.

3). The research on cytokine induction of XZ-C traditional Chinese anti-carcinoma medicine for immunologic regulation and control

1. XZ-C4 inducing thecytokine factors

> (1) Through the experiments: XZ-C4 has many immune strengthening function; XZ-C4 can induce cell factors in the host and have closely relationship to the cell factors.

> (2) XZ-C4 can inhibit the reduction of the white blood cells, granulation cell and platelet.

> (3) XZ-C4 can have the direct function on GM-CSF production from granulation cell (GM) through IL-1β, also increase TNF, IFN ect all of kind of the cell factors, which are possible the indirect function.

> (4) XZ-C4 can increase the Th1 cell factors, which were decrease in the cancer patients. There are the curative effects on the anemia and the white blood cells decrease due to the chemotherapy.

> (5) The experiment analysis showed that XZ-C4 not only protect the bone marrow function, but also the direct function on the tumor cell division.

In brief, XZ-C4 can induce the tumor division and natural death through the autocrne which produce all of kind of factors. The autocrne is the secretory things from the host to affect the hosts' function. XZ-C4 probability will become the induction therapy to the tumor division in the future.

2. XZ-C4 inhibiting the tumor development and metastasis

The malignant development is defined as tumor cells accepting invasion and metastasis characters during the proliferation. Cancer research need to have good repeated animal models. Then the good repeated animal model was made from the mice fibrosis cancernoma QR-32. QR-32 cannot proliferate after inoculation in the skin, and will completely disappear; there were no metastasis lump after injecting into the veins. However, if QR-32 were injected with Gelatin sponge together under the skin in the mice, the QR-32 will become the proliferating tumor cells QRSP.

In vitro culturing QRSP and then transfer into another mice, even if there is no foreign thing, the tumors will grow such as the lung metastasis will happen after injection in the vein.

XZ-C4 were used in the animal models to search the effects of the tumor development. To divide this animal models into two steps: the process from QR-32 to QRSP(early progress) and from the QRSP to tumor(later progress). After using XZ-C4, the tumor development will be inhibited in these two models, especially the former will be inhibited significantly. And this has relationship with the dose of the medication.

On the survival experiment the animal models of the inoculation of the QR-32 AND Gelatin sponge died during 65 days, however in XZ-C using animal models the mice surviving 150 days was 30%.

XZ-C4 can increase the immune effects and reduce the side effects of other anticancer medication.

This research proved that XZ-C4 have inhibition of the cancer progression function and inhibit cancer invasion and metastasis.

4). XZ-C immunomodulatory anticancer medicine toxicology studies

XZ-C1 can be long-term use. Acute toxicity experiments showed that: 100 times the adult dose to mice fed (10g / kg body weight) were observed at 24, 48, 72, 96 hours, 30 purebred mice without a death. The median lethal dose (LD50) is difficult to make and is a branch quite secure prescriptions.

According to WHO "cancer medicine and acute toxin Classification Standard" assessment patients with different measurement, different forms of treatment, changes in the peripheral blood, liver and kidney function in order to understand its toxicity and adverse circumstances, xz-c medicine oral taken in more than 6000 cases, continuous medication at less 3 months, some for years, a small number of patients have no abnormal phenomenon before and after treatment to check the blood, WBC, RBC, Hb, PLT; most had blood improvement of Hb. RBC, WBC, PLT. In patients with advanced many of our specialist clinics in order to control the tumor, the patient took this drug long-term so that long-term using XZ-C1,4 3-5 years, the patient didn't have metastasis and non-proliferation, the disease condition is stable, and lived with cancer. Adhere to long-term medication can often stabilize condition, inhibit cancerproliferation, improve the quality of life and prolong their lives, did not show toxicity, we insist on a longer-term experience serving XZ-C medicine and can help prevent cancer after radical short and long term recurrence and metastasis.

5). XZ-C immunomodulatory anticancer active ingredient in traditional Chinese medication

XZ- C1,4 is a compound consisting of 28 Chinese herbs. The extraction work of total effective ingredient compound is extremely difficult, the technology is complex and it was exceedingly difficult to extract the active ingredient compound. Active ingredients of single herb can be extracted. Thus, XZ- C series drugs except XZ- C1 outside is boiling agent, and the rest are used every herb of fine powder powder or capsules, in order to remain independent of each herb's active ingredients, and thus play its antitumor effects, powders of mixed fine powder, the active ingredient can remain independent of each drug, the drug is boiling chemical change, inevitably changing the active ingredient of the drug, making it difficult to know the active ingredients after boiling.

But in all the prescription the active ingredients of various drugs are:

1. Alkaloids

2. Glycosides: there are saponins and glycosides

In the formula each herb has anti-tumor active ingredient, for example prescription Ganoderma lucidum, its anti-tumor component A is Ganoderma lucidum polysaccharides, antitumor effect is: with a hypodermic method, graft inoculation 7 days of S_{180} ascites carcinoma to mouse right groin, at a dose 20% mg / kg, 10 / day's the inhibition rate was 95.6-98.5%; for the treatment of leukopenia, the recent efficiency is 84.6% and increases WBC 1028 / mm³; in the formula Ganoderma anti-tumor component B is fumaric acid (Fumaric acid). Its anti-tumor effect was to 60mg / kg; for mice inoculated with S180 gavage, 10 days the tumor was weight, the inhibition rate was 37.1% -38.6% body weight of mice did not decline.

Another example is the prescription holly child, its anti-tumor components of ursolic acid (Ursolic acid). Its anti-tumor effect on liver cancer cells in vitro has a very significant inhibition rate, can prolong life Ehrlich ascites carcinoma in mice. Pharmacological experiments show holly sub flooding agent capable of inhibiting certain animals transplanted tumor growth. This product contains oleanolic acid, with enhanced immune function, increased peripheral leukocytes, enhanced phagocytosis of reticuloendothelial cells, increase which white blood cells by radiation-induced reduction and has the role of cardiac diuretic and hepatoprotective effect.

Another example is the prescription of Sophora, its anti-tumor component A Sophocarpine. Its anti-tumor effect: In vitro experiments showed that Sophocarpine Ehrlich ascites tumor cells have a direct killing effect: mice transplanted U14, S180 inhibition rate of 30 to 60%. Clinical application has certain effect; Sophora antitumor component B Oxymatrine, its anti-tumor effects: for S180 mice have significant activity, 500ug per day and 250 ug administration, a total of five days, the treatment and control groups, respectively tumor weight 26.1% and 57.9%.

3. Another example is the prescription of bamboo ginseng, its anti-tumor component A, as β-Elemene, its anti-tumor effects: the goods on the ECA, ARS and other two kinds of ascites cancer have significant anti-graft tumor effect on YAS and S180 ascites also effective. Its anti-tumor components; ginseng total polysaccharides, its anti-tumor effects: animal experiments show; total ginseng polysaccharides on immune function has a stimulating effect on Ehrlich ascites tumor cells in mice at 400-800mg / kg dose, with significant inhibition. Ginseng polysaccharide on many tumor cells without direct killing effect, its anti-tumor effect may be due to the adjustment of the body's immune function so that cancer-bearing host enhanced antitumor capacity. Its anti-tumor component C is ginsenosides (Ginsenoside): S180 has a certain extent of, in 100, 120mg / kg dx7 when / its tumor weight inhibition was 36.4%, ginsenosides may act directly on cancer cells to grow restrained; also available through effects on metabolism and regulation of immunity, so that the body's resistance to disease increased, so that the tumor growth was inhibited. Workers acid ginseng extract has the inhibition for Marine, sarcoma S180, lung cancer T55.

Chapter 4 The research situation of Immune regulation anti-cancer Chinese and Western medications

1. Anti-cancer Function of cell immune system

As we all know, the occurrence and prognosis of cancer development and treatment are decided by two contrast factors: the biological characteristics of cancer cells and the host restrictive ability to cancer cells. If these two are balance, the cancer is controlled; if they are imbalance, cancer will develop.

What are the biological characteristics and the biological behavior of the cancer cells? The previous chapters in this book have been outlined respectively. Under normal circumstances, the host itself against cancer cells has certain constraints defense capability, but in cancer the defense capabilities of these constraints are suppressed and damaged in different degrees so as to lead the loss of the immune surveillance of cancer cells and cancer has immune escape, making cancer metastasis.

1. The human body anticancer mechanism and its influencing factors

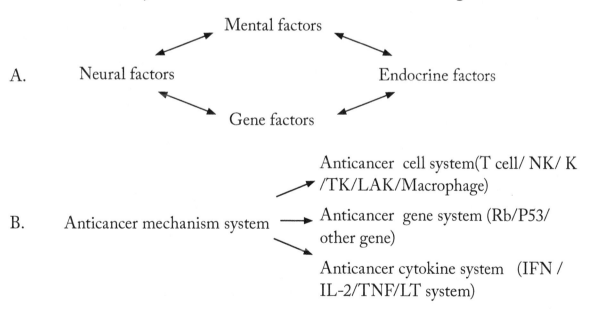

C.

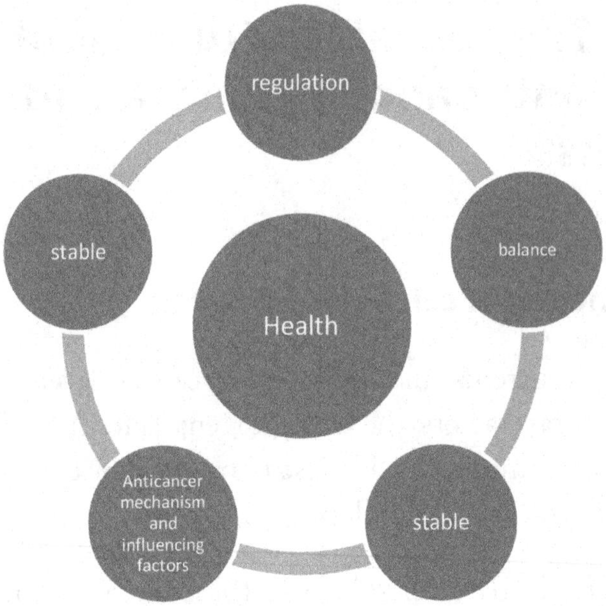

Figure 1 Anticancer mechanism and its influencing factors schematic diagram

The human body has a complete anti-cancer immune system: the anti-cancer immune cells series; anticancer cytokine family; humoral immune series; a series of anti-cancer gene.

Anti-tumor immunological mechanism of the body can be divided ①Cell-mediated immune: including T lymphocytes; NK natural killer cells; K cells; LAK cells; monocyte-macrophages. ②Humoral immune : contains B cells; anti-tumor antibodies. ③ cytokines: interleukin-cell lines have; IFN; TNF; CSF and the like.

These human inherent anti-cancer system and immune substances are their own material in vivo. How biological response modifiers mobilize, activate and enhance the anti-tumor effect occupies an extremely important role in the anti-cancer and anti-metastatic therapy and will have vast work prospects.

Therefore, we have to study which are anti-cancer cells, which are anti-cancer cytokines, which humoral immune can be activated to enhance the anti-cancer metastasis in the human body.

Here, we first review several biological therapies at the history of the 20th century in the treatment of cancer which have impressive results.

In the 1930s, Willam Coley and their successors Coley Nauts treated the advanced cancer with "Coley toxins". More than 200 cases of various types of cancer patients can be analyzed, which more than 30 cases were cured, and life more than 30 years. In the early 1980s Guesada and others treated hairy cell leukemia with IFN-a, which actually made the treatment effective (complete remission /CR + PR/ partial remission) reach over 90%.

In the mid-1980s Rosenberg and others treated patients with advanced metastatic cancer who cannot be treated with other methods with LAK / IL-2. Some patients could be PR(42/228 patients) and CR (9 / 228 cases).

"Biological Therapy" (biotherapy) is also known as "biological regulation therapy" (bioregulator therapy). "Anti-cancer system" is quite complex in our body. From a structural and functional point it is a fairly large network system and under this system a number of members constitutes a "network learning system."

Because of the rapid development of molecular biology, molecular immunology, molecular immunology pharmacology, genetic engineering, basic and clinical research at the molecular level, "cancer establishment" continues to expand and depth, the prospects of its anti-cancer metastasis extremely lure people.

Currently, the research of molecular biology on anti-cancer immunotherapy, are mainly focusing on the "four sub-systems": "anti-cancer cell therapy," "anti-cancer cytokine therapy", "anti-cancer gene therapy" and "anti-cancer antibody therapy."

The basic characteristics of these molecular biology and molecular immunotherapy are: all of formulations of molecular biology and immunotherapy used are "theirselves" in vivo. The fundamental difference from chemotherapy is: it not only did not carry out the role of the damage for the normal body tissue cells, especially the function of cells of the hematopoietic system and the structure and function of the immune system, but mainly there are the regulation and it enhances the role of the immune response; as we all know, radiotherapy and chemotherapy are completely different. Chemotherapy is a kind of non-selective "treatment injury", both killing cancer cells also killing normal cells, which damage the body's normal tissue cells, bone marrow and immune system structure and function suffered serious damage and leads to serious consequences.

Biological therapy is through the regulation of biological response mechanism to make life stable and balance. American scholar Oldam (1984) proposed biological regulation (BRM) theory, which later on this basis, proposed the concept of biological therapy of cancer.

Immune regulation mechanism of life is very important. Immune structure and function are extremely complex and its essence is to identify themselves by tolerance to their own body and removing others to maintain a stable internal environment. Immune defense, immune surveillance and immune homeostasis are three basic types of functions that bodies identify themselves, intolerance to foreign. From the basic point of biological function, immune regulation is one of the basic biological therapies.

On development of cancer there has always been two different views: one view, the tumor occurrence and development are a basic defense mechanism against any restriction body "independent process" so that the treatment for the tumor focused on itself emphatically, few pays attention to the regulation of the immune system; **another view is that the tumor occurrence and development are controlled by a variety of factors in vivo, particularly by the regulation of immune factors "involuntary procedure" or "controlled process", are subject to immune surveillance. The cancer cells escape the immune surveillance so that cancer was able to develop.** Based on these two different views there are two completely different proposition. The former believe that cancer is a largely unaffected by the body's defense mechanism for any restriction "independent process", which targets the treatment with simply killing cancer cells (regardless of the immune status) which the methods of treatment are radiation therapy and chemotherapy.

Cao guangwen and Du ping presented an important concept which it is about as cancer biotherapy core foundation - the concept of "cancer establishment". And in vivo "cancer establishment" is a fairly large network system, the current basic and clinical research on the anti-cancer organization is expanding and depth, work of anti-cancer treatment has an extremely important role and broad prospects.

About network functionality issues concerning anti-cancer mechanism, currently more study is cytokine network structure and function, the other sides also studied less. This is called as "cytokine network", simply said, various cytokines in structure and function have certain correlations.

2. Anti-tumor effect of various immune functions

The cause of the tumor is very complicated, there are environmental factors, but also the organism internal factors, particularly with the gene mutation, oncogene expression and the decreased immune function.

Modern immunology proposed that immune system has three major functions: the immune defense, immune stable and immune surveillance. There is great significance in the anti-tumor. Immune defenses can resist bacteria, viruses, parasites and other pathogens infection. Immune surveillance function can eliminate mutant cells and prevent tumor occurrence, if the immune dysfunction or loss of immune surveillance monitor can lead to cancer.

After the body normal cells have cancer, cancerous cells on the membrane surface express tumor antigen and the host can recognize such antigens and produces immune response to attack and to exclude tumor cells. Anti-tumor immune response has many ways: both acquired immune response and natural immune response; both cellular immune response and humoral immune response ; both immune cells and immune molecules.

(1). anti-tumor effect of cell-mediated immune

What anticancer human immune cells may be activated, enhanced to do the anti-cancer cell metastasis? Immune cells of participating in vivo anticancer effects are the following:

1). Anti-cancer effect of cytotoxic lymphocytes

Cytotoxic lymphocytes(CTL) play a major role in the anti-tumor immune and have specific cytotoxicity to the same kind of autologous tumor cells and is one kind of anti-tumor lymphocytes subject to MHCI class and (or) class II antigen restrictions. Human CTL cells are CD_4 and CD_8. CTL cells in peripheral blood and spleen have high amounts; thoracic duct, thymus and bone marrow contain a certain amount. The ability of proliferation and accumulation in tumors localized is stronger and the body is more sensitive to radiation and chemotherapy drugs such as cyclophosphamide. CTL is an important effector cell in situ treatment of cancer.

Under certain conditions CTL can produce IL-2, IL-4, IFN, etc., to activate other immune cells, such as anti-cancer killer macrophages, NK cells and anti-B-cell joint anti-tumor effect. Such CTL has a potentially important role in anti-cancer and anti-metastasis.

2). Anti-tumor effect of natural killer cells(NK cells)

NK cells are a group of broad-spectrum anti-NK cell tumor cells, killing activity does not require prior sensitization antigen, do not rely on antibodies, does not depend on the thymus, but also no MHC restricted. The main role is to monitor and to remove cancerous cells. Clinical observations: if NK cell activity is deficient, the incidence of malignant tumors is significantly increased. NK cells are important parts of early anti-cancer immune surveillance.

NK cells bind with tumor cells through tumor cell surface receptor to release perforin protein (Perform, PF) or cytolysin piercing on the tumor cell membrane so that cancer cells die within a fluid outflow. NK cells can release natural killer cell factor (natural killer cell factor, NKCF), this factor can lyse tumor cells. NK cells have a small number, only about 3% of lymphocytes so that it have smaller force for later and larger tumors.

In addition, NK cells produce IL-2, TFN-y and TNF-a, enhance the anti-tumor effects of other cellular and humoral factors.

Distribution of NK cells in organs and tissues is the highest concentrations in peripheral blood and spleen, followed by lymph nodes and peritoneal cells. NK cells is also in the lamina propria alveoli, sinusoidal, intestinal epithelium, skin and bronchial wall, interstitial, esophagus, reproductive tract lymphoid tissue. Low NK cell activity is in bone marrow, thymus undetectable NK activity. NK cells accounted for 5% to 7% of the total number of peripheral blood lymphocytes. NK activity among individual patients is quite different and the level of NK activity in vitro and in vivo is often associated with anti-cancer effect. Therefore, NK activity is often used as a strength and prognosis of cancer immunology indicators and assessment body's anti-cancer therapy response. NK activity was reduced or deficiency often occurs in cancer metastasis. NK activity is often associated with improvement or deterioration of the condition in parallel.

Given the important role of NK cells in anti-tumor immunity, so look for a strong enhancement of biological therapy anti-tumor activity of NK preparation is important. Some micro-organisms or their products, such as BCG, Corynebacterium parvum (Corynebacteri-urn Parvwm, CP) and certain cytokines such as IL-2, IFN, immune adjuvant interferon inducer can significantly enhance NK activity. IL-2 and IFN-y combination of NK cell activity enhancement are stronger than a single factor activation. Multiple cytokines enhance the role of NK activity and eliminate residual cancer cells, reducing metastasis and relapse rates. In addition, we developed medicine XZ-C immune regulation agents which can activate NK, IFN-Y.

3). K cells

K cells are in human peripheral blood, spleen and peritoneal cavity, but not much in the thoracic duct and lymph nodes. Advanced cancer patient's serum contains large amounts of free tumor antigen which antigen binds tumor antibody so that K cells can not bind to the tumor cells, and therefore can not play a role in killing tumor. Remove the free tumor antigen, the addition of anti-tumor antibody, or with a non-specific immune stimulants, can enhance K cell activity.

Anti-tumor effect K cells without prior sensitization, do not need to complement participation, but requires the presence of anti-tumor antibodies, so K cells is one of the main anti-tumor antibody effector cells biological therapies.

4). LAK cells LAK cell is the most important modern biotechnology anti-cancer cell. In 1980 Rosenberg and his colleagues found T cell growth factor (TCGF) can short-term induce mouse spleen cells which can give a strong anti-tumor activity. Human peripheral mononuclear cells (PBMNC) can significantly kill a variety of human tumor cell under IL-2 induced. In 1982 Grimn called this kind of IL-2-activated cells which can kill tumor cells that NK cell cannot kill as Lyrnphokine-activa-ted Killer(LAK) cells. LAK cell is a group mainly consisting of mixed lymphocyte with LGL body which is activated by IL-2 cytokines into anticancer cell ; it not only kills the same kind of passaged tumor cells, more importantly, can kill itself.

LAK cells can kill broader spectrum of tumor than NK cells, which LAK cells can kill tumor cells that NK cells cannot kill.

In fact LAK cells are IL-2-activated NK cells and T cells which have similar activity to IL-2-activated NK cells.

From a clinical and practical points all of cells, which are activated into anti-tumor cells by IL-2 cytokines, can be called LAK cells.

5). Macrophages Macrophage plays an important role in tumor immunity. It itself is a kind of effector cells capable of dissolving the tumor cells. If there is significant macrophage infiltration around tumors, the tumor spreads in the lower metastasis rate, the prognosis is better. Conversely, when macrophage infiltration around tumors is small, the rate of tumor metastasis will be highter. Prostaglandin E can inhibit the secretion of TNF gene transcription from macrophages, which antagonist was indomethacin and may counteract this effect.

6). Anti-tumor effect of monocyte-macrophage Its anti-tumor immunity, unless involved in recognizing an antigen and presented the antigen information to T cells and B cells, as well as participatory role in killing tumor cells antigen. Pathological biopsy tip: there are a lot of tumor monocyte-macrophage infiltration around the tissues, especially in primary and metastatic tumors. If the incidence of patients with a high degree of infiltration, tumor spread and metastasis is low, the prognosis is good; on the contrary, if there is no obvious monocyte-macrophage infiltration surrounding tumor tissue, metastasis rate of tumor spread is high, prognosis is poor.

Monocyte-macrophage tumor cell killing pathways are nonspecific:

(1) An activated macrophage can contact with the tumor cell directly and play a direct killing effect.

(2) The release of TNF and IL-i and other cytokines.

(3) The generation of reactive oxygen species, such as H_2O_2.

(4) The release of lysosomal enzymes and proteolytic enzymes play killing effect.

(5) The release of arginase. L-arginine is an amino acid essential growth of tumor cells. Mononuclear cells stimulates macrophages to release massive arginase and to decompose arginine so as to inhibit tumor growth.

7). Anti-tumor effect of neutrophils

Massive neutrophil can be observed as aggregation and infiltration around the tumor tissue. After activation neutrophil releases: ① reactive oxygen species; ② fat derivatives; ③ cytokines such as IFN, TNF and IL-i, these substances have tumoricidal activity.

Anti-cancer effects of neutrophils: one inhibiting tumor growth, the second is to play a role in killing. Killing time is several hours similar to macrophages, but longer than the time required lymphocytes and NK cells. Although neutrophils life is short, but are huge amounts so that anti-tumor effect must be paid attention. Neutrophils are non-specific anti-tumor effectors and have effects on a variety of tumors.

(2) Anti-tumor effect of humoral immune

In cancer patients serum, anti-tumor antibody can be found, but cannot be detected in all cancer patients. Serum antibody is negative in the majority of progressive or metastasis patients; after surgery or radiation therapy, some patients may turn negative into positive.

Anti-tumor antibodies are divided into protective and closed two: the former is beneficial; the latter is harmful.

1. Protective antibodies

The existing of protective anti-tumor antibodies is closely related to tumor growth and decline. A month or one week before metastasis, serum anti-tumor antibody titer tends to fall, or from positive to negative. There are three kinds of protective antibodies: cytotoxic antibodies, lymphocyte-dependent antibody and cytophilic antibody.

(1) Cytotoxic antibodies: These antibodies need complement participation to kill tumor cells, they are mostly IgM or IgG class.

(2) Lymphocyte-dependent antibody (LDA): such antibodies are mostly IgG, after binding to tumor antigens, which Fc fragment binds lymphocyte surface Fc receptor, the lymphocytes and tumor target cells attach to play a killer role. Such lymphocytes are antibody-dependent killer cells, i.e., K cells.

(3) Cytophilic antibody: It is IgG class antibodies and is macrophages specifically kill tumor way. Unlike activated monocyte-macrophage non-specific cytotoxicity, when addicted to cell antibodies present in body fluids, monocyte-macrophage cells surround the tumor to form a large rosette.

2. Closed factor

Animals and cancer patients have serum blocking factors, it may be proved by experiments. Closed factor is closely related to the presence of tumor ; after tumor is resected, closed factor disappears. If the tumor is blocking factor, the tumor appears relapse. Closed factor has specificity and blocks the same type of autologous or allogeneicfor tumor tissues, however, doesn't block different classes of tumor tissue.

3. The unblocking factor

After tumor resection, not only blocking factor disappears from the serum, and the serum also appeared closed factor antagonist, called deblocking factor (unbiocking factor), deblocking factors also have tumor specificity.

(3) Anti-tumor effect of human cytokine

Which anti-cancer cytokines can be activated, enhanced with anti-metastatic cancer cells in vivo? Cytokines against viruses, parasites, bacteria and cancer immune response in cells plays an important role in the body. It is in clinical trials for cancer treatment and other aspects of bone marrow regeneration. Therefore, cytokine research has a significant increase and there are lots of papers related to the structure and function of cytokine published in the last 10 years. Here is a brief elaboration for interleukins, colony stimulating factor, tumor necrosis factor, interferon and cytokine growth factor 5 categories.

1. Interferon (IFN)

In the 1930s it was discovered that virus-infected cells can protect surrounding cells from virus infection. In 1957 Isaacs and Lindenmann discovered a protein produced by the cells while the body cells are damaged by a virus or stimulation is an interferon. A few years later people realized that the interferon can resist cell differentiation and have immune regulation. Interferon belongs to the cytokine with a variety of biological functions, now known interferon which is divided into three categories: α, β and γ. IFN-α mainly is from leukocytes; IFN-β is mainly from fibroblasts; IFN-γ is mainly from T lymphocytes.

IFN has anti-proliferative effect on some tumor cells. Its anti-cancer effects may be related to immunoregulatory activity. It increases the activity of NK cells and macrophages.

The main formulations of interferon are: ① a drug name Interferon-alfa-2a, trade names Roferon R -A; ② drug name Interferon-alfa-2b, trade names Intron R -A

Clinical application of interferon: IFN-a is mainly used for ① blood system tumors and lymphomas: for hairy cell leukemia (HCL), chronic myelogenous leukemia, essential thrombocythemia, multiple myeloma, non-Hodgkin's lymphoma. ② solid tumors: Kaposi's sarcoma, renal cell carcinoma, metastatic melanoma. IFN for hematologic malignancies and solid tumors have the effect of slowing its progress; however only part of the role and transient effects.

2. Interleukin (IL)

Interleukin is human immune system natural ingredients, which are a class of cellular kinase, a chemical ingredient is protein, and is a group of molecule family. It mainly works on signal transduction of the immune system and the main function is immune regulation and immune modification. The originally definition of Interleukin is immune system signal transduction between cells. IL is secreted by white blood cells. When they bind to the receptor on the cell membrane, the target cells are activated.

Complex balance between cell activity and immune regulation is kept by the coordination of secretion of IL and immune system cells.

To date, only IL-2 and IL-11 for clinics, their therapeutic effects of cancer treatment and stimulation of hematopoietic cells are under clinical observation.

(1) Interleukin-2 (IL-2):

This lymphocyte line first is described in 1976. It is a T cell growth factor, mainly is produced by activated T helper cells and has a strong regulation immune function.

Biological activity of IL-2: IL-2 is an important material in the body to produce an immune response, which promotes proliferation of all T cel subsets, increases the activity of the cytotoxic T cell lymphocyte, NK cell and monocyte. Lymphocyte in the blood after activated is called LAK. IL-2 can help B cell growth, also promote the release of IFN-a, GM- CSF, TNF.

From 1984 it started to try recombinant IL-2 to treat various malignancies. There are multiple cases reports that IL-2 alone or combined with LAK cells were used to treat renal cell carcinoma and malignant melanoma. In May 1992 FDA approved that IL-2 is used to treat adults with metastatic renal cell carcinoma.

Recombinant IL-2 has been used as a single agent, or in combination with LAK cells, TIL cells, other biological regulatory factors, and other combined chemotherapy for cancer therapy.

(2) IL-4 : IL-4 is produced mainly by activated T cells. ① The effect on B cells: it can stimulate the growth and differentiation of resting B cells, stimulate B cells to replicate DNA, become a B cell growth factor. ② The effect on T cells: it can stimulate T cell growth, increase the production of IL-2, promote the proliferation of cytotoxic T cells and activate LAK cells. IL-4 promote Til growth, increase the cytotoxic effect on melanoma cells.

The clinical application of IL-4: IL-4 clinical trial has entered Phase II renal cell carcinoma, mainly, melanoma and chronic lymphocytic leukemia, Hodgkin's disease and the like.

(3) Interleukin -12 (IL-12): IL-12 has immunomodulatory and anti-tumor effect. Monocytes is mainly source for IL- 12. Its main role is to: stimulate the activity of T cells and NK cell proliferation; to induce T lymphocytes and NK cells to release IFN-y.

The clinical application of IL-12: the stage I, II clinical trials have been finished on the treatment of metastatic renal cell carcinoma and melanoma.

3. Tumor necrosis factor (TNF)

In 1975 Old etc isolated a material produced by activated phagocyte cell, monocytes and lymphocytes in the contact to toxin, called tumor necrosis factor (TNF). In 1984 TNF gene was cloned so that people can get a lot of recombinant TNF.

The biological effects of TNF: In vitro tests showed that TNF effect on cells is cytotoxicity, and can affect tumor microvasculature, resulting in the center of the tumor necrosis. In particular, TNF can induce the expression of tissue factor vascular endothelial cells and promote the formation of fibrin deposition and thrombosis.

In the anti-tumor effect of TNF, T lymphocytes play important role. Many observers prove that TNF and IFN-γ have a synergistic anti-tumor effect.

TNF has been tested in the treatment of melanoma, colon cancer, non-small cell lung cancer, ovarian cancer, but unfortunately none of them showed a clear reduction or therapeutic effect.

TNF and IFN-y work together, IFN-γ can increase the expression of cell surface TNF receptors, thus increasing the effect of TNF on cells. TNF and IL-2 together can treat all types of cancers, its strategy is IL-2 can stimulate cytotoxic lymphocyte activity and TNF can expand the effectiveness of anti-tumor. The side effects of the two drugs have emerged and only one case of breast cancer and one case of renal cell cancer in combination therapy have improved after exacerbations.

4. Hematopoietic growth factors (HGF)

HGF is also known as colony stimulating factor in the past because in vitro it can induce specific cell clones formation.

HGF effects on normal hematopoiesis: blood cells are made from pluripotent stem cell (PPSC). PPSC has small number within the bone marrow and can differentiate into any blood cell. In the bone marrow, each one PPSC split into two sub-cells, one will go to differentiation pathway; another return to the cell bank to maintain a static state. PPSC grows and develops in the sinus-like gap around stroma in the bone marrow.

(1) Neutrophils: a granule cells, total white blood cell count of 50% -70%, its maturation process has six steps, namely bone marrow blasts, before bone marrow cells, bone marrow cells, these three steps need 4-5d, then no mitosis, but continued to mature about 6d, and then released into the peripheral blood. Half of cells are free circulation; half of cells attached to the vessel wall. Cells circulating in the blood will

remove into the tissue after 6- 8h, where it can survive 2-3d. Generally the number of circulating cells is three times of the number of cells in the bone marrow so there is always reservation of neutrophils in vivo. Once serious injury, a lifetime of neutrophils is reduced to a few hours.

(2) Platelets: its ancestor cells are megakaryocyte colony forming units. In the bone marrow it is the megakaryocytic mother cell, and then differentiates into megakaryocytes which can release platelets. Platelets can form clots in injured blood vessel walls, while activation of the clotting factor. Platelets in the blood can survive 7-8d.

(3) Lymphocytes: lymphoid stem cells differentiate into pre-T or B lymphocytes. Pre-T lymphocytes mature in the thymus before becoming thymocytes, lymphoblastoid cells and T lymphocytes. They can mediate cellular immunity. They can freely circulate in the blood and peripheral tissues. When it is stimulated by antigen, T cell produces a variety of cytokines, which control specific immune response.

Pre-B lymphocytes mature after moving to the spleen and lymph nodes. When the antigen-antibody appear its response on the cell membrane, B lymphocytes has become mature, and eventually become plasma cells. Plasma cells secrete specific immunoglobulins, namely antibodies, responsible for humoral immunity. B lymphocytes accounted for 20%- 25% of total lymphocytes.

Blood cell growth factors control blood cell development by stimulating cell differentiation and maturation.

Particles colony stimulating factor (G-CSF) have been made to pre-clinical animal studies, such as G-CSF was administrated to accelerate neutrophil recovery after using 5-FU and total body radiation. Further research in monkeys show: intravenous injection of GM-CSF (granulosa cells of macrophage colony stimulating factor increased white blood cells after 24-72h.

In 1986 clinical trials started and FDA approved the use of G-CSF which can reduce the risk of incidence of infection in bone marrow cancer in patients receiving myelosuppressive chemotherapy in 1991.

2. Comparison of Traditional Chinese Medicine and Modern Pharmacology

Modern medicine also emphysizes the balacne of internal environments and our bodies have the regulation factors for the stablization of the internal environments which are

111

three systems: Neuoendocrine and immunoregulatory network (NIM) is a hotspot in immunopharmacology, and it is a kind of immunomodulatory system.

The traditional Chinese medicine is most significantly characterized by the emphasis on the overall concept, emphasizing the balance of yin and yang, that is, the balance of human internal and external environmental changes. If losing balance, the body appears as the disease.

There are a large number of herbs with immune function, especially Tonic Chinese medicine generally have the benefits of regulating immune activities. Typhoid Chinese medications generally have the benefits of regulating immune activity, known as immunomodulatory drugs, can cause non-specific immune response.

A lot of chinese medication researches showed that polysaccharides can increase natural killing cells(NK), macrophages (MΦ), cytotoxic T lymphocytes (CTL), T cells, LAK cells, tumor infiltrating lymphocytes (TIL), immune response, Interleukin (IL) and other cytokines to achieve the purpose of killing tumor cells. Although many polysaccharide alone has a certain anti-tumor effect, but the two immunostimulants including the combined effect two polysaccharides will be higher.

Because in our anti-cancer, anti-cancer metastasis in the course of research, and gradually found and recognized that the theory of Chinese medicine and our anti-cancer, anti-cancer metastasis concept, the rule there are similar or even very consistent.

Chinese medicine theory found	Our experimental study
A. Etiology	
righteousness	Tumor model: progressive thymic atrophy; immune function decrease; cancer cells continue division and proliferation.
B. Treatment	
The righting of this, get rid of cult	The goals of Drug Wester chemotherapy treatment must be to kill cancer cells (Qiuxie); we think: It should prevent thymic atrophy, promote thymocyte hyperplasia, improve immune surveillance, control transfer of cancer cells in the way

C. Drugs

Increase Tonic blood stasis

To find to enhance Immunity; the tradition medications of increasing the body resistance to disease eliminate the metastasis cancer cells, tumor thrombus so that it must be anti-thrombosis, anti-coagulation and improve blood flow; in western medicine it is called coagulation improving blood flow; in Chinese medicine it is called increasing blood stasis; both are matched.

3. Immune Function of Chinese herbal medication in patients with advanced cancer

1). The medication of improving immune function should be used in advanced cancer

A. The discovery from the tumor experimental research

The mice with advanced cancer has immunocompromised mice and thymus atrophy.

(1) In 1986 in our laboratory to manufacture tumor-bearing animal models removal of the thymus (THC) can be produced tumor-bearing animal models and injection of immunosuppressive agents can also contribute to the establishment of tumor-bearing animal models. Results of the study show that the incidence and development of cancer and immune function of the host and immune function of organs and tissues is certainly a significant relationship. No removal of the thymus is difficult to manufacture cancer animal models. Repeating several experiments, results were confirmed.

(2) Whether the prior immunocompromised then easy to get cancer, or cancer happens then lead immune function to decrease. The results of our experiments are: first, unocompromised and then tend to have a carcinoma; in the absence of immune function decline, the inoculation of cancer is not successful. The results of this study tips: to improve and maintain good immune function and to protect the immune organs Thymus (TH) can prevent cancer.

(3) The animal model of liver metastasis was divided into A and B groups, A with immunosuppressive agents, group B without our laboratory studies of cancer metastasis and immune relationship. Results: A group was significantly more than the number of liver metastases group B. The results suggest that: the transfer of immunization-related immune dysfunction or immunosuppressive agents, may promote tumor metastasis.

(4) In our laboratory of tumor impacting on the immune organs it was found that with the progress of cancer, TH namely cell proliferation was progressively blocked, volume was significantly reduced. These results suggest that: the tumor can inhibit TH, resulting in atrophy of immune organs.

The above experimental results prove: cancer occurrence, development, metastasis and host immune function decline have significantly affirmative relationship, mice with advanced cancer are immunocompromised and Thymus atrophy. Thus, in advanced cancer treatment should be used Increasing immune function drugs, but cannot be used to reduce or suppress the immune drugs.

B. The experimental study of searching anti-tumor immune regulation and control medications from the natural herbal medications:

Our results demonstrate that with the progress of the tumor the host has thymus atrophy so that we can use some ways to prevent the host Thymus atrophy.

In order to prevent the ongoing thymus shrinkls during the tumor development and to search for the methods of recovering thymus function and rebuilding the immune function, the author started to search for the anti-cancer medication of enhancing the immune function from the natural herbs. After long-term and in turn of selecting the efficient anti-cancer medication in the animal tumor models from 200 traditional herbs. The results showed that there are only 48 herbs which have the effective anticancer functions and at the same time have enhancing immune functions including 26 herbs which strengthen the phagocyte function or stimulate the increase of thymus weight in the animal immune organ thymus or increase the white cell counting ; promote the lymphocyte proliferation in the spleen to increase the transferring rate of the lymphocyte and strengthening the T cell function and NK cells activities and inducing IFN function and 152 herbs which don't have the results.

After combination of the components, we selected the effective combination and got rid of the unstable effective combination in the animal tumor models such as liver cancer, stomach cancer and S-180 etc so that further formed XZ-C immune regulation anti-cancer medication to protect the thymus function and protect the bone marrow and to improve the immune function. Based on the success of the animal selecting experiments, these were applied to the clinics. After 16 years of the huge clinical cases tests, XZ-C medication can improve the life survival qualities in the advanced cancer stages and increase the immune function and strengthen the ability of the body defense and improve the appetite and prolonged the survival time and the curative effects are significant.

2). The Experimental research of the effects of medication of righting training on inhibiting tumor and enhancing the immune effects on S180 mice

1). Objective:

Through 50 years of the research and practice of integrative cancer prevention and treatment, it was found that many traditional Chinese medication for the treatment of cancer have a certain effect; in particular, studies of the efficacy of traditional Chinese medication with righting training for the treatment of malignant tumors showed the medication with right training can enhance physique health and improve immune function, improve quality of life and prolong survival. But Chinese medicine treatment of tumors were observed in clinical experience, without experimental research. In order to explore whether the spleen, and kidney medication in Chinese medication with righting training can inhibit tumor growth or not, and therefore, the following experiment was done:

2). Methods:

  (1) Experimental animal: 160 Kunming mice, 5-6 weeks old, weighing 27±2.0g, each half of male and female.

  (2) Tumor-bearing animal models:

  S_{180} ascites tumor lines, $1X10^7X0.2ml$ tumor cells were seeded in the right forelimb armpit skin each of the mice.

  (3) The experimental groups:

The experimental animals were randomly divided into:

Group A: Yiqi treatment group ((n = 20);

Group B: blood double up treatment group ((n = 20);

Group C: nourishing yin treatment group ((n = 20);

Group D: Warming kidney treatment group ((n = 20);

Group E: ATCA mixture treatment group ((n = 20);

Group F: Xiaochaihutang treatment group ((n = 20); Group G: Compound Capsule treatment group ((n = 20); Group H: tumor-bearing control group ((n = 20). At the second day after inoculation in each group 0. 4ml / per mice /day of herbal was given by oral respectively in tumor-bearing mice; the control group was given with normal saline.

(4) The preparation of the traditional Chinese medications in each group:

200% of the crude drug concentration made through the change from the original recepes amounts into the modern way. And oral doses of the drug concentration above on the mices are the doses which were exchanged based on the normal human doses.

In this study, the traditional medications with the righting training the deficiency of qi and blood make up, nourishing yin, warming yang, supplementation and attack, ATCA agent, Xiaochaihutang and compound capsules and other medications were used to treat S_{180} mice.

(5) Observation: systematic observation of the time of tumor occurrence and tumor survival time, measured their serum protein content, the peripheral blood T lymphocyte counts and the weight of immune organs in each mice group.

3). Results

The medication with righting training and ATCA agent based on the major righting training component can significantly delay tumor appeared time, inhibition of tumor growth (A, B, C, D, E group inhibition rate was 40 percent, respectively, 45 %, 44.5%, 31% and 36%), to extend the survival time of tumor-bearing mice, (A, B, extend the lifetime of the CDE groups were 27.6%, 45% .38 5%, 25% and 26.5%). Quxie based Xiaochaihutang and compound capsules did not significantly inhibit tumor growth and prolong survival (compared to E group, P> 0. 05). Serum protein increases in A, B, C, D, E group ; A / G ratio increases, the peripheral T lymphocyte counts increase (compared with G group P <0. 05, B, C groups P <0. 01), thymic atrophy was significantly inhibited.

4). Conclusion

This study shows that the medication treatment with righting training or based on righting training can inhibit tumor and enhance immunity, can improve the level of the peripheral blood T lymphocytes in varying degrees and are more effective than with Quxie.

5). Discussion

(1) The role of inhibiting tumor and prolong survival of the traditional righting training Chinese medication.

Many cancer patients clinically shown "deficiency" symptoms, such as qi deficiency, blood deficiency, yin deficiency, yang deficiency and the like. Righting training should be adopted through traditional Chinese medication on the treatment. This study investigated the tumor inhibitory effect of righting training and supplementation and attack. The results showed that: Chinese medication wth righting training and ATCA with traditional Chinese medicine based righting training such as buzhongyiqi, qi and blood double up, nourishing yin yang, and warming renal can significantly delay the appearance of tumors in mice inoculated with time, inhibition of tumor growth and prolong survival time of tumor-bearing mice. From each group inhibition rate analysis: in the experimental group with qi-blood double up, the inhibition rate was 45%; in nourishing yin experimental group, the inhibition rate of 44.5%, followed by deficiency of the inhibition action is also up 40%, the effect is also good: Once again, ATCA agent inhibitory rate of 36%: but poor Warming kidney treatment group, the inhibition rate of 31%. The opinion with qi-blood double complement and treatment of nourishing yin should be adopted in terms of inhibition of tumor. From a prolonged survival rate analysis: in the group of supplement qi and blood it was 45%, which was the longest group with extending the lifetime; followed by nourishing yin group, it was up 38.5%, the effect is also good, as in the ATCA mixture treatment group with the supplement zhong and yiyang and warming supplement and yi yang and supplementation and attack it also can prolong survival, but less than in the nourishing yin qi and blood complement treatment groups. Based on Quxie of Xiaochaihutang, in the compound capsule treatment group in this set of experiments, it showed that they were not significantly inhibit tumor and cannot prolong survival of tumor-bearing mice and the effect was the worst. Therefore, from the extension of terms of survival term qi blood double up and nourishing yin blood treatment are preferred, followed by the deficiency of warming yang and supplementation and attack. From both inhibition of tumor and prolong survival analysis of both qi and blood complement the optimal places, followed by nourishing yin, then followed Buzhongyiqi and ATCA mixture, Warming kidney treatment was ineffective. As for Quxie of Xiaochaihutang and compound capsules, from the present experimental results, they have no significant effect.

In short, each righting training and the treatment based on righting training inhibit tumor growth and prolong survival role to varying degrees, and the treatment based on Quxie had no significant anti-tumor and prolong survival role.

This experiment showed that: the righting training medication or medications based on righting training treatment have very significant inhibitory effect, and can significantly prolong survival and improve quality of life for the smaller tumors, so clinically it becomes one of adjuvant therapy of postoperative radiotherapy and chemotherapy. In the literature Many reported that in the clinical the treatment of malignant tumors with the righting training has achieved good results and our experimental results further confirmed that supplement qi and blood, nourishing yin, buzhongyiqi etc other treatment can suppress tumors and prolong survival, which provide an experimental basis for the Integrative clinical treatment of malignant tumors.

(2) The effect of Chinese righting training medication on enhancing the immune effect.

This experiment showed that Chinese medications with the righting training and Chinese medications based on righting training treatment could improve the peripheral blood T lymphocytes in varying degrees, such as when the first four weeks, T lymphocyte levels were as follows: 41.5% in Buzhong group; 44.8% in qi blood double up group, 38.6% in nourishing yin group, 37. 5% in warming yang group, 35.6% in ATCA mixture group; the suppression of thymus atrophy, such as the first two weeks in the deficiency of blood double up, nourishing yin, yang Warming and AT-CA mixture treated group thymus index were significant differences with the tumor-bearing control group. Tip: anti-tumor effect of righting training may enhance immune function. Some people think that a lot of plant polysaccharides have immunomodulatory agents (immunenoclulator) performance, called anti-tumor polysaccharides, these polysaccharides cannot directly kill cancer cells, but it can activate the immune system to release cytokines which have anti-tumor effects or enhanced LAK cells killing effect on cancer cells. This drug with righting training is rich in plant polysaccharides, such as Zhao Kesheng reported: Astragalus polysaccharide extract, wherein the molecular weight was 20,000-25,000. The components has significant role in promoting in vitro secretion of tumor necrosis factor (TNF) in the normal and cancer patients peripheral blood mononuclear cells (PBMC). Chen Kai reported: traditional Chinese Fuzheng anti-tumor medication can promote natural killer cell activity and interleukin-2 (IL-2) activity, and promote T lymphocyte activation, and promote peritoneal macrophage phagocytosis in transplanted tumor S_{180} in mice, increased spleen and thymus weight. In short, the role of righting training on the human immune system is very complex, pending further observation and research.

(3) Chinese righting training medication can enhance the body resistance to disease, improve blood cells and build up their strength.

This experiment showed that: the righting training drug can increase serum protein in tumor-bearing mice, raise clearing / globulin ratio. Our clinical observations in cancer specialist clinics showed that: applications of $XZ-C_4$ immune regulation medications based on righting training in liver cancer, esophageal cancer, stomach cancer, colorectal cancer tumor can suppress cancer and increase immune function. Red blood cells, hemoglobin were higher, leukopenia was also suppressed. All of these describe that right training instinct enhance blood cells and proteins, increase body strength, improve resistance to disease.

One rule of righting training as a combination therapy of tumors has been widely used clinically. The results showed that: righting training drug treatment can delay tumor occurrence time, inhibit tumor growth, prolong survival time the tumor-bearing inoculated mice, enhance immune function and disease resistance, improve quality of life. It can provide experimental evidence for clinical anti-cancer medicine.

3). The immune function of Chinese herbal medicine for advanced cancer patients

Patients with advanced cancer is mostly deficiency and common immune dysfunction. Tonic righting medication can enhance immune function, the prevention and treatment of the patient's tumor immune dysfunction has important significance.

1)). Enhance non-specific immune function

(1) Can stimulate animal immune organs thymus, spleen to gain weight: Ginseng can increased 2.2 fold of thymus weight as the control group of young mice.

(2) Enhance phagocytosis of macrophage: such as ginseng, Codonopsis, Astragalus, angelica, medlar (Wolfberry), etc. can promote macrophage phagocytosis, especially the role of increasing qi drug is obvious.

(3) Increased peripheral leukocytes count: for example, ginseng, astragalus, Codonopsis, Rehmannia and Millettia etc can significantly increase white blood cell count.

2)). Enhancing cell-mediated immune function

(1) to promote lymphocyte proliferation: such as ginseng, can increase the number of lymphocytes; yams, mistletoe, etc. can increase the proportion of peripheral blood T cells.

(2) Increasing the lymphocyte conversion rate: such as ginseng, astragalus, Angelica, white fungus and other tonics, lymphocyte transformation rate were increased role.

(3) to enhance red blood cell immune function: such as astragalus, medlar (Wolfberry) can significantly increase the red blood cell C_{36} mice receptor (RBC-C_{36}) a rosette rate and RBC immune complexes (RBC-IC) rosette formation rate.

3)). Enhanced humoral immune function

(1) the promotion of antibody production: such as ginseng, Huang Jing, Cynomorium, Curculigo, cinnamon, Dodder, Cistanche deserticola are to promote the role of antibody production; they increase serum IgG, IgA, IgM and other antibody levels to varying degrees.

(2) Increasing the number of antibody-forming cells in the spleen: Longspur bud polysaccharide injection can production increased more than one time of antibody produced by the cultured mouse spleen cells; yam polysaccharides can significantly increase the cell numbers formed by mouse spleen, hemolytic plaque. However, some tonic medications have double-acting function of immune enhancement and inhibition.

4). The enhance function of the effect of Chinese herbal medication on immune function in tumor-bearing

In Chinese medicine, tumor formation and development are inadequate positive qi, and that positive qi deficiency associated with tumor occurrence, development, treatment and prognosis of the whole process. Righting training is a basic rule in the prevention and treatment of cancer medicine, and the most prominent is the body's immune function, particularly in the regulation of cellular immune function.

Modern studies have shown that occurrence, development and prognosis of tumor is closely related to cellular immune status in the cancer patients, the body immune function is suppressed and is in immunosuppression situation. This immune suppression is particularly evident in terminally ill patients or long after long treatment of chemotherapy or radiotherapy. Surgery, radiotherapy, chemotherapy can cause a decline in immune function. By Chinese medicine righting training to enhance immune function, thereby enhance the body cancer-fighting ability, improve the effectiveness of surgery, radiotherapy, chemotherapy, improve patient quality of life and prolong survival of patients.

1. The protection function of Chinese herbal medicines on immune organs

In the experiments of protecting immune organs and increasing the weight of immune organs it was found:

(1) Daily respectively fed mice with 15g / kg, 30g / kg extract Angelica and with 12.5mg / kg, 25mg / kg ferulic suspension for continuous 7d which could significantly increase mouse spleen and thymus weight.

(2) Gavage mice with Polygonum 6g (kg • d) decoction, continuous 7d can significantly increase thymus weight and also antagonized prednisolone-induced immune organ weight decreases.

(3) Littoralis polysaccharide 32mg / (kg • d), continuous 7 days can significantly increase thymus weight in mice by intraperitoneal injection.

(4) Cistanche deserticola decoction can significantly increase the weight of spleen and thymus with fed mice.

It must be noted that some herbs can reduce weight of immune organs and prompt immune organ atrophy, such as Hook, cicada, Puhuang, Sarcandrae, rhubarb, etc. Thymus atrophy, thymus cortical thinning, decreased cells and spleen weight was significantly reduced, splenic artery sheath surrounding the central lymphocytes (mostly T lymphocytes) decrease after fed 0.5g / d rhubarb decoction continuous 8d in normal mice. There is no significant effect on mice immune organs after perfusion medication 10mg / kg per day continuous 10d. Generally small dose had no effect, while large doses decreased.

2. The enhancement function of Chinese herbal medication on mononuclear phagocyte system

Polysaccharide, Glycosides and a variety of other ingredients in Chinese herbal medications can enhance the mononuclear phagocyte system, particularly macrophage activity, enhance its immune function. Anti-tumor effect of macrophages are activated by tumor antigen through the T cells release specific macrophages, activated macrophages specifically kill tumor cells: macrophage-mediated cytotoxicity kill tumor cells, such as by activating the macrophages to secrete tumor necrosis factor (TNF), proteolytic enzymes, interferon (IFN) and others directly killing or inhibiting the growth of tumor cells.

(1) Medlar (Wolfberry) polysaccharides (LBP): Wang Ling etc. summarizes the research of immunomodulatory LBP effects in the second phase of "Shanghai Journal of Immunology"(1995): LBP with 0.125g / (kg • d) mice with 5d can enhance macrophage phagocytosis that LBP has a certain immune function. Zhang yongxiang and other like researched LBP effects on mouse peritoneal macrophages in tumor cell proliferation inhibition activity.

(2) Velvet polysaccharide (PAPS): can significantly improve macrophage function in immunocompromised induced by Hydrocortisone, namely with 0.01ug / ml concentration it has promotion function and has clear dose-effect relationship. PAPS has the strongest effect in 1ug / ml concentration.

(3) Gypenosides: Gypenosides with 300mg / (kg • d) once daily for continuous 7d can significantly enhance the ability of peritoneal macrophage cells in normal mice. In the "Wenzhou Medical College,"(1990) Volume 20(1) Shou Zhi Juan reported that macrophages volume increases and phagocytic digestion increases in lung and the abdominal loose connective tissue when mice were fed by Gypenosides with 50mg (containing 1.21% total glycosides) once daily for a month later.

(4) ABPS: can induce the synthesis of IL-1 and tumor necrosis factor (TNF-α) in macrophages. ABPS 25mg / kg or 50mg / kg can improve the LPS-induced

IL-1 production by intraperitoneal injection. ABPS with 100mg / kg can promote the formation of TNF-α by intraperitoneal injection and it has the same strength role as BCG.

(5) Psoralen: with carcinogens Urethane cause lung cancer in mice, then intraperitoneally injection of psoralen 1mg / 20g the body weight, continuous 10d can significantly enhance lung cancer mouse peritoneal macrophage phagocytosis.

3. Chinese medication with enhancing the role of T cells immune function

T cells are very important in body's immune cells, not only will lead to specific cellular immune, and is involved in immune regulation, and other functions. Tumor cells are often accompanied by changes in cell surface antigens. Because of immune surveillance of T cells, T cells sensitized by tumor antigen can directly kill tumor cells or and release cytokines to kill T cell by directly or indirectly cytotoxicity.

(1) Epimedium polysaccharide (EPS): EPS with 100mg / Kg/ d for continuous 5d significantly increased peripheral WBC and T lymph cells by subcutaneous injection.

(2) Alfalfa Polysaccharides (MPS): in vitro can enhance lymphocyte proliferation induced by PHA, CONA, LPS and pokeweed (PWM). MPS 125mg / (kg · d) and 250 mg / (kg · d) significantly increased spleen lymphocyte index and the number of lymphocytes by intraperitoneal injection. MPS also partially antagonized lymphocytes decrease induced by cyclophosphamide in intraperitoneal injection.

(3) Medlar polysaccharide (Wolfberry) (LBP): can significantly increase the percentage of peripheral external T lymphocytes in mouse. LBP 5mg / (kgxd) increases peripheral blood lymphocyte count by abdominal injection for continuous 7d. The control group was 65.4%, 81.6% for the treatment group, but increasing the dose does not continue to improve this effect. In T lymphocyte mitogen CONA inducing conditions, a small dose of LBP (5-10mg / kg) can also cause lymphocyte proliferation which means LBP can significantly promote T cell proliferation.

(4) Moutan: 12. 5 / kg and 25g / kg doses orally can significantly improve the mice's T lymph cell transformation. Radix paeonail rubra(TPG): 25g / kg dose orally can significantly improve mice IL-2 activity. Wulingzhi: dose 12.5g / kg and 25

g / kg not only can significantly improve the T lymphocyte function in mice, but also 25g / kg dose also significantly increased IL-2 activity in mice by Gavage.

It must be noted, herbs also have to inhibit T cell immune function, such as Sophora, turmeric, Hook, Millettia, rhubarb, etc. which reduction of T cell immune function must be caution.

4. The role of traditional Chinese medication on LAK cells

(1) Wind polysaccharide in a certain concentration range can be significantly increased IL-2-induced LAK cell killing activity.

(2) The sea buckthorn increases blood circulation. In tumor-bearing mice sea buckthorn juice (3g / kg) can significantly improve their spleen NK cells and LAK activity by injected intraperitoneally.

(3) Cao wenguang etc. found that three kinds of traditional Chinese medications such as APS, PAS and LBP could significantly promote the proliferation of mouse spleen cells with 5- 30mg / kg intraperitoneal injection in C57BL / 6 mice and. The spleen cells were $2X10^6$ / ml with 125-1,000U / ml of rIL-2 induced 4d, APS group found that injections of spleen cells LAK activity of the group increased by 70%) - 120% compared with normal saline; injection PAS group increased by 20 % -90%; injection LBP group by 26% -80%.

(4) Cao wenguang etc treated 79 cases of advanced cancer patients which didn't have good response to radiotherapy and chemotherapy with traditional Chinese medicine LBP combined with LAK, IL-2 from February 1992 to November 1993. LBP with oral dose 1. 7mg / kg, LAK total doses 1.2-32X 10^{10}, IL-2 with 3. 4- 4. 8X10^7U / person, specific programs in the conventional therapy is stopped after a month, give LBP 3 weeks after injection riL-2, giving LBP 4 week After a large number of patients with autologous PBL isolated LAK cells in vitro, reinfusion after various inspection, and then continue to give LBP and work L-2, 1 weeks. Results : 75 cases of evaluable patients, LAK / IL-2 combined with the efficacy of LBP group (36.36%) than single with LAK / IL-2 effect group (18%), the former combined LBP group before and after treatment and NK activity of PBL 500U / ml IL-2 induced the LAK activity increased level significantly higher than the latter alone LAK / IL-2 group. Show LBP could significantly promote NK and LAK cells antitumor activity.

The regimens of strength spleen, warm yang, supporting kidney, YiQi, Yangyin etc increase LAK activity in vivo.

5. Immune function regulation of traditional Chinese medication on red blood cell (RBC)

In 1981 according to adhesion phenomena of RBC and the facts of type I complement variant (CR1) combining with immune complexes (IC) on the surface of RBC American scholar Siegel and others put forward to the concept of "red cell immune function", illustrated not only the respiratory function of red blood cells, and is involved in a variety of immune and immune regulate in the body: such as the removal of circulating immune complexes, and promote phagocytosis, immune regulation of lymphocyte. The red blood cells is involved in the production of IFN-7, IL2 antibodies and the regulation of natural killer cells (NK cells), lymphokine-activated killer cells (LAK cells) and phagocytic immune cells and so on.

(1) It was found that Astragalus (Astragalus polysaccharide, APS) enhances the activity of erythrocyte C3bR attached to the tumor cells and immune function in cancer patients in vitro. APS enhances erythrocyte immune function in cancer patients.

(2) In the group of Trichosanthes root(TCS) treatment and of untreated group in Ehrlich ascites carcinoma in mice it was found that in the untreated group RBD-C_3bR rosette rate was significantly lower than the normal group, the treatment group RBC-C_3bR rosette rate significantly higher than the untreated group and slightly higher than the normal group, which means mice RBC-C3bR activity was significantly decreased in the cancer mice and Trichobitacin can increase RBC-C_3bR activity significantly.

TCS influence on mice erythrocyte SOD activity: After the mice inoculated with cancer cells to 11d, the treatment group erythrocyte SOD activity was significantly higher than the untreated group and the normal group. Late tumor-bearing mice decreased erythrocyte SOD, this experiment shows Chinese medication TCS can restore and enhance the activity of SOD.

TCS influence on the ability of immune adhesion of red cell to tumor cells: with Ehrlich ascites tumor cells as target cells, to determine the TCS effect on the capability of the adhesion of immune in mice red blood cell to breast tumor cell, it was found 11 day after tumor cell inoculation tumor erythrocyte rosette rate(11.90±5.00)% in non-treatment mice was significantly lower than the normal mice (22.13 ±6.28)%; while in treated mice tumors erythrocyte rosette rate(26. 54± 7.27)% was slightly higher than the normal group was significantly higher than the untreated group.

TCS's effect on erythrocyte immune function in cancer patients: it have also a significant enhancement of the adhesion ability of the red blood cells to tumor cells in cancer patients. Tests found that cancer patients directly enhance rosette rate of RBC-C_3bR effect which there is a significant difference with normal saline (NS) group, and this role of the promotion has dose-dependent manner.

5). Types of biological medicine and its component response regulator (BRMS) action

Chinese medicine has a very important characteristic which has the role of two-way adjustment for biological therapy which can restore the body immune function to the normal direction.

In 1983 Jingjianping found that Astragalus can significantly increase IL-2 in "spleen false" mice model, but have no effect on normal mice.

In 1991 Xungxiaolin etc studied the effects of Millettia, FruitofPurpleflowerHolly, Psoralen Chinese medication on IL-2 production in mouse spleen cells and found that these drugs in three groups such as immunocompromised, hyperthyroidism, normal showed increased, inhibition, no influence which reflect double-acting medicine. Besides traditional Chinese medicine on the body due to the impact of anti-tumor substance and the amount thereof are closely related. Medlar at low concentrations can promote IL 3-secretion, but high concentrations inhibit IL-3 levels. When total glucosides of peony increase IL-2 production in the low concentrations by a dose-dependent. After the concentration exceed 12. 5mg, it will inhibit IL 2-secretion.

Chinese medication has been used in our country for thousands of years and many Chinese medications can have the roles of BRMS which the research of anti-cancer immune agents will have a bright future. Chinese medication by oral has mild adverse reactions. Compared with genetic engineering BRMS and exogenous IL-2, IFN TNF, the advantages of traditional Chinese medication similar to BRMS has the whole body anticancer role in the body immune system and can be repeatedly administered with non-toxic side effects, and is available for tumor, chemotherapy, radiotherapy-induced immune dysfunction, boost the immune cell activation so that endogenous cytokines can be released and cause inhibition of tumor growth.

In modern cancer treatment, Chinese medication can at least play a role in three areas: ① enhance the role of inherent anti-cancer member effect in the body, enhance the body's anti-cancer cell system (NK cells, TK cells, LAK cell factor); ② Some traditional Chinese medicine has a direct anti-cancer effect; ③ some medicine ingredients can reduce side effects of radiation therapy, chemotherapy, and reduce the inhibition to the white cells and help to recover, even increase radiotherapy and chemotherapy anti-cancer effect.

Thinking and reform of traditional therapy

Challenge the present cancer treatment and reform can develop

Chapter 5 Analysis and Evaluation of traditional cancer therapy

1. Analysis, Evaluation and Doubt of Systemic Intravenous Chemotherapy on Solid Tumor

Through reviewing, reflecting, summarizing and analyzing the experience in success and lessons from failure, I have gradually realize that systemic intravenous chemotherapy on solid tumor may be confronted with some important problems, which are worthy of reflection, evaluation and re-discussion.

Why the chemotherapy does not prevent the recurrence and metastasis and get the expected curative effects? Through repeated reflection, we doubt: whether it is reasonable and scientific or not to use route of administration of intravenous chemotherapy to treat the malignant tumor in stomach, intestines, liver, gallbladder, pancreas and pelvic cavity and so on. We think deeply about the route of administration, especially the one for the malignant tumor in the abdomen and find that it is necessary to research and discuss the route of administration over again, the same to calculation of the dose and the evaluation standard of curative effects.

1). Analysis and doubt of the route of administration for systemic intravenous chemotherapy of solid tumor?

The present chemical chemotherapy for tumor is mainly the systemic intravenous chemotherapy, the standard scheme of chemotherapy in the world, the united scheme or the single-agent scheme is mostly the systemic intravenous chemotherapy, the same to the treatment of leukemia, malignant tumor of the blood system, tumor of the lymphatic system, solid tumor, tumor of the abdominal cavity, malignant tumor of stomach, intestines, liver, gallbladder and pancreas and to the assistant chemotherapy after operation or perioperative assistant chemotherapy.

1. Analysis of route of administration and medication of cytotoxic drug for intravenous chemotherapy for solid tumor:

In systemic intravenous chemotherapy, the intravenous drip enters the blood circulation, flows back to the right ventricle via venous blood, and then enters the arteria pulmonalis, after it is oxygenated with blood in lung, it flows into left ventricle via pulmonary vein and then is transfused into the aorta via bender and enters the systemic artery system for systemic circulation. Then it is distributed to the systemic organs with the arterial blood in viscera. At this moment, the chemotherapy drug enters the extracellular tissue fluid via interspace of capillay wall and then comes into play after entering the cancer cells.

As to the systemic intravenous chemotherapy, after the drug is distributed by the systemic blood, only a tiny minority of cytotoxic drug for chemotherapy enters the external organs of tumor cells and a tiny minority of drug enters the cancer cells, with slight curative effects.

Intravenous injection of chemotherapy drug via forearm vein →right ventricle →pulmonary artery→ oxygenation of pulmonary alveoli→ pulmonary vein→ aorta →systemic artery system (the drug is transported to the systemic viscera and is distributed in the whole body) →arteries of viscera→ veins of viscera →venae cavae→ right ventricle→ recirculation as above.

Analysis: as above-mentioned, the drug is spread in the whole body and distributed to all viscera, in this way, the systemic viscera obtain the cytotoxic drug, however, the body surface area or volume of the solid tumor only accounts for a very little ratio of the systemic body surface area or volume, for example, even through one carcinoma of stomach as large as one adult's fist, accounts for a very little ratio of the volume of an adult. Therefore, the carcinoma of stomach as large as one adult's fist obtains a tiny minority of cytotoxic drug in the chemotherapy of systemic intravenous injection, resulting in very little curative effects or roles. Meanwhile, most of the cytotoxic drug for chemotherapy is transported to the normal histiocytes of the viscera (including heart, liver, spleen, lung, kidney, brain, bone marrow, blood, lymph and immune organ), all of which receive the cytotoxic drug for chemotherapy, resulting in side reaction. The more the times of chemotherapy, the larger the dosage, the more the drug combination, the more serious of the accumulative side reaction, even resulting in loss of immunologic function and endangering the life. The patient takes a risk of endangering the life, however, does it have curative effects on the cancerous protuberance? The carcinoma of stomach as large as a fist only can obtain a very tiny minority of dose for chemotherapy entering the cancer cells as per the body surface area, in this way, the curative effects are very little and it is impossible to realize the good curative effects.

Some patients think by mistake that the large side reaction represents the curative effects, the larger the reaction, the better the curative effects, therefore, they mistake that the reaction kills the cancer cell, but they hardly realize that the reaction kills the normal cells: it is the reaction that kills the active normal cells with normal proliferation, such as bone marrow cells, immunological cells and mucous membrane cells of the stomach and intestine and the hair, resulting in decrease of white blood cells and decrease of blood platelets. Meanwhile, no one knows whether the cancer cells are killed by the chemotherapy and how many cancer cells are killed. However, it is known that it kills the normal cells just because the decrease of white blood cells and blood platelets only indicates the completion of the chemotherapy, no one knows whether it has curative effects or not.

Therefore, we analyze the reason why the chemotherapy cannot prevent the recurrence and metastasis is possibly that the route of systemic intravenous chemotherapy does not realize the curative effects you hope and expect, the local cancer lesion is applied with a tiny minority of dose, since a very tiny minority of drug enters the external tissue fluid of the cancer cells and only a minute of dose can enter the cancer cells and takes curative effects.

An example of 5-FU, the common chemotherapy drug: 5-FU intravenous chemotherapy 1000mg/d x 5=5000mg, 85% is catabolized by DPD enzyme in the liver without any therapeutic effects; some of the rest 15% is excreted through the kidney in form of drug prototype, some enters the cells and takes curative effects through anabolism. Given the latter is 8% and the locality with easy recurrence and metastasis of carcinosis accounts for 5% of the volume of the whole body, the effective availability of 5-FU is only:

5000mg x 8% x 5%=20mg (0.4%).

In another word, when intravenous drip is used for systemic chemotherapy, chemotherapy drug 5-FU infused via intravenous drip is 5000mg, after distributed in the whole body by the viscera, the available 5-FU really reaching the cancer lesion is only 20mg, that is to say, only 0.4% of the drug reaches the cancer lesion and is utilized. The drug takes the curative effects in the cancer cells. The rest, namely 99.6% of the chemotherapy drug takes the untoward reaction in the normal cells. In other words, only 0.4% of the chemotherapy drug plays a role in killing the cancer cells while 99.6% of the chemotherapy drug kills the normal cells of the patients with active proliferation, namely bone marrow cells, epith epithelial cells of mucous membrane of the stomach and intestine, hair, white blood cells, blood platelets and immunological cells and so on, resulting in degression of immunologic function, inhibition of hematopiesis of bone marrow cells, emesis, alopecia and obvious decrease of white blood cells and blood platelets.

According to the reports of the literatures, the metabolic pathway of 5-Fu:

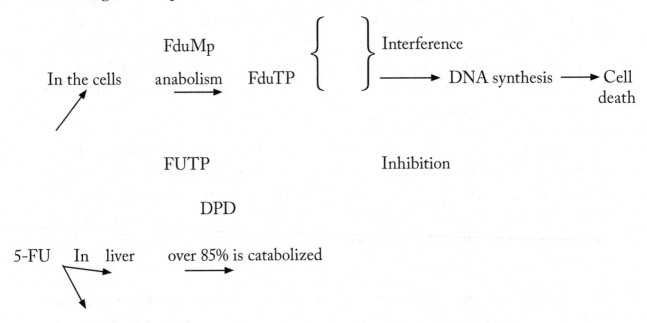

In the kidney excreted in form of drug prototype

In systemic intravenous chemotherapy, how many chemotherapy drugs can reach the cancer cells and play a role in killing the cancer cells? With an example of the above-mentioned 5-FU, the patient is intravenously injected with 5000mg in 5 days, however, the one really reaching the cancer cells and playing a role is only 20mg, only accounting for 0.4% of the injected chemotherapy drug, the rest of the injected chemotherapy drug, namely 99.6% has the side effects on the normal cells with active proliferation in the whole body in clinical menifetation, namely bone marrow cells, epithelial cells of mucous membrane of the stomach and intestine and immunological cells, the systemic side reactions include arrest of bone marrow, reaction of gstrointestinal tract and toxic reaction of heart, lung and liver; the local toxic reactions include toxic reaction of skin and alopecia and so on.

In systemic intravenous chemotherapy, how does the cytotoxic drug for chemotherapy work from blood to cancer cells intravenously transfused? The chemotherapy drug is distributed and applied in the whole body, finally the chemotherapy drug enters the external tissue fluid of the cells via the interspace of capillay wall and then comes into play after entering the cancer cells.

In systemic intravenous chemotherapy, after the chemotherapy drug enters the vein, the drug is necessarily distributed in the body fluid, among the moisture in the human body, about 5% is blood, 15% is the external tissue fluid of the cells and 40% is intracellular fluid. The chemotherapy drug in blood is circulated and utilized in the whole body and distributed with the blood in the viscera. When the chemotherapy drug is in the external tissue fluid, it is absorbed and metabolized respectively by the viscera. When the chemotherapy drug enters the cells, the drug takes curative effects in the cancer cells while it takes side reaction in a large number of normal cells.

As above mentioned, we should objectively and calmly analyze the advantages, the disadvantages, the gain and the loss of the route of administration of systemic intravenous chemotherapy for the solid tumor? Which are the advantages? And the disadvantages? What the patient gains? And losses? All of which shall be seriously reflected, analyzed and evaluated.

2. It shall be discussed and doubted whether the route of administration of cytotoxic drug to kill the cancer cells of the solid tumor and the systemic intravenous drip are reasonable and scientific or not?

The above-mentioned systemic intravenous chemotherapy is used for all types of leukemia, leucoma and malignant tumor in the blood system, which is reasonable just because the malignant tumor of the blood system and the malignant tumor cells of the malignant leucoma of the lymphatic system are distributed in the systemic blood system or lymphatic system, in this way, they shall be applied with drug through the intravenous drip, which is reasonable and scientific just because there are so many cases and experience in successful treatment.

However, as to the carcinoma for solid tumor, the drug entering the tumor is minute, it plays a minor role in killing the cancer cells, it has obvious side reaction in damaging the systemic proliferative cells. The chemotherapy drug transfused through the route of administration to solid tumor only can kill a tiny minority of cancer cells while most of it kills the normal proliferative cells of the host, resulting in pains from the side reaction of chemotherapy undertaken by the patients.

At present, there are so many solid malignant tumors adopting the systemic intravenous administration route for the assistant chemotherapy after operation or perioperative assistant chemotherapy. Through intravenous drip, the chemotherapy drug enters the right ventricle via the caval vein, enters the lungs via pulmonary artery, enters the left ventricle through the pulmonary vein and then is distributed in the whole body through the aorta, in this way, the chemotherapy drug reaching the cancer lesion is very little, most of the drug is distributed in the whole body and kills the normal cells, especially the immunological cells, hematopoietic cells of bone marrow, causing the patients to be severely damaged; meanwhile, it does not play a remarkable role in the solid tumor. Over half a century, it has been all the same, although it has not taken the expected effects, so many patients have suffered from the pains from the side reaction of the chemotherapy drug widely killing the normal cells. The clinicians should seriously reflect, analyze and evaluate the route of administration, which is unadvisable, unreasonable and unscientific. We shall try to apply the drug to the specific locality instead of applying drug in the whole body and we shall research it and try to correct, reform and innovate it.

II. Analysis and doubt of calculation method of the dose of systemic intravenous chemotherapy drug for solid tumor

1. Based on the above-mentioned systemic intravenous administration route, the medication is calculated as per the calculation method of leukemia, since the leukemic cells are distributed in the systemic circulatory system, the administration must cover the systemic blood system. The malignant lymphocytes of leucoma is also distributed in the systemic lymphatic system, the administration must also cover the systemic lymphatic system, the blood system and the lymphatic system are distributed in all organs, tissues and skin in the whole body, therefore the administration shall be calculated as per body surface area or volume. This kind of route of administration, calculation of dose, pharmacokinetics and bioavailability is reasonable and scientific, which conforms to the distribution of the cancer cells.

2. Since the systemic intravenous chemotherapy has taken good curative effects and experience in all types of leukemia, leucoma, epithelioma of chorion, some malignant moles, blastocytoma Wilms tumor and so on, it has been widely applied to the solid tumor of the viscera in the whole body and the assistant chemotherapy after operation, although we have accumulated much experience and obtained some achievements, we have not had our wish fulfilled just because the death rate has been not reduced, the recurrence and metastasis has been not prevented, indicating it is unreasonable to apply the calculation method to dose of the leukemia and it does not conform to the actual conditions of the solid cancer, therefore, its reasonableness and scientificalness shall be doubted and it shall be further researched for reforming and innovation.

3. Since the carcinoma of the solid tumor is restricted to the viscus before remote metastasis, it is necessary to distribute the drug to the viscus in chemotherapy, however, the drug for systemic intravenous chemotherapy is distributed in the whole body, it necessarily needs relatively more dose. However, the chemotherapy drug is the cytotoxic drug, large dose necessarily leads to large toxicity, which cannot be withstood by the patient, so the calculation of dose for systemic intravenous chemotherapy cannot be calculated as per pharmacodynamics namely how much dose is needed to kill a certain number of cancer cells, but as per the tolerance dose of the patient to the cytotoxic drug just because the patient cannot withstand it if it exceeds the tolerance dose of the cytotoxic drug as the too large toxicity will endanger the life.

In the recent 30-40 years, the systemic intravenous chemotherapy is widely used to the solid tumor or the assistant chemotherapy after operation and there have been various international chemotherapy standard schemes. the schemes and the guides indicate the kind of drug, the dose mg/m^2, from which day to which day, iv or others, indicating how many days are a cycle. The schemes are universal, no matter the side of the solid tumor, no matter whether the solid tumor is ablated or not, the schemes are all the same, the same to the calculation of the dose, which are not individualized. Since the dose determined for each scheme is determined as per the tolerance dose of the cytotoxic drug undertaken by the patient instead of the effective dose. It is calculated as per the distribution of the systemic intravenous chemotherapy in the whole body, therefore, the calculation of the dose for solid tumor and the assistant chemotherapy after operation is not reasonable and scientific just because the normal tissues of the viscera shall not be killed by the cytotoxic drug, which shall be seriously analyzed, individualized, further researched and reformed.

III. Analysis and evaluation of curative effect evaluation criteria of systemic intravenous chemotherapy for solid tumor

1) The evaluation criteria of curative effects on solid tumor at present include:

1. Size of tumor: it shall be measured in every examination.

(1) Shrinkage of measurable volume of tumor and/or metastatic lesion: indicating the degree of shrinkage with the arithmetic product of the max. diameter (cm) and its diameter (cm) of the tumor;

(2) As to the tumor with immeasurable size, the method for improvement of disease is the calcification of osteolytic tumor again, as to the celiac tumor that cannot be easily measures shall be expressed with the estimated shrinkage value.

2. Remission stage: the remission stage shall begin from the treatment. In both checks in the treatment stage, the tumor grows up once again, the arithmetic product of its orthogonal diameters increases over 25%. The remission stage is calculated in days, weeks or months.

3. Evaluation criteria of size of solid tumor

CR (complete remission; evidently effective): the tumor disappears entirely, lasting over 4 weeks;

PR (partial remission; effective): the arithmetic product of two diameters of the tumor is shrunk to over 50%;

MR (middle remission): the tumor is shrunk to over 25% and below 50%;

NC (or S, stable, unchanged): the tumor is shrunk to below 25% and enlarged to below 25%;

PD (or P, progressive; deteriorative): the tumor is enlarged to over 25% or new lesion appears.

2)Analysis and discussion

1. The above-mentioned curative effect criteria of systemic chemotherapy for solid tumor is summarized in three points: size of tumor, remission and remission period.

Chemotherapy and radiotherapy only kill the differentiated and matured tumor cells rather than the stem cells of the tumor accounting for 0.1%~1.0% of the tumor cells. The remained stem cells of tumor are differentiated and proliferated once again, forming new tumor, with the clinical menifetation of recurrence and metastasis of tumor as well as the failure of treatment, resulting in death of the patient.

At present, although the chemotherapy drug for clinical application can shrink the tumor, the effects are commonly temporary and it cannot obviously prolong the life of the patient. Therefore, the curative effect evaluation criterion is referred to as remission, the remission stage is calculated in days, weeks or months, for example, the complete remission only means the tumor disappears entirely, lasting over 4 weeks, indicating it may recur after 4 weeks. What is meant by remission? I understand it as follows: we rope an animal, then untie it for two hours and then rope it again, in this way, the untying is referred to as remission, the two hours of untying is the remission stage, obviously, remission is not the treatment objective of the patient, the patient is hospitalized for chemotherapy, undertaking the pains and the risks from the side reaction of the cytotoxic drug for chemotherapy, only getting a temporary remission at most, which is apparentlyteh requirements and treatment objective of the patient hospitalized for chemotherapy, which shall not be the objective of clinical treatment.

2. Why chemotherapy only can play a role in remission? Because:

The cytotoxic drug for chemotherapy only can kill the differentiated and matured cancer cells rather than the undifferentiated or immature stem cells or the ones to be differentiated and matured, the chemotherapy drug kills the differentiated and matured cancer cells at this time, however, after a time, the undifferentiated and immature cancer cells are gradually differentiated and matured, the tumor cells are uninterruptedly and progressively divided, proliferated and cloned, one is divided into two, and two into four, in this way, it is multiplied in form of geometric progression, at the same time, the period of effectively killing cancer cells of the patient through chemotherapy drug is only 1~5 days of intravenous drip, that is to say, it only lasts 5-6 days for taking the effects on killing the cancer cells, the so-called cycle of 3-4 weeks only means that the white blood cells and the blood platelets with bone marrow inhibited can be recovered within 3-4 weeks and withstand the second chemotherapy.

Since the chemotherapy drug only can kill the differentiated and matured cancer cells rather than the undifferentiated stem cells of the tumor or the ones being differentiated, the chemotherapy only can merely alleviate the symptoms, but it cannot treat the root cause, it only can be regarded as the assistant treatment, but not as the radical treatment because the principles of chemotherapy do not conform to the biological characteristics and behaviors of the cancer cells. Although chemotherapy can temporarily shrink the tumor, it cannot obviously prolong the life and one of the reasons why the treat fails is that the tumor cells loss the drug resistance, maybe another reason is the existing therapeutic methods cannot effectively kill the stem cells of the tumor, the treatment of cancer through chemotherapy may be said that "no prairie fire can destroy the grass, it shoots up again with the spring breeze blows". Why? Because the grass is burn, but the root is remained, only some matured cancer cells rather than the stem cells of tumor to be differentiated and matured are killed, the stem cells of tumor will be continually divided and cloned in form of geometrical progression.

The judgment of the curative effects on tumor shall not regard the size of the tumor as the standard: the objective of existing tumor chemotherapy and radiotherapy is mainly to reduce the volume and number of the tumor cells just because they often determine the curative effects by means of the capability of shrinking the tumor, in fact, "the big" does not mean "the bad" and "the small" does not mean "the good". The clinic judgment of chemotherapy at present, no matter the clinic or the sickroom, is mainly based on CT and MRI as well as space occupation, as a matter of fact, the space occupation is not the size of the solid tumor because the peripheric tissue of the solid tumor may affect the space occupation. I am a surgeon and I have been engaged in medicine practice for 54 years and performed over 5000 radical and abscission operations for cancers at breast or abdomen. The size of the tumor seen in the operation has not been always consistent with the one reported in CT and MRI. In addition, although some solid tumors are as large as a fist even larger than a fist, when they are incised, the cancer cells inside is not dense while there are so many interfibrillar interstitial tissues; although some solid tumors are only as large as a table tennis, when then are incised, there are so many highly malignant cancer cells inside, the latter is more malignant than the former. Therefore, I think "the big" does not means "the bad" and "the small" does not means "the good", which cannot be regarded as the standard. We also find from a large batch of tumor-bearing animal models in the lab that although the hypodermically inoculated experimental tumors of some tumor-bearing experimental mice are very large, the cancer cells of the central tissue of the transplanted solid tumor are unlike to the peripheral cancer cells, the mode center is mostly aseptically necrotic or liquefied while its periphery is the active cancer cells, although its volume is increased, the malignancy is low.

The solid tumor has the drug transmission blockage, which in the huge solid tumor results in drug resistance or does not realize the curative effects. Some anti-tumor drugs have very high anti-tumor activity to various tumor cells in culture dish, some even has 100% inhibition rate., which are clinically used to treat malignant tumor in the blood system or the child cancer, with satisfactory curative effects, however, these drug cannot obviously reduce the rate of death of the adults caused by the most common solid tumor (such as carcinoma of stomach, hepatic carcinoma, carcinoma of large intestine, carcinoma of lung, breast carcinoma, carcinoma of pancreas, prostatic carcinoma, esophageal carcinoma, brain carcinoma and so on).

It can be found through comparison of the malignant tumor in the blood system with the solid tumor that the former can directly contact the single cancer cell in the blood just because it omits the step of districting the drug in the tumor tissue. Therefore, it can be concluded that the drug transmission has some factors in the solid tumor that can cause the drug to produce the drug resistance.

The above-mentioned systemic intravenous administration route, medication, calculation of dose, calculation as per body surface area and curative effect evaluation criteria have been used in the world over half a century, forming the internationalized chemotherapy standard scheme, various guides or idiomatic usages. However, its curative effects cannot be satisfactory, it neither reduces the rate of death from cancer nor prevents the tumor recurrence or metastasis while the patient may undertake the pains and risks of side reactions from chemotherapy.

Through in-depth thinking, review, reflection, analysis and evaluation, Profession Xu Ze summarizes his clinical experience and lessons of treatment of patients over 54 years, puts forward the above-mentioned questions, evaluates, discusses and doubts the route of administration, medication, calculation of dose and curative effect evaluation criteria of systemic intravenous chemotherapy for solid tumor especially the tumor at abdomen and pelvic cavity. Since the above-mentioned questions exist, it is necessary to further research them and improve the traditional therapeutic method based on the traditional approaches as well as update the concept and understanding, make progress in reforming and have the courage to innovate. The innovation must have the challenge to the traditional concept to overcome the disadvantages, correct the defects to make it more perfect. It shall be reformed and innovated.

2. The Suggestion of Reforming the Systemic Intravenous Chemotherapy for Solid Tumor to Intravascular Chemotherapy in Target Organ

Through probing into the route of administration of systemic intravenous chemotherapy for solid tumor, we propose to reform it to the intravascular administration route in target organ and reform the systemic intravenous chemotherapy of solid tumor (especially the tumor of liver, gallbladder, pancreas, spleen, kidney, lung, uterus, ovary, abdominal cavity and pelvic cavity) to intravascular chemotherapy in target organ. Why?

Just because we have deeply taken cognizance of its disadvantages. This cognizance has been deepened and strengthened step by step through reviewing, reflecting, analyzing, evaluating and doubting a large number of cases and then the truth has been found gradually. Over the past half a century, million of cancer patients have undertaken the side reaction of chemotherapy once and again after receiving the chemotherapy, only to stilly bear the pains without any other way just because they want to kill off the cancer cells so that they can get well and be full of vim and vigor.

I. Evaluation of Problems and Disadvantages of Systemic Intravenous Chemotherapy for Solid Tumor

(I) Evaluation of the route of administration of systemic intravenous chemotherapy for solid tumor

The route of administration, not the specific targeting administration, distributes the cytotoxic drug in the whole body through the general blood circulation. In this way, it does not have a definite object for administration, but administers drugs in the whole body, resulting in:

1. The diseased cancer lesion area is very small (accounting for very small ratio of the body surface area of the whole body) only can obtain very little cytotoxic drug, resulting in very little action and curative effect.

2. However, the disease-free normal tissue in the whole body is damaged by the reaction of 99.6% of the cytotoxic drug. The normal tissue in the whole body does not need the cytotoxic drug, but it obtains a large number of cytotoxic drugs. However, the cytotoxic anti-cancer drug has relatively toxicity to the tissue with relatively rapid proliferation, such as the toxicity of alimentary canel, hemopoietic system, heart, liver, spleen, lung, kidney, nervous system and endocrine system, in this way, so many patients cannot receive the treatment or have to interrupt the treatment. Killing the tissue with relatively rapid proliferation in the whole body leads to harm to the patients instead of benefits to the patients.

3. The medication of this route of administration, does not have a definite object for administration, but the blind administration, which is non-targeting administration. Without the definite object, it only distributes and administers the drug in the whole body, as a result, the cancer lesion obtains a minute of cytotoxic drug while the area of the tissue in the whole body damaged by the cytotoxic drug is very large, resulting in bad curative effects, large side reaction and many and heavy complication, so the medication is unreasonable and unscientific.

4. With the above-mentioned medication, the cytotoxic drug administered in chemotherapy does not greatly attack the cancer cells, but only attach the cancer

cells slightly (0.4%) while the normal tissue is greatly attacked in an all-round way by the cytotoxic drug (99.6%), at the same time, the cancer patient has low immunologic function by nature, now the cytotoxic drug in chemotherapy kills the hematopoietic cells, immunological cells, T lymphocyte, blood cells and blood platelet of the bone marrow again, resulting in further drop of immunologic function, the cytotoxic drug in chemotherapy attacks and kills the hematopoietic cells and immunological cells of the bone marrow once and again, resulting in the future drop of the immunologic function, in this way, one disaster comes after another, some cytotoxic drugs even urge the breakdown of the immunologic function.

(II) Elevation of calculation of dose for systemic intravenous chemotherapy for solid tumor

1. Since the systemic intravenous chemotherapy for solid tumor is not the specific targeting administration, but blindly distributed in the whole body, it necessarily needs much dose of cytotoxic drug; furthermore, it needs the combination of multiple drugs, in this way, it is possible to make the cancer lesion with very small area obtain the dose for remitting and shrinking the cancer lesion. The reason for large dose is that the 99.6% of the dose is absorbed by the whole body while only 0.4% is absorbed by the local cancer lesion. As a result, the relatively larger the dose, the larger and the more obvious the side reaction, resulting in remarkable drop of white blood cells and blood platelets, sometimes it also needs drug for increasing white cells, so it is unreasonable to calculate the dose.

2. At present, the systemic intravenous chemotherapy for solid tumor is the experience and the method obtained from the treatment of leukemia, however, as to the treatment extended to the solid tumor, its guiding ideology is to administer the drug as per the calculation of the body surface area of the whole body, which is unadvisable. Why? Because the leukemic cells are distributed in the general blood circulation system, in the organs and tissues in the whole body, the target to be treated exists in the general blood circulation system, therefore, it is reasonable and advisable to adopt the systemic intravenous chemotherapy and conforms to the targeting treatment. Because the target cells of the leukaemia are distributed in the general blood circulation system, so it is reasonable and advisable. However, since the solid tumor is limited to a certain organ, its target to be treated is mainly a certain organ suffering from cancer, so it shall adopt the route of intravascular administration in the target organ and specific targeting administration, in this way, it can greatly reduce the

dose of cytotoxic drug, as well as greatly reduce and eliminate the side reaction of the cytotoxic drug.

3. The calculation of the dose of systemic intravenous chemotherapy for solid tumor as per the body surface area is not based on therapeutical does by which how many cancer cells can be killed but on the tolerance dose of the organism to the cytotoxic drug. It is unknown whether one chemotherapy and two chemotherapies kill the cancer cells and how many cancer cells are killed by the chemotherapy. It is unknown. Whether there are cancer cells in the body of the patient? And where? It is unknown. Only one chemotherapy is carried out and only one task is accomplished.

(III) Evaluation of curative effect evaluation criterion of systemic intravenous chemotherapy for solid tumor

In a word, the curative effect evaluation criterion of systemic intravenous chemotherapy for solid is mainly embodied in three points: size of tumor, remission and remission time. As to the size of tumor, it is mainly based on CT, MRI or type-B ultrasonic, however, all of the images only reflect the size of occupation. As to the size of occupation, in our opinion, "the big" does not mean "the bad" and "the small" does not mean "the good". In addition, most of the occupations are short-term, the reason has been mentioned above.

2. Remission and remission time. Why the remission is regarded as the curative effect evaluation criterion and why the remission has a certain period? Apparently, the remission is not the objective of treatment or the treatment requirement of the patient or the objective of determination of treatment of the doctor just because the patient pays a certain price after several chemotherapies and only obtains a short-term remission. However, at present, the tumor medicine cannot heal all cancers (namely non-recurrence and non-metastasis) for a long time. Then, to say the latest, remission is better than the failure to remission. It is practical and realistic. Why it only can remit the cancer? Because the cytotoxic drug only harms the cancer cells and destroys their DNA rather than killing all cancer cells, which is only the first order kinetics. In addition, the reaction duration of cytotoxic drug only lasts 24h~48h even 72h after drug injection, after several days, the cancer cells will also be divided, proliferated and cloned in geometric progression, one into two, two into four and four into eight. Since the cytotoxic drug cannot kill the stem cells of the tumor, after administration for chemotherapy, the stem cells of tumor are still divided, proliferated and cloned. So in out opinion, killing the cancer cells does not conform to biological characteristics

and behaviors or multi-link and multi-step of the metastasis of cancer cells, it only can regulate and control the cancer cells and prevents their division, proliferation and clone rather than the simple killing.

(IV) Evaluation of side reaction of systemic intravenous chemotherapy for solid tumor

Why the side reaction is so large? Just because this kind of route of administration needs so much dose or has to adopt combined administration. In order to remit and shrink the cancer, it has to determine the tolerance dose of the patient as the dose, in this way, the reaction is necessarily large and the damage is large, the distribution mode of this kind of route of administration leads to large dose or combined administration, otherwise, it is difficult to realize the curative effect criterion of shrinkage, in fact, it is avoidable to administer 99.6% of the cytotoxic drug to the normal tissues, in other words, it is avoidable to reform this route of administration to the specific targeting administration. If it is reformed to intravascular administration in the specific target organ, naturally, the side reaction will become little or be eliminated.

II. We Propose to Reform Systemic Intravenous Chemotherapy for Solid Tumor to Intravascular Chemotherapy in Target Organ

Since the above-mentioned problems are in existence, they shall be further studied. We should continue to improve the traditional curative therapeutic method as per the traditional idea, in the meanwhile, we should update the idea and the understanding, make progress in reforming and have the courage to innovate. Innovation, must challenge the traditional idea instead of replacement, it shall overcome the disadvantages, correct the defects so as to make it more perfect. Innovation, shall open a new path to overcome the cancer. Therefore, we specially propose the new idea, new concept and new principles of anti-cancer as well as new treatment mode and adopt organic integral new treatment mode to reform and innovate the traditional problems based on the biological characteristics and behaviors of cancer as well as the immunologic conditions of the host and the multi-link and multi-step of metastasis.

(I) Necessity, reasonableness and scientificalness of reform the systemic intravenous chemotherapy for solid tumor to intravascular chemotherapy in target organ

As above-mentioned, the route of administration of systemic intravenous chemotherapy is not the specific targeting administration but the blind general distribution, which is unreasonable and scientific distribution, so it must be reformed. The cancer lesion is limited to the local of the viscera, so it is necessary to adopt the specific targeting administration with clear target, which is reasonable and scientific. As to the systemic intravenous chemotherapy, since most of the cytotoxic drugs are administered to the general normal tissues, if the drugs are administered to the target organ, it can save the dose administered to the whole body, in this way, the dose can be greatly reduced, thus the side reaction is greatly reduced even eliminated, so the chemotherapy even may have no toxicity.

Analyze the source and formation of the side reaction of chemotherapy and probe into the method to eliminate the side reaction. Through review, reflection and analysis, we deeply realize that the source, the blind distribution of the cytotoxic drug in the whole body by the systemic intravenous chemotherapy for solid tumor, is unreasonable. In order to shrink the tumor, it necessarily increases the dose, resulting in unavoidable side reaction.

The increased dose of cytotoxic drug does not entirely react on the cancer lesion, but mainly on the whole body to damage the normal histiocytes while these general normal tissues do not need the cytotoxic drug, however, they get most of the cytotoxic drugs in fact, which is unreasonable. It is necessary to study and reform it.

In view that its source and formation is based on the blindness of the route of administration of systemic intravenous chemotherapy, resulting in increased dose and combined administration and leading to unavoidable side reaction, so the solution is to reform the route of administration.

How to reform the route of administration?

Professor Xu Ze proposes to reform the systemic intravenous chemotherapy for solid tumor (especially the tumor of liver, gallbladder, spleen, pancreas, stomach, intestine, uterus, ovary, pelvic cavity and abdominal cavity) to intravascular chemotherapy in target organ, in this way, the drug is administered to the specific target and then to the cancer lesion of the target organ, necessarily leading in the greatly decreased dose; the reduction of dose of cytotoxic drug necessarily leads to the reduction and elimination of side reaction. The elimination of side reaction of the traditional chemotherapy, makes millions of cancer patients free from the pains and risks of side reaction of chemotherapy and benefits the patients.

Professor Xu Ze holds: the intravascular administration in the specific target organ, reduces the dose, improves the curative effects, eliminates the side reaction, necessarily leading to great reduction of medical charge, saving billions of medical

charges and expenditures (in RMB Yuan) for the state and the patients and being advantageous for settling the problems of being difficult and expensive in taking medical treatment.

Over half a century, millions of cancer patients have been deeply damaged by the side reaction of the chemotherapy, therefore, this reform will benefit millions of cancer cells, which is a great pioneering undertaking and an original innovation and promotes the further development of the oncology in the 21ˢᵗ century.

(II) It is necessary to firstly study and make clear where the target is so as to carry out the intravascular chemotherapy in target organ; it is necessary to study and make clear where the cancer cells are so as to kill the cancer cells with cytotoxic drug in chemotherapy? In this way, it can have a definite object.

The primary lesion of the solid tumor is in the organ, for example, the stomach cancer lies in the stomach, the liver cancer lies in the liver, the lung cancer lies in the lung, the intestinal cancer lies in intestine, that is to say, the primary cancer lesion lies in the organ, even if it meets with metastasis in the advanced stage, its primary cancer lesion is still in the organ.

Where are the cancer cells? The cancer cells of stomach cancer, intestinal cancer, liver cancer, lung cancer and so on are mainly in the portal system and meet with metastasis via the portal system. An example of liver cancer: the main blood supply of liver cancer is from the hepatic artery, the most primary route of the metastasis of liver cancer is the venous system in the liver. The metastasis of liver cancer in liver is the most common metastasis mode, the cancer cells invade the branch of the portal vein, form the cancer embolus in the portal vein, continually extend to the hepatic portal until the left and right branch of the portal vein and its beam are blocked by the cancer embolus, the deciduous cancer cell balls are floating in the portal vein and are spread to the liver through blood.

The hepatic vein wall is thin and receives the blood flowing back from the cancer lesion, so it is easy to be encroached and the cancer embolus is formed in the hepatic vein, sometimes, the embolus can reach to inferior vena cava and to right atrium and then meet with metastasis via the lung.

The liver is one of the organs meeting with metastatic carcinoma most commonly. According to information of pathologic anatomy, among the cases of the patients who die of the malignant tumor, about 40% meet with the liver metastasis and its incidence rate is next only to lymphatic system. The liver metastasis of malignant tumor of gstrointestinal tract is the most common.

The liver receives the dual blood supply from portal vein and hepatic artery, the liver metastasis can come from the portal vein circulation and systemic circulation, that is to say, the cancer cells enters the systemic circulation via pulmonary capilliary station. The blood supply is complicated, about 90%of the blood supply is from the hepatic artery.

The administration along the route of hematogenous metastasis of cancer cells for tracking and killing shall follow the flow direction of the tumor vein, the chemotherapy drug follows the flow direction, killing the cancer cells in metastasis with small dose. As to the cancer cells, the cancer cell groups and micro-metastasis cancer embolus in metastasis, it is only necessary to kill $10^{4\cdot5}$ cancer cells with eth cytotoxic drugs for chemotherapy, the rest $10^{4\cdot5}$ cancer cells can be eliminated by the immunological cells and immunological surveillance in the blood circulation of the organism. According to the plan, it is satisfactory for the dose to kill $10^{4\cdot5}$ cancer cells, the dose cannot go so far to kill too many immunological cells. To kill some cancer cells and to protect the immunological cells from being damaged excessively as well, shall be judged with the sign of not affecting the drop of white blood cells and blood platelets. The viscera and organs in the abdomen, such as stomach, rectum, colon, liver, gallbladder, pancreas, uterus and ovary and other tumor-producing vein gather at the portal vein system, therefore, the target organs of tumor at the abdomen shall focus on the portal vein system and hepatic artery.

III. The Suggestion of Reforming the Systemic Intravenous Chemotherapy for Solid Tumor at the Abdomen to the Specific Method and Approach of Intravascular Chemotherapy in Target Organ

(I) Intravascular administration for chemotherapy in target organ

1. Administration via arterial route

    (1) The chemotherapy pump shall be arranged in the hepatic artery;

    (2) Hepatic artery interventional therapy, embolism + chemotherapy;

    (3) Interventional chemotherapy perfusion of bronchial artery;

    (4) Interventional chemotherapy perfusion of internal iliac artery;

(5) Interventional chemotherapy of arteria pancreatica;

(6) Interventional chemotherapy perfusion of gastric artery;

(7) Hepatic artery chemotherapy pump through laparotomy.

2. Administration via portal vein route

(1) Portal vein chemotherapy pump through laparotomy;

(2) Omentum venous pump through laparotomy;

(3) Subcutaneous chemotherapy pump through laparotomy via mesentery vein;

(4) Subcutaneous deep vein conduit chemotherapy pump: can be used in the treatment of malignant tumor of the intestines and stomach tract.

Surgical interventional chemotherapy for tumor patient has been widely applied, now the subcutaneous chemotherapy pump for drug delivery system is mostly adopted at present and it is a good route of administration for tumor chemotherapy, which can be divided into three classes: venous duct chemotherapy pump; ductus arteriosus chemotherapy pump and celiac duct chemotherapy pump, compared with the peripheral vein chemotherapy and artery interventional chemotherapy, it has a lot of advantages.

3. Administration via target organ at the abdomen

Oral administration: oral administration→ stomach→ vena coronaria of stomach (left vein and right vein of stomach)→ splenic vein→ portal vein, for example, oral administration of Xeloda.

Oral administration: oral administration→ stomach→ lymphatic vessel under gastric mucosa →lymph node around the stomach→ lymph node behind peritoneum→ cisterna chyli→ thoracic duct, for example, oral administration of Brucea emulsion.

Rectal suppository: rectal suppository (a few of chemotherapy drug) → venae intestinales → vein under mesentery → portal vein.

Route of administration for the target organ of lung cancer:

A. vein of antibrachium → superior vena cava → double lungs

B. Portal vein conduit or pump → liver → hepatic vein →lower caval vein → right ventricle → double lungs

C. Oral administration: oral administration → portal vein →liver →lower caval vein → right ventricle → double lungs

(II) Paying attention to arterial interventional administration

An example of liver cancer: since the onset of liver cancer is insidious, when the patient see a doctor, it is mostly in intermediate and advanced stage, followed by other factors such as high combined hepatocirrhosis rate, relatively low surgical removal rate and high recurrence rate after operation, most of the patients need non-operation therapy. At present, among the non-operation therapies with positively curative effects, interventional therapy is most widely used.

Its indication can be used to the liver cancer in different stages and it is better for the liver cancer in early and intermediate stage. These suffering from serious icterrus, voluminous ascites, serious damage to liver function and widespread metastasia shall be abstained from contraindication.

Generally, the first period of treatment of interventional therapy of liver cancer needs 3-4 times, with the interval of 2-3 months. In principle, the next interventional therapy shall be carried out only after the general condition and liver function of the patient are basically recovered over 3 weeks.

Interventional therapy

Since the interventional therapy will damage the normal tissue especially the liver and the immune system of the organism synchronously, the organism needs a certain time for recovery to understand the second interventional therapy, in the interval of interventional therapy, it shall nourish the liver, improve the immunity and adopt the complex treatment. In Shuguang Tumor Clinic of Shugang Tumor Research Institute, in the past 16 years, all the patients of liver cancer receiving the interventional therapy administer XZ-C medicine after operation and they take oral administration of XZ-C_{1+4+5} for protecting the chest, improving the immunity, protecting the bone marrow, enhancing hematopiesis, protecting liver and great curative effects have been made. Most of the patients have been in good condition and have had good appetite, their symptoms have been improved, their survival quality has been improved, and most of them have had an obviously prolonged survival period.

(III) Paying attention to the route of administration of chemotherapy pump in portal vein

It is necessary for the specific targeting administration for target organ to understand where the target organ of the cancer cells is. The tumor-bearing vein of stomach cancer, colon and rectal cancer, gallbladder cancer, pancreas cancer, cancer of pelvic cavity and oophoroma flows into the portal vein system, therefore, the cancer cells, and the ones in metastasis are flowing into the portal vein system, therefore, attention shall be paid to the chemotherapy pump in portal vein for targeting tracking and killing the cancer cells.

Chemotherapy pump in portal vein is remained in the portal vein after exploration of laparotomy or remained in the lower omentum vein after laparotomy; or remained in the drug delivery system in the mesentery under the direct vision of the laparotomy.

Chemotherapy pump embedded in portal vein body, also called implanted drug delivery system or subcutaneous embedded drug delivery system, is a kind of drug subcutaneously embedded for local perfusion, which is used for the guiding chemotherapy of cancer and oriented local perfusion chemotherapy for preventing the recurrence after removal of tumor. The drug can directly enter the target organ through drug pump and conduit, improving the lethality and the curative effects to cancer cells and reducing the side reaction of chemotherapy. It is reported by the literature that when the density of the local chemotherapy drug is increased one time, the lethality to the tumor can be increased 6-12 times. This system can increase several times of the density of the local drug. At present, this system is widely used for the clinic at home and abroad and great curative effects have been made.

In a word, as above mentioned, the systemic intravenous chemotherapy for solid tumor, only has a few of drug reaching to the cancer lesion while most of the cytotoxic drugs react on the normal histiocyte in the whole body, especially, they are relatively toxic to the tissue with rapid proliferation such as hemopoietic system of bone marrow, immune system and alimentary system and have the side reaction, however, these normal tissue, not needing the cytotoxic drugs, obtains a large number of cytotoxic drugs, which is unreasonable.

As to the chemotherapy through intravascular administration in the target organ, the drug is directly sent to the target organ via the conduit, the cytotoxic drugs obtained by the cancer lesion are all drugs administered, which is reasonable and scientific, greatly reducing the dose for chemotherapy. The specific targeting administration, reduces the does, improves the curative effects, reduces or eliminates the side reaction. In this way, it improves the curative effects, eliminates the reaction, resulting in the reduction of expenses. It is advantages for settling the problems of being difficult and expensive in taking medical treatment. Since it reduces or eliminates the side reaction, necessarily reducing the medical charge and saving billions of medical expenses and expenditures.

3. Review and Analysis of Clinical Cases of Postoperative Adjuvant Chemotherapy for Carcinoma

People have been struggling with the cancer for hundreds of years. Surgical operation of traditional treatment has been developing for over 100 years, radical treatment for 80 years and chemical treatment for 60 years. But until now, the cancer is still rampant in the crowd, and the three treatments produce little effect. Also its morbidity is increasing year by year and mortality remains high. According to the statistics of 1995, 7 million people around the world have been found with cancerous protuberance every year, and 5 million of them die from cancerous protuberance. In 1996, 1.8 million people had cancer in our country, and 1.28 million of them died from it. In terms of the mortality, tumor ranks first and becomes the most serious illness of threatening the human health. In 1975, U.S. government announced to deploy vast manpower and materials for "the declaration of war on cancer". This was the first time that conquering a disease was treated as the national policy. They attempted to use strong national power to conquer the tumor. But the courses of many events are independent of man's will. In 1993, when American Cancer Society was summarizing research progress since "the declaration of war on cancer", they found that the result of $25 billion financial input for anti-cancer instead was not optimistic, with morbidity rising 7% and survival rate only up 4%. Our academic world and clinicians should calmly, objectively, matter-of-factly and seriously review, analyze, summarize, self-evaluate and rethink our decades of practical cases. We need to sum up experience and lessons of success and failure in the fight against cancer during the half century. We should ask why the traditional treatment does not reduce the mortality obviously. What problem does the traditional treatment have actually? What exactly is the flaw? How should we improve the traditional treatment and correct its shortcomings to make it more perfect?

While continuing to enhance effects of traditional surgical operation, radical treatment and chemical treatment with traditional train of thought, we should open up a new way and look for a new route to conquer the cancer.

According to the writer's analysis of patient history derived from 54 years' medical practices, chemotherapy and radiation must be further practiced on clinical foundation research, and also on analyzing, summarizing, evaluating and rethinking therapeutic effect of verification on clinical cases. The radical or chemical treatment must be tried to eliminate the damage to the host. It is essential to further complete it, improve the treatment of killing off tumor cells but damaging the body, even just damaging the body. Then how to grasp the principle of proportionality is very important. How to evaluate the medical quality for cancer? The writer considers that the medical quality equals the therapeutic effect. The therapeutic effect of tumor for cancer patients should be the good life quality and very long survival time, but not merely the tumor shrinkage or remission. The effect should relieve the patient's pains and prolong the patient's life.

In view of the recurrent relapse and metastasis after surgical radical operation, therefore, postoperative adjuvant chemotherapy has been prevailing universally after the 1980s. While cancer experts have different perspectives whether postoperative adjuvant chemotherapy has arrested relapse, or whether it has prevented metastasis. Specific research report has not yet appeared. According to a group of case reports for five-year follow-up results of postoperative adjuvant chemotherapy or radiation patients by British Stomach Cancer Group, this cancer group adopted mitomycin and fluorouracil to provide adjuvant treatment for the first group patients in 1976. But the result showed that this treatment didn't benefit the postoperative patients. Therefore British Stomach Cancer Group carried out adjuvant treatment research for another group of patients again.

British Stomach Cancer Group adopted prospective, randomized, controlled grouping research for 436 sdenocarcinoma of stomach patients, whose postoperative staging was phase II to phase III. The 436 postoperative patients were respectively treated by radiation or combined chemotherapy of mitomycin, adriamycin and fluorouracil treatment (MAF). During five-year follow-up, 372 patients died, in which 45 patients died from surgical complications and 327 patients died from tumor relapse. In this randomized grouping research, 145 patients adopted surgical operation. 153 patients accepted adjuvant radiation, and the range of irradiation included hilus lienis and porta hepatis region, also the radiation dose was 4500cGy. Another 138 patients accepted combined chemotherapy (MAF Treatment). Mitomycin was 4mg/m^2; adriamycin was 30 mg/m^2; fluorouracil was 600 mg/m^2. The three drugs were all intravenous injections, and the treatment cycle was 8 cycles, which three weeks were one cycle. Overall two-year survival rate of this group was 33% (31%~35%), and five-year survival rate was 17% (13%~21%). Compared with the survival rate of patients only adopting surgical operation, the survival rate of patients accepting adjuvant treatment had no increase. The five-year survival rate of patients only adopting surgical operation was 20%, rate of surgery and radiation was 12%, and rate of surgery and chemotherapy was 19%.

Thus, surgical operation remains to be the standard treatment for sdenocarcinoma of stomach. The adjuvant treatment measure should be limited within certain field of research.

The writer of this book sorts, analyzes, evaluates and rethinks the following part of the cases (cases with personal inquiry of medical history, medical examination, diagnosis and treat, complete observation) with nearly ten-year personal clinical diagnosis and treatment.

I. Failure Cases of Postoperative Adjuvant Chemotherapy to Arrest Relapse

Case 1 Patient Wei ××, female, fifty, Changsha Hunan, engineer

Diagnosis: Cystosarcoma phylloides of left breast had serious malignant change and relapse. In July 1996, the patient was found the enlargement of lump in her left breast. The puncture of the lump diagnosed that the lump was fibroma. In October 1996, the left breast was removed. Pathological examination: cystosarcoma phylloides of left breast, level II. Since December 19, 1996, the patient began to accept VAD treatment for chemotherapy and get chemotherapy once every three weeks. The second chemotherapy was on January 16, 1997. Constantly, the third chemotherapy was on February 24, 1997; and then the fourth chemotherapy on March 6, 1997; the fifth chemotherapy on April 8, 1997; the sixth chemotherapy on April 29, 1997. On July 2, 1997, type-B ultrasonic examined that there was a 15mm×12mm sized lump in the similar 9 o'clock position of the right breast. Considering the relapse and metastasis, the patient came to the anti-cancer coordination group (Hubei Group) for outpatient treatment, adopting traditional Chinese and western medicine combination treatment.

Surgery ①Chemotherapy ② ③ ④ ⑤ ⑥ Relapse   XZ-C Treatment

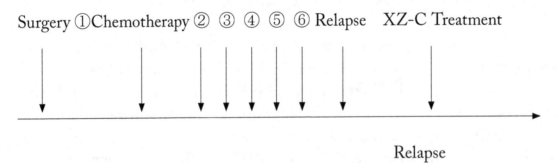

Relapse

Analysis: This patient had one-year postoperative chemotherapies continuously, defining once every month and five days one time. The treatment was standard systematic chemotherapy. But after stopping chemotherapy for two months, the tumor appeared local relapse. That explained that the chemotherapy failed to arrest relapse.

It was speculated that chemotherapy might cause the continuing decline of patient's immunity functions beyond retrieval. The tumor lost the immunoregulation and made rest tumor cells set into the cell cycle. Then the tumor was induced. It prompted that long-time continuous chemotherapy must attach importance to protect the host and confront side effects of chemotherapy drugs to avoid the damage for the host. Although chemotherapy killed off tumor cells, it damaged the body at the same time.

Case 2 Patient Yang ××, female, fifty-four, cadre, Honghu

Stomach cancer relapsed after surgery. The pain of superior venter had continued for one year. The result of stomachoscopy was stomach cancer. On August 26, 1997, the patient accepted radical operation for stomach cancer. The radical operation was $_2$B1 type. There was a 8mm×5mm sized lump in the lateral side of the lesser curvature of stomach, which caused the pyloric obstruction and enlargement of lymph nodes on the side of the arteria coeliaca. The patient began to accept postoperative chemotherapy after a month. MMC and 5-Fu were seven days one time and the intervals between two times were three weeks. There were total six times in September, October, November, December 1997 and January, February 1998. After that no other treatments were adopted. In January 1999, the patient appeared swallow obstruction and emesis. On February 24, 1999, the patient accepted the stomachoscopy. Front and back of gastric remnant which closed to anastomotic stoma swelled and developed pathological changes. There were mucosal erosion and ulcer. Stomach cancer patient had the postoperative relapse. On March 4, 1999, the patient came to the anti-cancer coordination group (Hubei Group) for XZ-C$_{1+4+2}$ treatment.

Surgery ①Chemotherapy ② ③ ④ ⑤ ⑥ stomachoscopy XZ-C Treatment

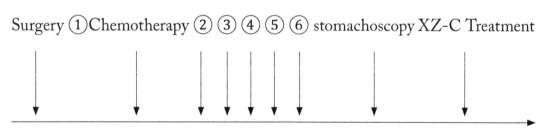

Relapse XZ-C$_{1+4+2}$

Analysis: This patient had six-time postoperative chemotherapies, defining once every month and seven days one time. The sixth chemotherapy was in February 1998. Until January 1999, the patient appeared swallow obstruction. The result of stomachoscopy was the postoperative relapse of stomach cancer. In this case, the patient had six-time postoperative chemotherapies continuously. It prompted that postoperative adjuvant chemotherapy failed to arrest relapse.

Case 3 Patient Li ××, male, forty-two, Shanxi, cadre

On November 18, 1997, the patient was found left-liver space occupying lesion through CT in 161 Hospital. On December 2, 1997, the patient accepted the left-liver lateral lobectomy. After 20 days, the patient began to accept postoperative chemotherapy. The chemotherapy drugs were 10mg/dl with intravenous injection and 20mg of hydroxycamptothecine with intravenous injection every other day in two weeks. A course was 15 days. And then the patient needed to repeat the last course after resting 15 days. Before chemotherapy, SGPT was 77μ. After chemotherapy, SGPT was 500μ. In the operation, chemotherapeutic drugs above the chemotherapy pump of portal vein (no chemotherapy pump in the artery) were injected into the organism through the pump. Before the operation, AFP was 200μ. After the operation, AFP was 200μ. In April 1998, the patient accepted the third chemotherapy in the hospital. Chemotherapeutic drugs were injected through the pump. The chemotherapy adopted the high dose pulse therapy, using 6mg of MMC, 200mg of carboplatin and 750mg of 5-Fu. Before chemotherapy, AFP was 180μ. After chemotherapy, AFP was 302μ. On May 19, 1998, the patient accepted the fourth chemotherapy, using the chemotherapy pump as the third time. On June 30, 1998, the patient accepted the fifth chemotherapy with pump. When the AFP was 219μ, it should be detected every other day. On July 28, 1998, the patient accepted the sixth chemotherapy, adopting the high dose pulse therapy through the pump. The reexamination showed that AFP>363. In early August 1998, the examination found that there was a 4cm sized lump under the incision of abdominal wall. On August 27, 1998, the lump was removed in tumor hospital. On September 29, 1998, the patient accepted the seventh chemotherapy with pump. After chemotherapy, the reexamination of type-B ultrasonic, CT and intrahepatic widespread metastasis showed that there were many ball shadows and metastases. In December 1998, the patient accepted hepatic artery embolism and pulmonary intervention in the general hospital of a military region. The examinations found that there were lumps equivalent to the size of an adult fist and infant's head in epigastrium and right abdomen. The lumps were stiff. On March 1, 1999, the patient came to the anti-cancer coordination group (Hubei Group) for outpatient treatment, adopting traditional Chinese and western medicine combination treatment and XZ-C$_{1+4+5}$ series treatment.

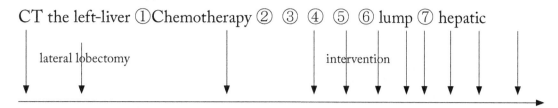

CT the left-liver ①Chemotherapy ② ③ ④ ⑤ ⑥ lump ⑦ hepatic

lateral lobectomy   intervention

Relapse of intrahepatic
incision of widespread
abdominal wall metastasis

Analysis: This patient suffered from cancer of the liver. After the left-liver lateral lobectomy, the patient had seven-time postoperative chemotherapies continuously, defining once every month. The seventh chemotherapy showed the intrahepatic widespread metastasis and pulmonary metastasis. It prompted that postoperative adjuvant chemotherapy failed to arrest relapse and prevent metastasis.

Case 4 Patient Xiang ××, male, forty-three, cadre, Chongyang

In June 1994, the disease of this patient was treated as gastroenteritis. Until December, the X-ray examination in city hospital showed that the patient suffered from intestinal obstruction. In early January 1995, the emergency operation explored the disease as a transverse colon tumor. Then the tumor was removed, adopting the end to end anastomosis. Pathological examination showed that the tumor was a malignant tumor. In February, March, April, May, June, July 1995, the patient had six-time postoperative chemotherapies continuously, defining five days one time. In January 1996, the colonic neoplasm of anastomotic stoma was found. The patient accepted the radical excision. At the end of December 1997, the tumor of anastomotic stoma was found again. On March 31, 1998, the patient accepted the palliative excision. In September 1998, another 5.6cm×4.6cm sized lump equivalent to the size of an adult fist was found between stomach and caput pancreatic. On November 24, 1998, the patient underwent an operation again to remove the lump. Those lesser tubercles, such as the omentum, were difficult to be removed completely. And the operation could only remove big ones. In 1996, the patient once accepted four-time postoperative chemotherapies in Tumor Department, defining five days one time. And the patient also took Doxifluridine orally for two months. In April, May 1998, the patient accepted twice chemotherapies. And as well, the patient took two courses of traditional Chinese medicine dispensed by Wang Zhenguo of Shenyang. But the course didn't work. Then the patient took one course of Shijiazhuang Chinese medicine. The course also didn't work. On November 13, 1998, the patient came to the anti-cancer coordination group for outpatient treatment, adopting traditional Chinese and western medicine combination treatment, $XZ-C_{1+4}$ treatment and $XZ-C_2$ treatment. In November 1999, the patient accepted the reexamination, which showed the stable condition.

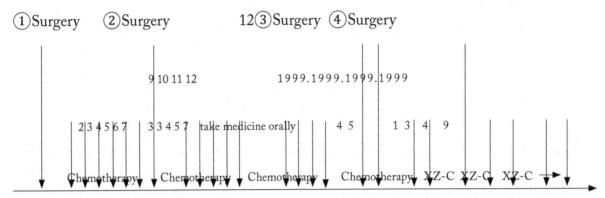

Analysis: This patient underwent the colon cancer operation of removing the tumor. After that, the patient had six-time postoperative chemotherapies continuously, defining once every month and five days one time. Five months later, the colonic neoplasm of anastomotic stoma relapsed and was removed by surgery. During the one year after operation, the patient proceeded with postoperative chemotherapies monthly and continuously. The tumor of anastomotic stoma relapsed and was removed again. The patient proceeded with postoperative chemotherapies. This case prompted that chemotherapy failed to arrest relapse and prevent metastasis. In November 1998, the patient came to the outpatient department for traditional Chinese and western medicine combination treatment, and also took traditional Chinese medicine of $XZ-C_{1+4+2}$ immunoregulation series chronically and continuously. After taking medicine orally, the patient's condition was improved. In November 1999, the patient accepted the reexamination, which showed the stable condition.

Case 5 Patient Li ××, male, fifty, cadre, Hanchuan

Diagnosis: Rectum cancer relapsed after surgery.

In December 1994, the patient underwent a radical operation for rectum cancer. The operation was Dixon type. The length of rectum cancer lesion was 12cm. The patient had six-time postoperative chemotherapies continuously, defining once every month and seven days one time. The condition was good after operation. On April 30, 1998, the patient accepted the colonoscopy examination. There was a lump at the area of rectum, having 10cm distances to the anus. The 3cm×3cm sized lump had a rugged surface and swelled towards the intracavity. The biopsy of four living tissues showed that the cell had became allotypic gland cell. On June 25, 1998, the patient suffered from the incomplete intestinal obstruction. Then on July 9, 1998, the patient underwent the Hartmann operation and partial cystectomy. The surgery proved it the recurrent rectum cancer, which had involved the bladder. The patient had five-time postoperative radiotherapies for pelvic cavity with accumulated dose of 5000CGY (from October 12, 1998 to November 13, 1998). The patient also had postoperative chemotherapies for one month. The chemotherapy drugs were 5-Fu and calcium leucovorin (five days, once a day). Since the proctoscopy examined the relapse of rectum cancer in May 1998, the patient came to the anti-cancer coordination group for the traditional Chinese medicine treatment of XZ-C immunoregulation series, which was adopted to control the relapse and metastasis. On November 28, 1999, the patient accepted the reexamination. After taking the medicine orally, the patient regained a high spirit, a good appetite and enough physical strength, which showed the stable condition. The patient continued to live normally without any discomfort.

1994.12 1995.1—1995.6 1998.4   1998.6   1998.7   1998.10—11

Surgery ① ② ③ ④ ⑤ ⑥ Colonoscopy Intestinal Obstruction Surgery Radiotherapy Chemotherapy

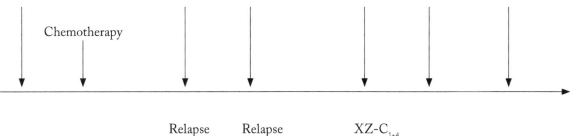

Analysis: After a radical operation for rectum cancer, the patient had six-time postoperative chemotherapies continuously, defining once every month and seven days one time. Two years later, rectum cancer appeared the local recurrence and widespread metastasis. Then the patient continued to accept the chemotherapy, but the rectum cancer relapsed again. It prompted that postoperative adjuvant chemotherapy failed to arrest relapse and prevent metastasis. After the relapse in April 1998, the patient came to the anti-cancer coordination outpatient department for the traditional Chinese medicine treatment of $XZ-C_{1+4}$ immunoregulation series. After taking the medicine orally, the patient's condition was stable and improving. The patient had been persisting in taking the XZ-C medicine for over one year and was being in good health.

Case 6 Patient Luo ××, female, housewife, Gongan county

In September 1994, the patient found a lump in the left breast. The local hospital scanned the lump as a fibroma. In September 1995, because of the enlargement of the lump (5cm×5cm×3cm), the patient underwent a radical operation for breast cancer in the district hospital. Pathology: infiltrating ductal cancer of right breast, ER (+), P.R (+), removal of one subclavicular lymph node and two axillary fusional

lymph nodes. After the operation, the patient accepted chemotherapies with CMF treatment for one week. On December 6, 1995, the patient accepted chemotherapies with CAF treatment for one week. On December 26, 1995, the patient accepted chemotherapies with CAF treatment for one week again. From February 5, 1996 to March 30, the patient accepted radiotherapies. In August 1996, the patient continued to accept two courses of chemotherapies, defining three weeks of one course. In September 1997, a lump was found in the right axilla. There were tubercles under the prethoracic skin again. The breast cancer appeared relapse and metastasis. Then the patient came to the anti-cancer coordination outpatient department for the traditional Chinese medicine treatment of XZ-C immunoregulation series. On January 4, 1998, the patient began to take XZ-C medicine during the outpatient treatment. After taking 45-day medicine, the patient's condition kept stable. In October 1998, the patient accepted the reexamination in the outpatient department, which showed the stable condition. There was a tubercle equivalent to the size of the little finger in the top part of right axilla. Above this tubercle, there was another tubercle equivalent to the size of a rice grain. But it had no more growth.

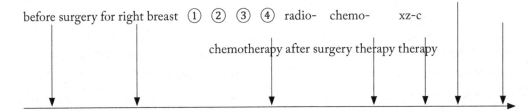

Analysis: The patient suffered from the breast cancer. Before the surgery, the patient accepted one-week chemotherapies. After the surgery, the patient accepted postoperative chemotherapies, defining once every month and one-week one time. But the treatment failed to prevent metastasis, diffusion and progression. In January 1998, the patient came to the outpatient department and took 10-month traditional Chinese medicine of immunoregulation. The patient's condition was stable. The breast cancer had no more progress. The general condition was improving.

Case 7 Patient Yang ××, female, fifty, Hankou, technical cadre

Diagnosis: Rectal adenocarcinoma relapsed after surgery.

In June 1996, the patient was diagnosed with rectum cancer for diarrhea. On July 11, 1996, the patient underwent a radical low anterior resection operation for rectum cancer. In the operation, the tumor located under the reflection, which was 5cm×4cm and invaded the muscular layer. The lymph node under the mesentery developed obvious enlargement. The patient recovered well from the operation. Nine days after the operation, the patient accepted chemotherapies of 5-Fu and MMC series. After leaving hospital, the patient took Mifulong orally. On October 4, 1996, the patient accepted chemotherapies in a tumor hospital and then left it. From August 17, 1996 to October 5, the patient accepted three courses of chemotherapies with ELF treatment. From January 14, 1997 to February 3, the patient accepted the third chemotherapies in a tumor hospital of MMC and 5-Fu series. After the chemotherapy, the patient began the attack of diarrhea more than ten times every day. From May 1997 to July 1997, the patient took Mifulong orally. On February 4, 1998, the patient had a return visit for the rectal examination. In the area of the anastomotic stoma, the tubercle could be touched. The rectum cancer relapsed. The patient accepted eight chemotherapies again and 21 radiotherapies. Then the patient had hematuria and diarrhea. It showed that the patient suffered from the radioactive cystitis and radioactive rectitis.

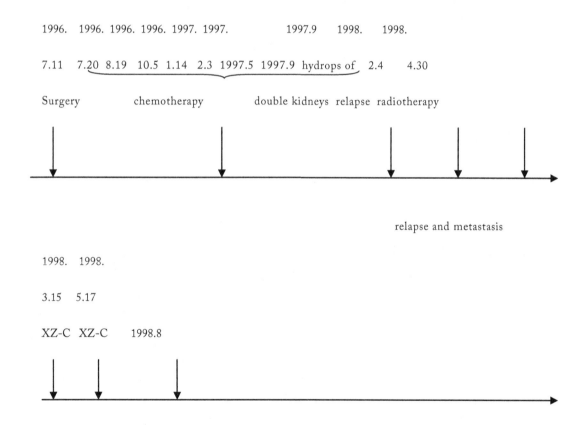

(Afterwards there was no more chemotherapy and radiotherapy. The patient had been accepting XZ-C$_{1+4}$ and brucea fruit latex treatments alone for one year. The patient's condition was stable.)

Analysis: This case was the rectal adenocarcinoma. After the radical operation, the patient accepted chemotherapies continuously. On February 4, 1998, the rectum cancer relapsed in the area of the anastomotic stoma. The patient had accepted continuous and multiple chemotherapies, involving intravenous chemotherapies and oral chemotherapy drugs. But it failed to arrest the relapse of rectum cancer in the area of the anastomotic stoma. After finding the relapse, the patient accepted radiotherapies and chemotherapies continuously again. These treatments also evoked the radioactive cystitis and other complicating diseases. The treatments failed to prevent the progression of recurrent cancer.

On March 15, 1998, the patient came to the anti-cancer coordination group for outpatient treatment, simply adopting the traditional Chinese medicine of XZ-C immunoregulation series and brucea fruit latex for enema. After taking the medicine, the patient's general condition was getting better. And the spirit and appetite were improving. The patient had chronically been taking the traditional Chinese medicine of XZ-C immunoregulation series for eighteen months. The condition of illness was stable. The tumor had been controlled, and it was stable with no more progression. The patient's condition was getting better markedly.

Case 8 Patient Xu ××, female, fifty-six, Macheng

Diagnosis: Lymph nodes of the left ventral groove metastasized. The adenocarcinoma of anal canal relapsed.

For the blood-stained stool, three blood examinations showed that the patient suffered from the cancer of anus. On February 25, 1997, the patient underwent a Miles-type radical operation for cancer of anal canal. The appendages of ambo-uterus were removed. Lymph nodes of the left perineum and ventral groove were cleaned. The patient had six-time postoperative chemotherapies. The first chemotherapy was on May 24, 1997 with MMC+5-Fu treatment. The second chemotherapy was on July 2, 1997. The third chemotherapy was on August 13, 1997. The fourth chemotherapy was on September 17, 1997. The fifth chemotherapy was on February 8, 1998. The sixth chemotherapy was on November 15, 1998. Since September 1997, the patient began to have the feeling of swell, distention, burn and urodynia in the area of anus. On April 14, 1999, the detected value of CEA was 5.8mg/ml. On April 16, 1999, the patient came to the anti-cancer coordination group for the traditional Chinese medicine treatment of immunoregulation. The patient had the feeling of swell, ache and tenderness in the area of anus. There was a very high chance that exfoliated survival cancer cells had relapsed.

1997.2.25

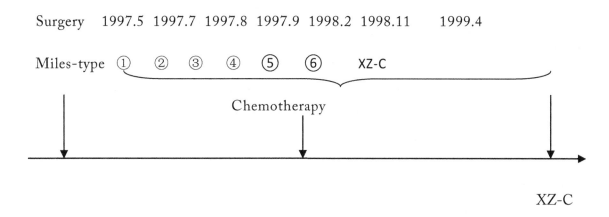

Surgery   1997.5 1997.7 1997.8 1997.9 1998.2 1998.11   1999.4

Miles-type ①   ②   ③   ④   ⑤   ⑥   XZ-C

Chemotherapy

XZ-C

Analysis: After the Miles-type radical operation for cancer of anal canal, the patient accepted chemotherapies of six courses continuously. In September 1997, the patient began to have the feeling of ache and tenderness in the area of anus. And the feeling of pain became doubly intense. It was obvious that exfoliated survival cancer cells were proliferating and relapsing. The poisonous drugs for cancers cells in continuous chemotherapies failed to totally destroy these exfoliated survival cancer cells. Thus, these cancer cells revived again, proliferating and relapsing in partial place.

Case 9 Patient Xiong ××, male, forty-two, worker, Wuhan

Diagnosis: Rectum cancer relapsed after surgery.

In March 1998, for the blood-stained stool, the disease of this patient was treated as "hemorrhoid". In May 1998, the proctoscop biopsy examination showed that the patient suffered from rectum cancer. On May 29, 1998, the patient underwent a Miles-type radical operation for rectum cancer. The postoperative plug was poorly differentiated rectum cancer. The cancer cells had invaded to the full-thickness of intestinal wall, involving the adipose tissue around the rectum. The lymph nodes around the rectum also had metastases (16/17). The patient accepted the postoperative chemotherapies. The first chemotherapy was in June 1998, adopting the MMC+5-Fu treatment for five days. In July 1998, the patient accepted chemotherapies for twelve days (pelvic cavity, front and back of abdomen) with twenty-four times. And then the second chemotherapy was in September 1998, adopting the MMC+5-Fu treatment for six days. The third chemotherapy was in November 1999, adopting the same drugs as the second chemotherapy for five days. On November 2, 1998, the patient accepted the reexamination of type-B ultrasonic. There was no abnormality in the pelvic cavity. In February 1999, the patient began to feel pain in the area of anus. The examination of type-B ultrasonic still showed no abnormality. In March, the CT examination showed that there was a lump in the deep part of pelvic cavity (the area of anus). On March 15, 1999, the patient accepted the radiotherapies of pelvic cavity for fifteen days. In the following five days, the patient had the chemotherapies. And then the patient proceeded with radiotherapies for six times. During the radiotherapies and chemotherapies, the patient was treated by XZ-C4 to fight against the toxic side effect and protect the chest and marrow for hematopoiesis and immunization. There was no untoward effect in the whole process. Since November 1998, the patient had been using the XZ-C series for the traditional Chinese medicine treatment of immunoregulation. The condition of the illness was stable and getting better.

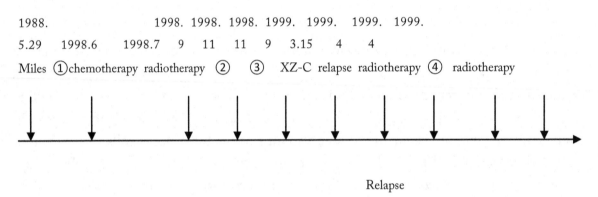

1988.			1998.	1998.	1998.	1999.	1999.	1999.	1999.
5.29	1998.6	1998.7	9	11	11	9	3.15	4	4
Miles	①chemotherapy	radiotherapy	②		③		XZ-C relapse radiotherapy	④	radiotherapy

Relapse

Analysis: After the Miles-type radical operation for rectum cancer, the patient accepted chemotherapies and radiotherapies continuously. Three months later, the CT examination showed that there was a lump in the deep part of pelvic cavity. The patient began to have the feeling of ache in the area of anus. The rectum cancer relapsed in partial place. It prompted that postoperative continuous chemotherapy failed to prevent the local recurrence.

Case 10 Patient Zhang ××, female, forty-four, married, Hankou

Diagnosis: Infiltrating ductal cancer of right breast relapsed after surgery.

In October 1997, the patient underwent the radical operation of mastocarcinoma for breast cancer (above 5㎡). Twenty days later, the patient accepted intravenous chemotherapies for eight days with CMF treatment. In December after leaving hospital, the patient accepted radiotherapies for twenty-five times. After that, the patient accepted the chemotherapies again. In February, March, April, May and June 1998, the patient accepted chemotherapies for six times, defining once every month. In April 1998, at the lower end of the incision, a tubercle about the size of a bean could be touched. Since then, the skin tubercles grew more and more. Now eczematoid lesion was diffusing around the skin incision, and the cancer cells had been metastasizing through the whole body. There was a cauliflower-shaped ulcer (3cm×3cm) in the middle part of incisional scar. On February 3, 1999, the patient came to the anti-cancer coordination group for outpatient treatment, adopting the traditional Chinese medicine treatment of XZ-C immunoregulation series and brucea fruit latex treatment. The condition of the illness was stable.

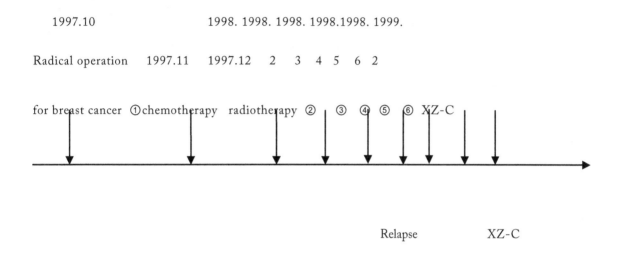

Analysis: After the operation for breast cancer, the patient accepted chemotherapies and radiotherapies continuously. Six months after the operation, when the patient was accepting chemotherapies, the cancer relapsed in partial places and the cancer cells metastasized through the whole body. It prompted that postoperative continuous radiotherapies and chemotherapies failed to prevent relapse and metastasis.

Case 11 Patient Yang ××, female, forty-three, accountant, Henan Luoshan

There was red mucus in the stool for one month. Then on December 23, 1997, the patient accepted the fibercoloscope examination. There was an irregularly shaped new growth (3cm×5cm) at the ascending colon of the blinding end, which had 100cm to the fibercoloscope. The surface of the new growth was rugged and anabrotic. The pathological test proved it villoglandular adenocarcinoma. On December 30, 1997, the patient underwent the radical operation for colon cancer to remove the right hemicolon. In the operation, it could be found that there was a 4cm×4cm sized lump in the juncture between the blind gut and the ascending colon. The lymph nodes of the mesocolic root enlarged. The cancer cells had no metastases to the liver. Pathological test showed that villoglandular adenocarcinoma (part of mucinous adenocarcinoma) had invaded to the full-thickness of intestinal wall. Twenty-two lymph nodes had no metastases. The patient accepted postoperative chemotherapies for six times, defining once every

165

month. The first chemotherapy was on November 26, 1998, continuing for eight days with FAP and hydroxycamptothecine. The second time started from February 12, 1998. A month later, the third time proceeded. The fourth time was on April 25, 1998 with FP treatment. The fifth time was on May 27, 1998. And the sixth time was on June 27, 1998. The chemotherapy continued for eight days. The patient had mild side effects. The white blood cell count (WBC) was 2100. On January 4, 1999, the patient accepted chemotherapies for ten days with MMC and hydroxycamptothecine. From February 1, 1999 to February 10, the patient accepted the tenth chemotherapy. In April 1999, the fibercoloscope reexamination showed the anastomosis ulcer of the colon. And the cancer relapsed in the anastomotic stoma. Then the patient came to the anti-cancer coordination group for outpatient treatment, adopting traditional Chinese and western medicine combination treatment, i.e. XZ-C$_{1+4}$ and brucea fruit latex. The condition of the illness was stable and getting better.

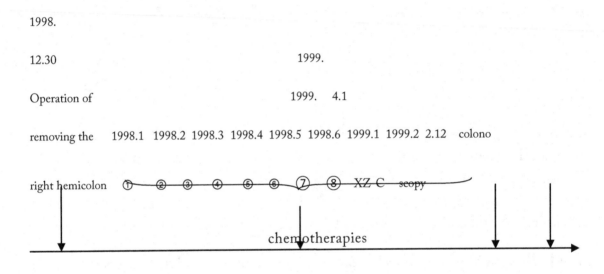

Analysis: After the radical excision for adenocarcinoma of ascending colon, the patient accepted chemotherapies for eight courses, defining one course of one month and eight days of one course. After the eighth course, the fibercoloscope reexamination showed the recurrence of anastomotic stoma. It prompted that postoperative continuous chemotherapies with eight lengthy courses still failed to prevent relapse.

Case 12 Patient Fu ××, male, twenty-four, demobilized soldier, Henan, Hu Aibin

Diagnosis: The carcinoma of colon relapsed after surgery.

Medical History: In February 1996, the abdominal pain was falsely diagnosed as appendicitis. Then the patient underwent the operation of removing the appendix. Pathological examination of appendicitis showed no inflammation. After the operation, the patient still felt pain in the abdominal region with recurrent paroxysmal pain. And it was treated as the spasmolysis of intestinal adhesion. Until December 1996, the patient underwent the operation of abdominal laparotomy in 153 Hospital of Zhengzhou because of intestinal obstruction. The operation showed that there was a tumor in the right hemicolon. Then the patient underwent the radical excision for right hemicolon. The pathological report was as follows. The patient suffered from the carcinoma of colon. Half month after the operation, the patient began to accept chemotherapies. The first chemotherapy started from January 1997 and continued for five days with the intravenous injection (iv). And the chemotherapy drugs were 5-Fu+cis-platinum+MMC. The second chemotherapy was in March 1997. The third time was in May. The forth time was in August. The fifth time was in October. The sixth time was in December 1997. In the following year, the patient accepted the chemotherapy every three months. The seventh time was in March 1998. The eighth time was in June 1998. The ninth time was in September 1998. The tenth time was in December 1998. (In 1997, there was one time every two months with a total of six times. In 1998, there was one time every three months with a total of four times.) The eleventh time was in October 1999. In January 1999, the patient began to feel pain and constantly pain in the lumbosacral portion. In August 1999, the patient began to feel pain in the abdominal region and have the abdominal tympania. And there was mucus in the stool. On November 14, 1999, the patient came to the anti-cancer coordination outpatient department for XZ-C$_{1+3+4}$ treatment. On November 15, 1999, the patient underwent a colonoscopy in the general hospital of Chinese People's Liberation Army (301 hospital). The examination showed that there was a recurrent tumor in the region, having 10cm to 30cm distances to the anus. Pathological examination showed that this tumor was the anaplastic adenocarcinoma.

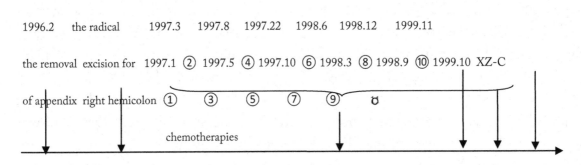

Analysis: This patient suffered from the carcinoma of colon. After undergoing the radical excision for right hemicolon, the patient accepted chemotherapies for eleven times continuously, defining two courses of one month in the first year after the operation and one course of three months in the second year after the operation. Until the tenth chemotherapy, the patient began to feel pain in the abdominal region. Retroperitoneal metastases appeared. The left colorectal cancer relapsed. Relapse and metastasis appeared while the chemotherapies were continuing. It prompted that postoperative adjuvant chemotherapy failed to arrest relapse and prevent metastasis.

II. Failure Cases of Postoperative Adjuvant Chemotherapy to Prevent Metastasis

Case 13 Patient, Xu ××, male, fifty-two, peasant, Xinzhou

Diagnosis: The hepatic metastases happened after the operation of carcinoma of anal canal.

The patient suffered from the carcinoma of anal canal. On September 23, 1997, the patient underwent the Miles-type radical operation. The tumor had 2cm from the anus, having the size of 3cm×3cm×2cm. The pathology was squamous cell carcinoma of anal canal. The patient accepted the postoperative chemotherapies once a month. There were five days per month for intravenous injection with carboplatin+5-Fu in October and November 1997. There were also five days per month for intravenous injection with MMC+5-Fu in December 1997, January 1998, February 1998 and March 1998. In April and May 1998, the patient switched to the oral route of Ftorafur-207 tablets.

In June 1998, the type-B ultrasonic showed no abnormality. But on January 8, 1999, the type-B ultrasonic showed that there were multiple occupying nidi in the liver. The biggest nidus had the size of 8.2cm×8.6cm, diagnosed as intrahepatic metastases and retroperitoneal lymphatic metastases. There were several lymph nodes with the size of 2.1cm×0.5cm.

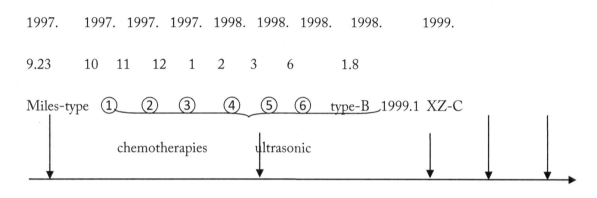

intrahepatic metastases
and retroperitoneal metastases

Analysis: This patient underwent the Miles-type operation. And the operation means was right. After the operation, the patient accepted chemotherapies once a month for six times continuously. Then the patient took the chemotherapy drugs orally for two months. The carboplatin, MMC and 5-Fu failed to prevent carcinomatous metastases. The tumor was the carcinoma of anal canal. But the first metastasis was hepatic metastasis. It prompted that continuous and systematical chemotherapies after the operation still failed to prevent hepatic metastases.

Case 14 Patient Yu ××, male, fifty-seven, worker, Nanchang

On October 22, 1995, the patient underwent the Miles-type radical operation for rectum cancer in a central hospital of Nanchang. After operation, the patient accepted the first chemotherapy was on December 5, 1995 with intravenous injection of 1000mg of 5-Fu once a day (d_1, d_2, d_3, d_4) and intravenous injection of 6mg of MMC (d_1). The second time was on February 2, 1996 with the same FM treatment as the first time. The third time was on March 18, 1996 with the same treatment. The fourth time was on May 24, 1996. The fifth time was on August 14, 1996. The sixth time was on September 14, 1996. All of the chemotherapies adopted the FM treatment. After the chemotherapies, the patient underwent the CT examination. On December 28, 1998, the report showed three points: ①fatty liver and metastatic liver cancer, ②colorectal cancer metastasis, ③polycystic kidney and calculus of kidney. On December 25, 1998, the type-B ultrasonic found the space occupying lesion of liver.

On December 30, 1998, the patient came to the anti-cancer coordination group for outpatient treatment with $XZ\text{-}C_{4+5+3}$. The examination showed that a lump in the form of bar could be touched in the right liver and the lump was hard. On January 20, 1999, the type-B ultrasonic in a central hospital of Nanchang found several tumors of unequal size about 4cm×2.1cm, 2.2cm×1.8cm and 2.0cm×1.7cm in the liver. There was a metastatic liver cancer with the size of 3.0cm×2.9cm in the right liver. On February 20, 1999, after taking the $XZ\text{-}C_{1+4}$, the patient's condition was stable and the patient regained a high spirit, a good appetite. The liver was functioning normally. The patient could walk on the street as a normal people. The symptom had an obvious improvement.

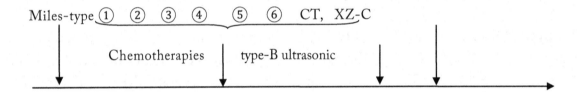

1995. 1996. 1996. 1996. 1996. 1996. 1998. 1998.

1995.10　12　2.2　3.8　5.24　8.14　9.14　12.2　12.30

Miles-type ① ② ③ ④ ⑤ ⑥ CT, XZ-C

Chemotherapies　type-B ultrasonic

hepatic symptom $XZ\text{-}C_{1+4}+LMS$

Metastases improved obviously

Analysis: After the radical operation of rectum cancer, the patient accepted continuous chemotherapies for six courses. One year later, the hepatic metastases happened. It prompted that systematical chemotherapies failed to prevent metastases.

Case 15 Patient Guo ××, male, thirty-six, teacher, Wuhan

In October 1996, the patient suffered from gastric bleeding. Then the stomachoscopy showed that the patient suffered from the stomach cancer. The patient underwent the total gastrectomy in a general hospital. Two months after the operation, the chemotherapies started. The patient accepted once every two months, defining ten days of one time. The chemotherapy drugs were MMC and 5Fu with intravenous injection. This course lasted for one year (six times). In the second year, the patient accepted once every half year. The chemotherapies in 1998 were carried out once every three or four months. In September 1998, the patient accepted one time. Every time before the chemotherapy, the patient needed to undergo the examination of type-B ultrasonic. If the type-B ultrasonic showed that there was a problem, the type-B ultrasonic would be switched to CT. The patient underwent the CT examinations for five times successively, and the CT was strengthened. After the last chemotherapy in September 1998, CT showed that the cancer cells were metastasizing to liver and retroperitoneum. Then the patient underwent the photon knife (X-knife) treatment for one time and the interventional chemotherapy for hepatic vessels embolism. In October 1998, the sclera of the patient turned yellow. The CT showed that the nubbly lump of caput pancreatic was oppressing the bile duct. Then the patient underwent the radiotherapies continuously for three times in October, November 1998 and January 1999. The doses at a time were 4000 dela. The patient had an intense reaction with bad physiques and vomiting, and couldn't feed at all. The patient couldn't undergo it and stopped the treatment. On February 28, 1999, the patient came to the outpatient department of anti-cancer coordination group for traditional Chinese and western medicine combination treatment. At that time, the patient had been bedridden. The patient was not able to take in any food for the repeated nausea and vomiting. After taking the XZ-C drugs, the patient was getting better.

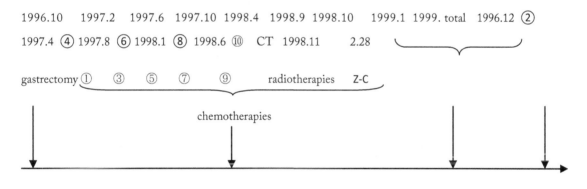

Analysis: After the total gastrectomy, the patient underwent the continuous chemotherapies and radiotherapies for a long time. After the last chemotherapy in September 1998, the CT reexamination showed the hepatic metastases and retroperitoneal metastases. It prompted that continuous and long-term treatments still failed to prevent metastases, even resulting in the failure of immunologic system and threatening the patient's life.

Case 16 Patient Cao ××, male, thirty-five, married, peasant

Diagnosis: The hepatic metastases happened after the operation of stomach cancer.

On June 28, 1996, the pre-operative diagnosis in the People's Hospital of Hanchuan certified it as the ulcer of gastric angles. The property of the illness was yet to be investigated. The patient underwent the massive resection of the stomach and the resection of great epiploon. The operation was B1-type anastomosis. The postoperative pathological report showed it the sdenocarcinoma of stomach. The cancer cells had invaded the full-thickness of stomach wall with lymphatic metastases of lesser curvature side (4/4). The lymph nodes of greater curvature side had reactive hyperplasia. The patient underwent the postoperative chemotherapies for four times in July, August, September and October 1996, defining once a month and three days every time. The chemotherapy drugs were 5-F and MMC. In September 1997, after the half month of swelling pain in right upper abdomen, the type-B ultrasonic and CT prompted that there were several low-density shadows in the right and left lobe of liver. Those were metastatic hepatic tumors and could be touched below the right costal margin of 3cm with pressing tender. On September 30, 1997, the patient underwent the interventional chemotherapy for hepatic artery. On October 5, 1997, the patient came to the anti-cancer coordination outpatient department, adopting the Z-C series for the traditional Chinese medicine treatment of immunoregulation. After taking the medicine orally, the patient regained a high spirit, a good appetite and enough physical strength. The lump below the right costal margin became soft and narrowing.

1996.6.28

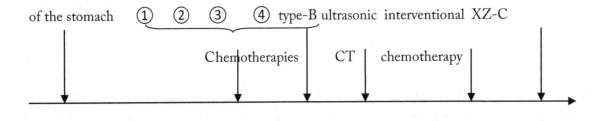

Analysis: After the operation of stomach cancer, the patient underwent the continuous chemotherapies for four times, defining once a month and three days every time. One year after the last chemotherapy, the CT reexamination showed that there were several metastatic lesions in the right and left lobe of liver. It prompted that postoperative adjuvant chemotherapies still failed to prevent metastases.

Case 17 Patient Li ××, male, fifty-five, Huangshi, second-grade actor

Diagnosis: The cancer cells metastasized to pancreas after the operation of stomach cancer.

In October 1995, the patient suffered from the epigastric discomfort. In November, the stomachoscopy in Huangshi Hospital diagnosed it as the stomach cancer. On November 27, 1995, the patient underwent the massive resection of the stomach. After the operation, the patient accepted five courses of chemotherapies with one course per month. In early May 1996, the last course ended. On June 4, 1996, the CT reexamination showed the space occupying lesion of pancreas. The patient began to have the abdominal distension and bad appetite. Then the patient came to the anti-cancer coordination group for outpatient treatment, adopting the XZ-C$_{1+4+2}$ series for the traditional Chinese medicine treatment of immunoregulation. After taking the medicine orally, the patient regained a high spirit, a good appetite.

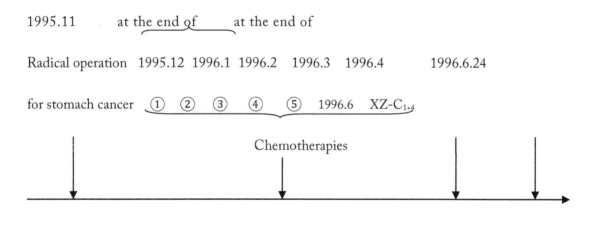

Analysis: After the radical operation of stomach cancer, the patient accepted five courses of chemotherapies with one course per month. After the five courses, the patient underwent the CT reexamination, finding the space occupying lesion of pancreas and metastatic carcinoma of pancreas. It prompted that postoperative chemotherapies still failed to prevent postoperative carcinomatous metastases.

Case 18 Patient Li ××, female, forty-five, Guangshui, teacher

Diagnosis: The stomach cancer relapsed and metastasized to ovary after the operation. The middle and down section of choledochus had solid space occupying lesions.

In April 1998, the stomachoscopy showed that there was a new growth in the body of stomach with bulb ulcer. On April 20, 1998, the patient underwent the total gastrectomy and lienectomy. Esophagus and empty intestine were connected by the end-to-side anastomosis. The pathological test showed that the patient suffered from the mucinous adenocarcinoma of stomach. The cancer cells had invaded the full-thickness of stomach wall with lymphatic metastases of lesser curvature side. On May 13, 1998, the patient accepted the first chemotherapy, adopting 1000mg of 5-Fu with five-day intravenous injections. On the first day the chemotherapy drugs were added with 10mg of Mitomycin. On June 3, 1998, the patient accepted the second chemotherapy with 10mg of Mitomycin. The third time was on July 1, 1998. The fourth time was on July 29, 1998. The fifth time was on September 9, 1998. The reexamination found the relapse. On December 24, 1998, the type-B ultrasonic showed the cancer of biliary duct and ovarian metastasis. On December 26, 1998, the patient came to the anti-cancer coordination group for outpatient treatment, adopting the XZ-C series for the traditional Chinese medicine treatment of immunoregulation. After taking the medicine orally, the symptom was improving, and the condition of the illness was getting better.

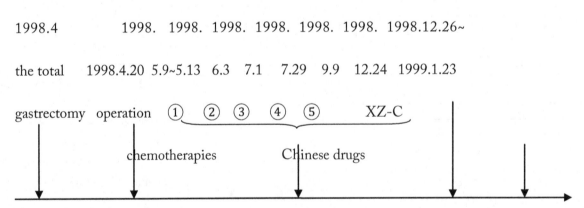

Type-B ultrasonic: relapse of cancer of biliary duct, ovarian metastasis.

Analysis: This patient suffered from the mucinous adenocarcinoma of stomach and underwent the total gastrectomy. After the operation, the patient accepted the chemotherapies once a month with five days per time. After the fifth chemotherapy, the type-B ultrasonic found the relapse of cancer of biliary duct and ovarian metastasis. It prompted that postoperative adjuvant chemotherapies still failed to arrest relapse and prevent metastasis.

Case 19 Patient Li ××, female, thirty-seven, worker, Yingcheng

Diagnosis: The rectum cancer cells metastasized to ovary after the operation.

Since 1997, the stool had been being with the blood. In June 1998, the colonoscopy showed it as the rectum cancer. On July 9, 1998, the patient underwent the anterior resection of the rectum (Dixon-type, anastomat). There were six-time postoperative chemotherapies. The first time was on July 27, 1998 with carboplatin and 5-Fu. The second time was on September 6, 1998. The third time was on October 2, 1998. The fourth time was on November 19, 1998. The fifth time was on December 25, 1998. The sixth time was on January 31, 1999.

On April 16, 1999, the patient came to the anti-cancer coordination group for outpatient treatment with the XZ-C series. In May 1999, the CT examination showed the rectum cancer cells metastasized to bilateral ovaries.

Chinese drugs for anti-cancer and immunoregulation

Analysis: After the operation of rectum cancer, the patient accepted continuous chemotherapies for six courses. Three months after the last course, the type-B ultrasonic

175

and CT found that rectum cancer cells metastasized to bilateral ovaries. It prompted that such continuous and long-term chemotherapies still failed to prevent metastases.

III. Cases of Chemotherapy Accelerating the Failure of Immunologic Function

Case 20 Patient, Xu ××, male, forty-two, cadre, Wuhan

Diagnosis: Lung cancer of right middle lobe

In February 1997, fluoroscopy of chest showed no abnormity. Because of the home decorating, the patient had contacted the marble powder bed for about one month. Then this patient began to have a complaint of the chest. On June 1, 1997, X-ray chest film showed the atelectasis of right lung. On June 13, 1997, the CT reported the lung cancer of median lobe and metastases of hilar lymph nodes. The examination of bronchofiberscope showed that each bronchus of the right side became narrower. The brushing biopsy showed it as the adenocarcinoma cell. Right now, the patient had no cough and emptysis. There was a lymph node about the size of fingertip in the right neck region. On June 13, 1997, the patient underwent the interventional therapy for one time. Because of the intense reaction, there was no more interventional therapy. On July 25, 1997, the patient began to accept chemotherapies for two times. The first time adopted the intravenous injection with a large dose of Adriamycin, Cyclophosphane, Cis-platinum and **Xierke**. On August 9, the white blood cell count (WBC) was 1100. Then the patient accepted the blood transfusion, adding with injections of interleukin-2, tumor necrosis factor and interferon. The second time was on August 20. The chemotherapy drugs were same as the first time with intravenous injection. On September 10, X-ray chest film showed no obvious pathological change. On September 11, the patient left the hospital. On October 10, 1997, Emission Computed Tomography (ECT) showed widespread metastatic tumor of bone of the whole body. On October 13, 1997, X-ray chest film showed the lung cancer of double lungs. The lesions increased significantly as compared with the past. After undergoing the reinforced chemotherapies of two courses, the lesions of double lungs spread. The cancer cells quickly metastasized to skeletons of the whole body. The immunologic function broke down. By the end of October 1997, the patient died from the failure of immunologic function.

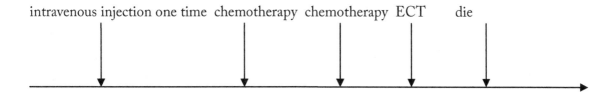

1997.6.13   1997.7.25   1997.8.20   by the end of

CT lung cancer of right lobe ① reinforced ② reinforced 1997.10.10 1997.10

intravenous injection one time chemotherapy chemotherapy ECT   die

The cancer cells metastasized to skeletons of the whole body. The immunologic function broke down.

Analysis: This patient suffered from lung cancer of right middle lobe. The left lung had carcinomatous metastasis. So the patient couldn't accept the operation. Since July 1997, the patient accepted the reinforced chemotherapies of two courses with four kinds of drugs. The patient began to vomit and couldn't feed at all. After the treatment, the immunologic function of the patient broke down. Emission Computed Tomography (ECT) showed that there were several dozen osseous metastases in the whole body. It prompted: ① the reinforced chemotherapies failed to prevent metastases. ② the reinforced chemotherapies severely suppressed the immunity, which led to the severe failure of immunologic function. The host lost the immune surveillance. The cancer cells immediately spread to the whole body. The osseous metastases resulted in the failure of immunologic function and shortened this patient's life.

Case 21 Patient Feng ××, female, fifty-one, Xiangfan, doctor

Diagnosis: After the operation of the breast cancer, the cancer cells metastasized to bones, liver and brain.

In February 1995, the patient underwent the modified radical mastectomy for the lump in the right breast. The patient suffered from the metastatic carcinoma of axillary lymph nodes (3/6). Pathology: infiltrating ductal cancer became partly hard. On February 19, 1995, the patient accepted the chemotherapy with the drugs of Adriamycin and Cyclophosphamide. On April 28, 1995, the patient transferred to Wuhan for eleven cycles of chemotherapies with CMF treatment. On May 21, 1996, the CMF treatment was switched to Xierke treatment in the eleventh cycle. The arrest of bone marrow became obvious. The white blood cell count (WBC) dropped to 300! Transfusion of 20g of leucocytes eventually made it come back to the normal value. The doctor gave express order that the patient couldn't accept the treatment after leaving hospital. On June 4, 1996, the Ct reexamination found metastatic carcinoma of the ninth rib. Then the patient accepted the radiotherapies without any chemotherapy. On July 7, 1997, the type-B ultrasonic found the metastatic carcinoma of liver. There was a tumor about the size of 3.2cm×3.9cm in the right anterior lobe of liver. The MRI and CT examinations diagnosed it falsely as radioactive hepatic lesion. On July 17, 1997, the angiography proved it as the metastatic carcinoma of liver. On July 28, 1997, the patient underwent the resection of the right anterior lobe of liver. And the patient was inserted a catheter into the hepatic artery for implantation of the drug pump. The chemotherapy drugs of epirubicin, cis-platinum and 5-Fu had been pumped successively for four times. On November 10, 1997, the type-B ultrasonic found that there were a metastatic carcinoma about the size of 3.4cm×3.3cm in the right lobe of liver and another metastatic carcinoma about the size of 1.7cm×1.9cm in the right anterior lobe of liver. The patient couldn't undergo the surgery, radiotherapy or chemotherapy any more. That was because none of the three treatments could prevent metastasis and extension. On November 16, 1997, the patient came to the anti-cancer coordination group for outpatient treatment, adopting the XZ-C series for the traditional Chinese medicine complex treatment of immunoregulation. After taking the medicine, the patient regained a high spirit, a good appetite. The general condition was improving. On March 17, 1998, MRI showed that there were multiple occupying nidi inside the calvarium. The cancer cells were metastasizing to the brain. Then the patient accepted the reinforced chemotherapies. After a course of reinforced chemotherapies, the patient gradually faded away.

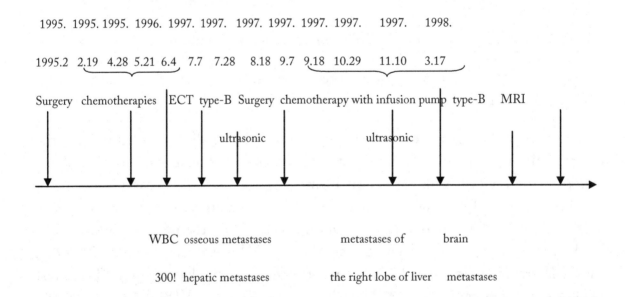

Analysis: (1) After the operation of breast cancer, the patient accepted the continuous chemotherapies, starting with short-course chemotherapies and proceeding with the eleven courses of chemotherapies. And then, the patient was injected with the chemotherapy drugs by the infusion pump. Although the patient continuously accepted the chemotherapies and other treatments without a stop, the cancer still ignored those treatments, slowly and gradually making the distant metastases through the whole body. Why did so many treatments fail to stop metastases and extensions? What kind of role and status did those chemotherapy anti-cancer drugs play and have in this case? The chemotherapies didn't produce the due effect, because after the chemotherapy the cancer cells immediately metastasized to bones, liver.

(2) The chemotherapy suppressed the immunologic function and marrow hematopoietic function. The question was whether the suppression would promote osseous metastases. The reinforced chemotherapies of this case once made WBC reduce to 300. The body's immunological function suffered the severe suppression. The cancer cells lost the immune surveillance and would inevitably have the further multiplications, extensions and metastases.

(3) Why were the chemotherapies of this case useless? The question was whether the chemotherapy drugs had the drug tolerance. If having the tolerance, the chemotherapy drugs of more than one year were totally useless. The drugs didn't produce the due effect on cancer cells. On the contrary, the normal cells of visceral organs in the patient's body, especially the cells of immune organ (Marrow was the central immune organ), ceaselessly suffered form the damage. Then the ability of the body resistance and immunological function severely fell off. It promoted multiplications, extensions and metastases of cancer cells. The chemotherapy not only failed to achieve the therapeutic effect, but also conversely had the adverse effect on attacking the ability of the body resistance and promoting the metastases and multiplications of the cancer cells.

(4) Why were the continuous chemotherapies of this case useless? The question was whether the selected joint chemotherapy drugs were not sensitive to the cancer cells of this patient. (The anti-cancer drugs couldn't accept drug sensitive test as the antibiotic. Thus the drugs were selected according to the experience with certain blindness.) When doctors couldn't get the curative effect, they would increase the dose, intensify the chemotherapy or switch to use the better chemotherapy drugs. In this way, it would produce the more severe immunological suppression, result the failure of immunological function and lead to the further multiplications of the cancer cells, which the cancer cells would present the multiplication like the geometrical logarithm. But the chemotherapy drugs couldn't increase exponentially with the toxic side effect. Thus the increasing speed and quantity of chemotherapy drugs would never be able to

catch up those of cancer cells. So the continuous chemotherapies still failed to control metastases and extensions.

Case 22 Patient Lu ××, female, forty-three, shop employee, Changsha

Diagnosis: The patient suffered from the carcinoma simplex of left breast. The cancer cells had metastasized to the back bone, pelvis and liver.

Medical History: (Omission).

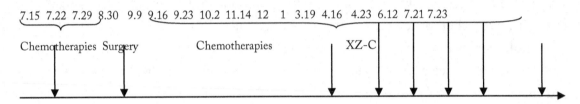

1996. 1996. 1996. 1996. 1996. 1996. 1996. 1996. 1996. 1996. 1997. 1997. 1997. 1997. 1997. 1997. 1997.

7.15 7.22 7.29 8.30 9.9 9.16 9.23 10.2 11.14 12 1 3.19 4.16 4.23 6.12 7.21 7.23

Chemotherapies Surgery   Chemotherapies   XZ-C

osseous metastases osseous hepatic metastases

destruction of lumbar multiple metastases

Analysis: This patient accepted the preoperative and postoperative chemotherapies continuously and chronically. After the operation, the patient accepted the chemotherapy once a month, defining five days every time. During the five months after the operation, there were over forty times of radiotherapies and eight times of chemotherapies. The patient underwent continuous multiple CT scans and ceaselessly continuous chemotherapies. But after eight months the cancerous protuberance widely metastasized and spread to skeletons of the whole body. Every time the patient accepted the radiotherapy or chemotherapy, she had to suffer the suppression, bone marrow suppression and the attack to the organisms of the body. The long-term and continuous chemotherapies were essentially the chronic and continuous attack to the immunologic function. The immunologic function of organisms and marrow hematopoietic function suffered such long-term and continuous damage that they couldn't restore the functions. Losing the immune surveillance, the cancer cells were bound to invade and metastasize widely to all of the visceral organs in the whole body.

The real effect of this case was that the treatment killed off tumor cells but damaged the body. It didn't turn out as it should be. In fact, the treatments failed to prevent carcinomatous metastases, essentially damage the function of immunologic and defensive system of the host, attack the ability of the body resistance and promote the invasion and dissemination of cancer cells.

Six months after the operation, metastatic carcinoma of bone appeared. Eight months after the operation, metastatic carcinoma of liver appeared. The radiotherapy and chemotherapy failed to prevent the progression of this disease. How to evaluate the therapeutic effectiveness that the radiotherapy and chemotherapy had on the patient? What kind of role and status did those treatments play and have?

Case 23 Patient Chen ××, male, Thirty-four, counterman, Wuhan

This patient had suffered from the repetitious and irritative dry cough without phlegm for three years. Then this disease was treated as bronchitis. In January 1997, X-ray film of the chest showed large compact shadows in the right upper lung. CT examination reported that there was a compact shadow about the size of 6cm×9cm in the right upper lung. And there was another sarcoidosis behind it about the size of 1.2cm×1.5cm. The sarcoidosis was the central type and had multiple metastases in the lung. On January 11, 1997, the patient underwent the exploratory thoracotomy. In the operation, it could be easily seen that the nidi had widely infiltrated and couldn't be cut off. The tissue slice showed it as the poorly differentiated adenocarcinoma in the right upper lung. Then the chest was closed. In February, March, April and May 1997, the patient accepted postoperative chemotherapies with the drugs of DDP and ADM for one course a month. On July 14, 1997, scanning reexamination showed the enlargement of lump in the right lung. Because the patient suffered from the headache for one week and felt dizzy. The CT scanning of brain showed the brain metastases. Then on July 22, 1997 and July 27, the patient successively underwent the r-scalpel operation for two times. The headache was eased and then disappeared. And on July 13, 1977, the patient came to the anti-cancer coordination group for outpatient treatment, adopting the drugs of XZ-C series. After taking the medicine, the condition of illness was stable. The patient regained a high spirit, a good appetite. The headache and vomit disappeared. The patient walked and talked as the normal people. Three months (one course) after taking the Wuhan Chinese herbal anticancer medicine of XZ-C series, the condition of illness had an obvious improvement. The patient had a rosy cheek, regained the physical strength and walked as the normal people. There was no cough or any kind of discomfort. The breathing sound of right lung faded out. Afterwards the patient accepted the chemotherapy in another hospital, continuously increasing the dose for reinforced chemotherapies. The white blood cell count (WBC) dropped to 300, which was an extremely low value. The immunologic function crocked up.

Analysis: This patient underwent the exploratory thoracotomy for the cancer of right lung. The nidi couldn't be cut off. Then the patient accepted the continuous reinforced chemotherapies. The cancer cells metastasized to the brain. After the r-scalpel operation, the headache disappeared and obtained satisfactory effects. With the immunoregulation treatment of XZ-C series, the general conditions of this patient were getting better obviously and the symptoms improved. But the continuous reinforced chemotherapies resulted in the failure of immunologic function.

4. Analysis, Evaluation And Reflection Of Clinic Practice Of Traditional Therapies

Three traditional therapies of cancel have made great achievements, which have making recognized contributions to cancer prevention and anti-cancer career of human. At the beginning of 21st century, as cancer is still at the top of the death rate, the traditional therapies have failed to inhibit and prevent the occurrence and development of cancer. Though many patients have accepted normal radiotherapies and chemotherapies systematically, the metastasis and recrudesce of cancer cell had been not prevented. The radiotherapies and chemotherapies have made many contributions and achieved a lot, however, they are still far away from the ideal requirements and objective demands in terms of domestic therapies of cancer. Why do the traditional methods fail to prevent the metastasis, diffuse and evolution of cancer? What is the reason for cancer metastasis during chemotherapies? Why can cancer metastasis be examined after chemotherapies? Are these drugs sensitive to cancer cells? Is there any drug resistance or not? What is the theory basis for the period of treatment arranged within 1 to 2years? Is there any cancer cell in patients' bodies after radiotherapies and chemotherapies? Which kind of chemotherapies can be used, local or general? What is the theory and fact basis? What are the curative effects of intensive chemotherapies as well as its influences and complications? Can the curative effects improve the quality of living and prolong the lifetime? Is there any need for chemotherapies? How to make the treatment modality? What are the effects of chemotherapies, positive or negative? Is there any possibility to accelerate the development and metastasis or diffuse of cancer cells?

Therefore, we should conclude the experience and failures of 50-year anti-cancer practice to analyze, reflect and evaluate by ourselves, in order to improve the research and the curative effects.

I. Concept of Cancer Cell Proliferation Dynamics and the Role of Chemotherapy Medicine in Cell Cycle

In this part, we will go on with the analysis, reflection and evaluation through the details of postoperative adjuvant chemotherapies of more the 6000 cases and their records of return visits.

From the point of Cancer Cell Proliferation Dynamics, having one chemotherapy every three or four weeks can hardly prevent cancer recrudesce and metastasis.

1. Basic Concepts of Malignancy Proliferation

As the object that the clinic chemotherapies are faced with is the cancer tissue rather than individual cell, the basic concept of proliferation dynamics should be described using cancer tissue as the representation of the malignant tumor tissue.

1. The collection of proliferative cells, refer to the proportion of the cancer cells that proliferate according to index in the whole cancer cells (meaning growth fraction GF). Different tumors have different growth fraction. Even one and the same tumor, the growth fraction of the prophase is higher, and different from that of the anaphase. Tumors with higher growth fraction grow rapidly and have higher sensitivity.

2. The collection of resting cells (cells of GO phase), which are the spare cells with proliferating capacity; however they don't enter the cell cycle temporarily. When the proliferative cells are killed by drugs, cells of GO phase enter into proliferating stage. Cells of GO phase have low sensitivity to drugs, which is the root of recrudesce during the treatment.

3. Collection of cells without proliferative capacity which are neither proliferative nor lost. Only a few such cells in the cancer tissue and they are insignificant in the chemotherapies.

The above three kinds of cells are in relative movements instead of standstill as the proliferative cells can change into the cells of GO phase, cells without proliferating capacity or even dead.

2. Cell Cycle

Cells of the collection of proliferative cells in cancer tissue are dividing and proliferating constantly. Cell cycle has been proposed for researching the growing process of individual cell in the collection of proliferative cells. Cell cycle refers to the entire process from the prophase of DNA synthesis to the accomplishment of mitosis. In recent years, with the advanced technologies such as flow cytometry, etc. we have achieved further researches on the proliferating cycle of cancer cells. The proliferating cycle of cancer cells can be mainly divided into four stages:

1. G1 phase meaning the prophase of DNA synthesis, is the stage letting the daughter cells from mitosis go on growing, in which the messengers mRNA and proteins are synthesized. The lengths of G1 phase of different kinds of cancer cells have great differentia from hours to days.

2. S phase meaning the synthesis of DNA, is the stage for duplicating DNA, in which the content of DNA is duplicated. In this phase, some other compounds such as histone, non-histone and enzymes relating to synthesis are also duplicated. It is worthy to note that the synthesis of tubulin has already begun in S phase. The length of S phase fluctuates between 2 and 30 hours, mostly more than 10 hours.

3. G2 phase meaning the anaphase of DNA synthesis or the prophase of division. In this phase, the DNA synthesis has finished and the preparation for cell division is processing, with the synthesis of the proteins and tubulins relating to cancer cell division, which lasts from two to three hours.

4. M phase means the stage of mitosis. Each cancer cell divides into two daughter cells. This phase is very short, only lasting from one to two hours.

The lengths of each phase can be measured by marking thymidines with 3_{HH}. The summation of G_1+S+G_2+M is the cell cycle time (TC). The TC value of acute medullocell is approximately 50~80 hours, in which G_1 phase is 20~60 hours, S phase is about 20 hours, G_2 is almost 3 hours and M is as short as 30 minutes. The TC value of albino rat L_{1210} leucocythemia is some 12.8 hours with M phase being an hour.

Thus during one-time chemotherapy, only making drugs acting on cells and experiencing the entire cycle for 50 to 80 hours, or the drugs for the chemotherapy acting on cancer cell or the cancer cells are soaked in the chemotherapeutant for 50 ~80 hours can kill the cancer cells in some phase. If using disposal catheter to inject drugs or during the chemotherapy, patients only accept 6~8 minute intravenous drip, maybe the drugs can not meet the most sensitive phase, that is to say, the desired curative effects can not be achieved. Just acting on some phase of cell proliferation blindly without selections fails to react on cell cycle.

Antibiotics G_+ or G- kill the bacterium G_+ or G- after contacting. Different from antibiotics, the chemotherapeutants can only react on the sensitive phase and make no effects on other ones. These two are completely different.

In terms of cell dynamics, the chemotherapeutants can be divided into two kinds according to sensitivity to malignant cells of each phase, cell cycle nonspecific agent (CCSNA) and cell cycle specific agent (CCSA)

1. Cell Cycle Nonspecific Agent There is no relationship between cell's sensitivity and its proliferating state. CCNSA can kill the cells of each phase through the entire proliferating cycle. Most alkylating agents and antibiotic drugs belong to this sort.

2. Cell Cycle Specific Agent Cell's sensitivity relates to its proliferating state. CCSA mainly reacts on some phase of the cell cycle, which is classified into two sorts; M phase specific drugs and S phase specific drugs.

    (1) M phase specific drugs mostly acts on mitosis, vegetable drugs like vinblastine and vincristine fall into this sort.

    (2) S phase specific drugs are used to inhibit the synthesis of RNA and proteins, most antimetabolite drugs such as methotrexate, 5- fluorouracil, purinethol and thioguanine and others belong to this sort.

CCNSA can damage tumors cells of each phases including G_0 phase without sensitivity. Cells of S and M phases in proliferation are the most sensitive to the drugs. These drugs include the metabolite(S phase) and the vegetable drugs (M phase) with the characteristic of schedule-dependent when giving drugs. At first, the curative effect of killing the tumor cells is proportional to the dosage, whose dose-effect curve presents exponential decrease. As the amount of cells in S phase or M phase is certain, there are no other benefits to add the dosage; in spite of the cells of S phase and M phase, others are not sensitive to this category of drugs.

For both CCNSA and CCSA, their effects of damaging cancer cells subject to the first order kinetics, that is to say it is impossible to kill all cancer cells but a definite proportion. Though patients accept drugs with high dose for several times, there are always some cells without sensitivity to the drugs. So, cancer cells always exist in the bodies, which can be only relieved rather than healed. This way can only prolong the lifetime instead of charming away (It is difficult to identify whether this therapeutic method can prolong the patients' lifetime or not for it is only considered from the aspect of killing cancer cells by drugs, however in terms of drugs' inhibiting immunity and the toxic side effects to marrow and liver, the living qualities and lifetime of the host cells are still faced with severe challenges).

As that the anticancer drugs damage the cancer cells subjects to the first order kinetics, generally it is difficult to find a perfect chemotherapeutic drugs to cure cancers. However, when the loads of tumors are below 10^6, it is possible to annihilate the cancer cells using XZ-C treatment by Chinese herbs for immunoregulation or immunological therapy.

That is the reasons why the postoperative adjuvant chemotherapies or palliative chemotherapy fail to prevent the recrudesce, the metastasis and the further diffuse of the tumors (Chemotherapies can not achieve the radical cure, so it is only palliative therapy, especially for solid tumors).

The curative effects of postoperative adjuvant chemotherapies for solid tumors are worse, however, we hold the idea that it is possible to gain better curative effects by using chemotherapies added with XZ-C Chinese traditional medicine for immunoregulation against the immunosuppression and toxic side effects to marrow and liver of chemotherapies.

II. Analysis, Reflection and Evaluation from the Angle of Inhibiting Whole Immunity by Chemotherapy

Why has not the quality of living been improved and the lifetime prolonged after postoperative adjuvant chemotherapies? Why does the cancer recrudesce and metastasize after chemotherapies or diffuse from head to foot, osseous metastasis happen immediately after chemotherapies for many patients? In terms of the destructing hosts' immunologic functions, chemotherapies cause the decrease in immunologic functions and immune monitoring capacity of the host cells, thus lead to the further development of cancer.

The immune system consists of immune organs, immune cells and immune molecules. Central immune organs, also called first level immune organs, are the place for the production, differentiation and maturation of immune cells, working as the leader of the circumferential immune organs. Central immune organs include the marrow and the thymus.

1. Thymus is located at the superior part of the mediastinum, back of the breastbone, and separated into two lobes, the right and the left. The size and the structure change

with the ages and the state of organisms, with the weight of 10~15g when born. After born, the thymus grows rapidly within 2 years which is the fastigium of the thymus activities. From then on, the thymus augments gradually and reaches the maximum during the adolescence, with the weight of around 30~40g. After the adolescence, the thymus begins to retrogress. On entering the agedness, most thymus tissue is replaced by the adipose tissue, but with some remaining functions. That the thymus is atrophying gradually as the organism is getting older after the adolescence is called physiologic atrophy of thymus, which is usually accompanied with the shrinking of cellular area in the lymph node. The animal experiment has proved that a newborn animal extirpated the thymus, whose lymphocytes in the circumferential immune organs T cellular area are sparse, has apparently reduced lymphocytes in its blood and the damaged humoral immunity function lacking the cellular immune function. The animal has the symptoms of immune deficiency, which may lead to death as the result of consumptive disease as the same as the consumption and exhaustion representations of the animal inoculated cancer. Reviewing the patients with clinic latecancer, their exhaustion deaths also present as the exhaustion of immune function. If embedded with thymus or the extract of thymus, this kind of patients can regain partial immune function.

The functions of the thymus: thymus is the principle organ that induces the T cells to differentiate and maturate, which has been proved.

(1) Thymus is the place for the differentiation and maturation of T cells. For an adult, the pre-T cells move from the marrow to the thymus, then grow and maturate in the thymus. After maturating, the T cells move out from the thymus with a certain amount (1%~2%) and settle in the circumferential lymphatic organs or tissue. Mature cells can present the antigen receptors and recognize the foreign antigens (pre-T cells cannot). In the anaphase of growth, T cells differentiate further into T cell subsets with different functions, T cell subsets with damage capacity (inhibiting) and adjuvant T cell subsets (inductivity), which explants from the thymus through blood or lympha, then settle in the thymus dependent area of the circumferential immune organs.

(2) Producing thymic hormone: the reticular epithelial cell on the thymus tissue can produce various kinds of thymic hormones, like thymosin, thymopoietin, thymic humoral factor, lymphocyte stimulating factor, etc. The mentioned dissoluble substance is the main component of thymic microenvironment and plays an important role in the differentiation and adjustment of T cells.

2. Marrow is the hematopoietic organ for human, as well as the birthplace of all kinds of immune cells. Though marrow is not lymphatic tissue, it possesses multipotential stem cells with strong differential potential. Marrow can differentiate into myeloid stem cells and lymphatic trunks cells. The former ones grow into erythrocytic series, granulocyte or B cells, and locate in the circumferential immune organs in the end. Moreover, except B and T cells, the lymphocyte cytokines precursors also achieve their proliferation, differentiation and maturations in the marrow, like K cells and NK cells. If the functions of the marrow are defective, it is possible to cause both the cellular immunity and humoral immunity defective. Injecting normal marrow can rebuild the immune functions, which indicates the importance of marrow in executing the immune functions.

The fundamentality of marrow is also regarded as the principle part of producing antibodies. The categories of the antibodies produced are lgG mainly and lgA secondly. As a result, marrow is the main place of immune response. The marrow can produce a large amount of antibodies tardily and continuously.

Circumferential immune organ, also called secondary immune organ, is the residence for T cells and B cells. At the same time it is the part for the immune response after the cells recognize foreign antigens. Lymph nodes, whose amount is about 500~600 in a human body, and spleens as well as other lymphatic tissue make up the secondary lymphatic tissue with complete structure, which locate in the non-mucous membranes mostly and distribute widely in the lymph channels. About 70% of the lymphocytes in lymph nodes are T cells and other 25% are B cells. The superficial cortex of lymph node which B cells settle in is called thymus independent areas, while the deep cortex area for T cells is thymus dependent areas. T cells and B cells in lymph nodes can enter into the blood circulation through postcapillary venules. Sensitized T cell and specific antigens produced by the T cells and B cells in the process of immune response gather in the lymph node medullary sinus and then discharge from the lymph efferents.

As a conclusion, the central immune organs include the thymus and the marrow; while spleen and lymph nodes are the circumferential organs.

We have observed when experimenting with the animal model of albino rat bearing tumor that tumors can excrete some special factor (called cancer-inhibiting-thymus factor temporarily) and act on the thymus, leading to the immune organ's atrophy and the decrease in immune functions. For the patients who are in the cancer procession, or with the metastasis of lymph nodes and the need of chemotherapies, cell poison of chemotherapies will inhibit the marrow severely with the decrease in WBC and the increase in PLT. For the special factor excreted by the tumors has inhibited the central immune organ thymus, the patients suffer the central immune organs' atrophy gradually, weakening and even losing its functions. Now as the cell poison attacks the marrow, patients' central immune organs are totally destroyed. For the circumferential immune organs are bearing the affects and metastases of tumor cells, some of their functions are weakened. Therefore, the patients' thymus, marrow, lymph nodes and other immune organs are damaged in such a way that the immune functions are already inhibited, plus that the chemotherapeutic drugs damage the immune organs, leading a further decrease in immune functions as one disaster after another. What are worse, efficient measures of protecting the host cells, immune organs and the immune functions are not taken, making patients put up with the further decrease in immune functions.

We can get such a conclusion by analyzing and reflecting from this point: chemotherapies must be added with immunotherapies, meaning that chemotherapies should combine with the XZ-C treatment by Chinese herbs for immunoregulation.

As XZ-C4 is used to increase immunity and protect thymus, while XZ-C8 is for hematopoiesis and protecting marrow, during chemotherapies XZ-C drugs must be taken, that is using XZ-C4 to protect thymus and XZ-C8 for marrow functions in order to protect the central immune organs and immune functions of the host cells. The above can help strengthen the chemotherapeutic effects and weaken the side effects of inhibiting immune functions by chemotherapies.

Since patients' immune functions are weak, the surgical operation for cancer may lead further decrease in the functions. While surgery is the principle occasion of forming the nidi of tumors with more cancer cells enter into the blood circulation, so during the peri operation, it is of great importance to improve the patients' immune functions during the complex treatment.

For the question how to control or even eliminate such cancer cells in the blood circulation, we consider that the immunotherapies must be essential in both preoperative and postoperative phases as well as during the operation. Using XZ-C treatment by Chinese herbs can improve immunity and redound to kill the cancer cells in the blood circulation making the lymphocytes immersed surrounding the cancer tissue, thus reducing the opportunities for cancer cells to metastasize.

After operations, immune functions are weakened and further decreased by the postoperative chemotherapies; therefore one of the key problems of taking chemotherapies as soon as possible after operations is to improve patients' immune functions in the prophase. We advocate that before operations or in the prophase after them it is applicable to use immunotherapies and XZ-C Chinese traditional medicine for immunoregulation which has been proved be able to protect central immune organs and strengthen the entire immune functions, to reach the mentioned goals. Making the patients' immune functions on the higher level to make up for the deficiency is benefic for the recovery, preventing the postoperative metastasis and recrudescence as well as the carcinomatosis and cancerometastasis resulting from the further decrease in immune functions.

III. Analysis, Reflection and Evaluation from the Angle of Drug Tolerance

Reviewing, reflecting and evaluating the postoperative adjuvant chemotherapy and curative effects, in many foregoing clinical cases, why does the postoperative chemotherapy fail to arrest relapse of tumor? Why is the postoperative chemotherapy incapable of preventing metastasis? Why do chemotherapeutic drugs injected into the patient have no damaging effect to solid tumor cells? We should reflect and consider whether the solid tumor processes drug tolerance.

Why does the solid tumor become resistant to drugs? One of the reasons is the drug delivery dysfunction in the tumor.

From the clinical standpoint, the drug tolerance means anti-tumor drug therapy causes apparent trauma to host normal histiocytes, but does not avail against the tumor cells. There is a positive correlation between damaging effects of anti-tumor drugs on tumor cells and the product of drug concentration and drug action time. But at the same time, those drugs often cause apparent trauma to normal histiocytes. That is, drugs kill both tumor cells and normal cells, having no selectivity of the two different cells. "Making no distinction between tumor cells and normal cells" or "destruction of good and bad alike", that is the fatal shortage of chemotherapeutic drugs. At the present time, it still has no pleased solution. Therefore the curative effects of most anti-tumor drugs are only in a limited extent which the human body can tolerate the trauma to normal cells.

In recent years, the clinical treatment level of anti-tumor drugs is also improving. Some malignant tumors (e.g. choriocarcinoma, infantile acute lymphatic leukemia and renal matricyte carcinoma, etc.) can individually apply the chemotherapy to cure. However, there are still many common malignant tumors, such as stomach cancer, liver cancer, non-small cell lung cancer and so on, still very resistant to anti-tumor drugs. Curative effects of using chemotherapeutic drugs alone are rather limited. Why do the chemotherapeutic drugs have little curative effects on solid tumor? On this question, it is necessary for us to develop a further study of mechanism of action and anti-tumor drug tolerance.

Currently, chemotherapeutic drugs have better effectiveness on tumor in blood system, but turn relatively poor effectiveness on solid tumor. Besides the reason of chemotherapeutic drugs having no or lower sensitivity to solid tumor cells, drug delivery dysfunction in the tumor is also the main reason:

1. Drug Delivery Dysfunction and Drug Tolerance

Tumor cells directly contacting with sufficient anti-tumor drugs is the prerequisite for chemotherapies to get curative effects. However, anti-tumor drugs must pass through a long way, overcome each obstacle and finally reach the tumor cells. During the drug delivery, a problem of any link is enough to generate drug tolerance.

Oral and Injection Drugs

↓←Absorption obstacle, blood vessel barrier

Absorbed into the bloodstream, near to tumor tissue

↓←Delivery dysfunction in the tumor

Delivery in the tumor (micrangium, stroma, tumor cells)

↓←Membrane transport obstacles

Drugs into the tumor

Delivery dysfunction of anti-tumor drugs in every link

Because of drugs delivery dysfunction in the tumor, the giant solid tumor cells generate drug tolerance, or the drugs cannot reach the curative effects. That is a very important question affecting the curative effects. At the meantime, it is an urgent problem that needs but has not yet been resolved. Some anti-tumor drugs show very high anti-tumor activity to various tumor cells in culture dish, and the suppression ratio of some drugs is up to 100%. With these anti-tumor drugs, Clinical treatment of malignant tumors in blood system and childhood cancer can also achieve satisfactory effects. However these drugs cannot obviously reduce adults' death rates from the most common solid tumors (e.g. stomach cancer, liver cancer, carcinoma of large intestine, lung cancer, breast cancer, prostatic cancer, pancreatic cancer, brain cancer and carcinoma of esophagus, etc.). Comparing the chemotherapeutic process between malignant tumors in blood system and solid tumor, the only difference is the former omits the step of drugs redistributing in the tumor tissues and directly contacts with individual tumor cell in the blood. Thus we can reason out that during drug delivery in the solid tumor, there are some factors which induce tumor cells to generate drug tolerance. Specifically, after anti-tumor drugs having been injected or taken by mouth, drugs deliver through blood to whole-body organs and tissues, some of which deliver to the targeted object- tumor tissues. If eliminating such a big solid tumor (abdominal surgery solid tumor, with hundreds or thousands of grams, even tens of kilograms), drugs have to be of high concentration, which is sufficient to eliminate each tumor cell of such a big solid tumor, to diffuse and distribute in the whole tumor. Then the drugs delivering through blood to tumor can contact with each tumor cell, which enable the chemotherapy to achieve curative effects. Nevertheless, the solid tumor often utilizes advantaged barrier to tackle against this diffusion process, which results in uneven and/or low concentration, even no drug distribution in the tumor. That leads to the drug tolerance of tumor.

There are mainly three mechanisms that the solid tumor applies to obstruct drugs to deliver in the tumor: ① Blood vessels of tumor have non-balanced distribution. Areas with fewer blood vessels cannot directly take drugs from the blood circulation. Thus some tumor cells fail to contact drugs directly. In other words, drugs cannot work on this part of cells; ② The pressure of tumor stroma rises abnormally, disturbing the diffuse, permeation and distribution of drugs in the tumor. ③ The structural anomaly of tumor vessels and high blood viscosity also affect the drug delivery in the tumor.

The penetrating power of some drugs to the tumor mainly depends on their structures. The malignant tumor generally consists of the following portions: ① Proliferative cells or tumor cells commonly account for less than half volume of tumor. ② Blood vessels zigzag back and forth through the tumor tissue, making up about 1% to 10% of the tumor's volume. ③ Collagens efficient matrixes fill up most space of the tumor tissue, which is much larger than extracellular matrixes in the volume of healthy tissue, and enclose the tumor cells to divide them from vascular structures. To determine the trace of drugs in the tumor, Kakesh K and the other people choose tumor cells which are singly into the artery and out of the vein to implant into the body of rodent (a), or optionally obtain this kind of tumor from patients, utilizing artificial circulation to maintain blood flow (b). The two models are used to measure the sum of drugs into and out of the tumor, and also calculate the absorptive amount. Later they adopt Sandison-Algire Tumor "Window Technique" to implant the tumor into the rabbit ear (c), mouse brain (d) or mouse skin of back, and place into the transparent apparatus. Then they use the microscope to directly observe new vascular development of the tumor tissue and the diffusion and distribution process of drugs in the tumor. The result displays that after twenty days of implanting the tumor into mouse skin of back, tumor peripheral regions have overgrown a labyrinth of vessels. But the tumor center loses the blood supply plentifully and appears white. Therefore the tumor is deprived blood vessels which deliver drugs directly to the central region.

On this account, if drugs are to approach toward each cell, they should firstly access to the blood vessels in the tumor, and then through the vessel wall enter in the stroma. Finally they have to difficultly pass through matrixes. But there are significant differences between vascular system in the tumor tissue and blood vessels in the normal tissue and organ. At the very start, tumor use existing blood vessels in this region to obtain blood. As tumors grow, eventually they produce "their own" minute vessels, which quickly branch, wind into curved shapes and gradually vary their growth directions. Consequently, some regions of the tumor present favorable blood vessels to supply rich blood, but others may be supplied with little or no blood. Such non-balanced distribution of blood vessels affects drugs distribution in the tumor. Regions which lack blood vessels cannot directly take drugs from the blood circulation. Therefore, in this region drug concentration is so low that it cannot produce the anti-tumor effect. Moreover, abnormal distorted branches of the vascular structure often slowdown the blood flow. High viscosity of blood in the tumor also slower the blood flow. Slow micro-circulating blood obstructs drugs delivery to regions where tumor vessels lack. These regions cannot (or seldom) obtain anti-tumor drugs. Thus, it's hard to produce anti-tumor effect.

The above non-balanced blood supply is the main reason for obstructing drugs diffusing in the tumor. And abnormal rise of interstitial pressure is also an important reason. The increasing pressures disturb drugs to flow among vessel wall, stroma and inside stroma, leading to the reduced concentration of drugs in the stroma.

The internal pressure distribution of tumor tissue is different from that of healthy tissue. The pressure of capillary network of healthy tissue is higher than that of stroma. The latter is about zero. However average internal pressures of the whole tumor stromata are almost equivalent to those of capillary network. The reason may be that the tumor grows in normal tissue, uses existing blood vessels and depends on the present lymphatic system to discharge excess liquid from stromata. As the tumor grows, its new blood vessels cannot produce their own lymphatic system. Moreover for inordinate hyperplasia of the tumor, its press causes abnormal vessels to vary in geometrical shape, reducing the blood flow rate and further increasing pressure in the capillary. Thus large amounts of liquid soak into stromata from blood vessels. Due to the lack of functional lymphatic system, exosmic liquid cannot be removed effectively.

The liquid is piling up until the internal pressure in stromata is equivalent to that in blood vessels. The internal pressure in the tumor is impressively high, exerting obvious influences on drugs infiltration and distribution in the tumor.

2. Membrane Transport Obstacles

Transport obstacle method of drugs entering to tumor cells is not entirely clear. It may have a close correlation with drug structures and physicochemical properties. Such drugs include methotrexate, phenylpropionic acid chlormethine, chlormethine, cisplatin, cytosine arabinoside, anthracene nucleus, vincristine, and son on. In addition, Drugs into the tumor cells need mediated transport by carriers. Therefore, affinity degree for carriers can influence transportation. In belief, drugs transport obstacle is the main reason for chemotherapeutic drugs tolerance of the tumor. To make the application effect of chemotherapeutic drugs in vivo equal to that of experiment in vitro, we have to surmount these obstacles.

3. Immunity and Drug Tolerance

The immune state before tumor patient accepts any treatment is of influence to drugs curative effects. Generally, the more complete the body's immunologic function, the better the patient's response to medication. Among patients who accept cytotoxic drugs therapies, the complete immunologic function before therapy is relevant to the better prognosis.

The animal experiments prove that elspar can kill most tumor cells in animals' bodies with suppressed immunologic function. But drug-resistant tumor cells survive, proliferate and finally kill the animals. In animals' bodies with better immunologic function, drug-resistant or surviving tumor cells will be destroyed by the immunologic system. When the host suffers from sensitization, the mouse fleshy tumor induced by chemicals can strengthen the anti-tumor action of cyclophosphane, but doesn't work for the host without sensitization. For patients suffering from acute granulocytic leukemia, chemotherapies combined with immunotherapies show better effects than those of single chemotherapies. Meanwhile, it's reported when the patient accepts non-small cell lung cancer chemotherapies, effects of chemotherapies combined with thymic peptides are better than those of single chemotherapies.

When some experienced doctors adopt medications to treat cancer patients, they also examine patients' immunologic function in detail. Facts prove that it has some values for designing chemotherapies. We have found that choriocarcinoma's "antagonizing against" chemotherapies is related to the gradual decline in immunologic function. If the immunologic function can restore, reusing the drugs which have been subject to the obvious antagonism is still in effect.

4. Metabolism and Drug Tolerance

Anti-metabolic drugs are a kind of drugs interfering with cell metabolism. Their chemical structures are often similar to required substances of nucleic acid metabolism, such as folic acid, purine and pyrimidine, etc. These drugs can utilize specific antagonism to interfere with nucleic acid metabolism, especially DNA synthesis. They also prevent cell division and reproduction, and then produce the anti-tumor effect.

All the clinical common anti-metabolic drugs except MTX, need to be converted to active structures by metabolizing, then they can really possess the anti-tumor effect. If the coloboma of activating enzyme leads to insufficient activation of anti- metabolic drugs, the drugs lose the ability of anti-tumor and anti- metabolism.

5. Dynamics of Cell Proliferation and Drug Tolerance

Tumor dynamics of cell proliferation has three fundamental concepts, i.e. ① Grouping theory of tumor cells; ② Cell cycle theory; ③ Heterogeneity theory of tumor cells.

1. Grouping theory of tumor cells It is represented based on the motion law of cell growth, proliferation and death, i.e. all the tumor cells are made up of three colonies, proliferative cell colony, resting cell colony and cell colony with non-proliferative capacity. Tumor cells of different colonies have different responsivity to chemotherapeutic drugs. ① Proliferative cell colony refers to continuous exponential proliferation of tumor cells. The tumor body grows quickly. Its chemotherapeutic drug susceptibility is also higher. ② Resting cell colony includes auxiliary cells, i.e. G_0 phase cells, which are temporarily not into cell cycle. When cells of proliferative phase are killed by drugs, resting cells can enter into proliferative phase. During this stage, internal drug tolerance of tumor cells is the recurrent root in the tumor therapy. ③ Cell colony with non-proliferative capacity has little significance in chemotherapies.

Understanding the grouping theory of tumor cells can help to design the optimal therapeutic schedule. In recent years, progresses in tumor chemotherapies are not some newfound effective chemotherapeutic drugs but are precisely the applications of dynamics of cell proliferation therapy that have designed plenty of high-level chemotherapies.

2. Cell cycle theory It is another fundamental concept of tumor dynamics of cell proliferation, which is represented based on studying individual cell growth in the

proliferative cell colony. The relevant information has been stated in above paragraphs. Proliferative cycle of tumor cells can be broadly divided into four phases: DNA pre-synthesis phase (G_1), DNA synthesis phase (S phase), DNA post-synthesis phase or division phase (G_2), mitotic phase (M phase).

According to anti-tumor drugs' selective acting on different phases of tumor cell cycle, in terms of the cell cycle theory, anti-tumor drugs can be divided into phase-specific and phase nonspecific chemotherapeutic drugs.

Cell cycle nonspecific chemotherapeutic drugs can only kill off cells in certain sensitive phase of cell cycle (usually as S phase). This is because that during the administration, some cells do not pass through the sensitive phase, so cells are insensitive to drugs. As to cell cycle phase nonspecific chemotherapeutic drugs, they can kill off cells in all phases of cell cycle, especially the rapid proliferative cells. For the rapid proliferative tumor, it has high growth ratio, short interphase and is sensitive to chemotherapies. For the slow-growing tumor, its growth ratio is low and interphase is long, which inevitably engender unbearable toxic side effect. By this time, the tumor often becomes resistant to chemotherapeutic drugs.

Facts have proved that for nidi of tumor cells below 10^6, their cells are totally in division cycle. While for nidi of tumor cells above 10^6, a certain proportion of tumor cells are often outside the division cycle. The "optimal" therapeutic schedule can either not treat the tumor. For there reasons, it can be concluded generally that S phase-specific chemotherapeutic drugs can effectively fight against the leukemia, and cell cycle nonspecific chemotherapeutic drugs are available to battle the solid tumor. Clinical trials have confirmed the above conclusion. Compared with leukemia and lymphoma, the solid tumor's resistance to chemotherapies is because its multiplication and division time is long, proliferative quantity is small and label index is low.

3. Heterogeneity theory of tumor cells It is another fundamental concept of tumor dynamics of cell proliferation proposed in recent years. It means that a primary tumor is composed of different cell subsets, which have varying drug susceptibility. Especially the different cell subsets between primary and infiltrative nidus (or metastatic nidus) remain far more diverse in the drug susceptibility. In the same host tumor, some cell subsets may be sensitive to a drug; while others possess internal drug tolerance. This theory has some values for clinical applications. At present, combined chemotherapeutic drug types have an increasing trend. It might be closely related to that theory.

Drug tolerance is a clinical question of vital importance. If one patient is resistant to this chemotherapeutic drug, but the clinician has no idea whether this patient has drug tolerance, then this clinician relies on the experimentalism and continuously adopts this drug to complete each course by intravenous administration or infusion through catheter and drug pump. Afterwards, the patient suffers from serious damage. Because of the drug tolerance, the chemotherapeutic drugs have no effect on the patient's cancer cells, but cause extremely serious damage to immunologic system, marrow hematopoietic system and toxic side effects of liver and kidney. The drugs even result in immunologic and marrow hematopoietic function failures, which lead to infection, bleeding, organ failure and finally cause death. So the clinician must seriously and prudently treat the multidrug resistance (MDR) question, and place great emphasis on patient's safety.

The fundamental goal of drug tolerance studies is to find the method or drug for overcoming the drug tolerance. So far it has made certain progress, and some drugs and methods have been developed in the clinic. But more methods are still in the preclinical study, even the contemplation stage.

China has the traditional Chinese medicine and herbalism. And the effective component in herbs, i.e. TTMP has been confirmed to reverse the adriamycin tolerance of mouse Ehrlich's ascites carcinoma. We have observed from the laboratory experiment: TTMP has certain anti-metastasis effects to the mouse's liver cancer cells metastases. Our developed medicine $XZ-C_4$ also contains a small quantity of TTMP. We believe that Traditional Chinese Medicine could find the highly original method to reverse the drug tolerance of clinical tumor.

5. CHEMOTHERAPY TO BE FURTHER STUDIED AND IMPROVED

I. Some Wrong Ways in Current Chemotherapy

1. Current chemotherapy emphasizes on only killing cancer cells and neglects to protect or even damage host cells

It is essential to attach importance to the interrelation and the interaction among host cells, tumors and drugs. Here chemotherapy is cytotoxic drug without selectivity, so it can not distinguish tumor cells and the normal with killing them together. The initial target of chemotherapy is to kill cancer cells; however, actually it also kills the proliferative cells of host cells that are damaged as a result. Especially, chemotherapy inhibits the immune system and medullary hemopoietic system of the host cells, which leads to the general decline in immune function. Consequently, that tumors are not monitored by immunity promotes the evolution of tumors. That is the reason why tumors are constringed or relieved temporary, but continue to increase and evolve after a while or even metastasize and relapse during the period of treatment. Therefore, there is one problem about chemotherapy that has not been paid much attention, namely taking no actions to protect host cells and their immune organs and immune function. The strategy of curing cancer is to destroy cancer cells protect autologous functions at the most.

2. Chemotherapy as cytotoxic drug can aggravate the inhibition on central immune organic

It is well known that consist of central immune organs and peripheral immune organs, the former ones are thymus and marrow, the later are spleen and lymph node.

When patients are in chemotherapy, their three immune organs suffer damage (see Fig. 19-1), which leads to the decrease in immune function. Literature and the experimental results by the author have proved that when cancer emerges, tumors can produce a kind of immunorepressive factor (called factor of inhibiting thymus by cancer temporarily) and make thymus atrophied gradually. At the same time, chemotherapy also inhibits marrow. For the patients with cancer, the inhibition of both thymus and marrow by the chemotherapeutic cytotoxic drug make the function of the entire central immune organs inhibited, which reduces the holistic immune function as one disaster after disaster.

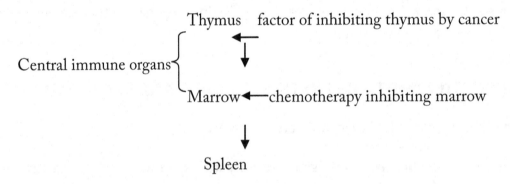

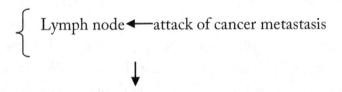

Fig. 5-1 the damage of immune organs during chemotherapy

Lymph nodes in peripheral immune organs as well as the areas around the focus, and lymph nodes in the process of metastasis are invaded by cancer metastasis and lost partial function, which lead to further decrease in immune function consequently. It is inevitable that tumors will evolve further, relapse and metastasize with weak immune monitor or even without it.

Due to the decline in the holistic immune function, the anti-infection ability is weakened, so chemotherapy can not continue. There may be serious complications during the process of chemotherapy, such as mycotic superinfection, viral and infectious infection. However, the antibiotics can not control them efficiently. As a result, the patients die of immune function prostration.

3. During chemotherapy general untoward reaction may occur due to the effect of cytotoxic

During chemotherapy, general untoward reaction can bring down immune function, and lead to arrest of bone marrow, hepatic and nephric toxic reaction, gastrointestinal response dysfunction, phalacrosis, etc. However, there is no positive and effective protection currently.

Inhibition of marrow is a usual clinic toxic reaction as marrow is the organ to store hematopoietic stem cells. It is mainly the dynamic effect of antineoplastics to the specific stem cells that chemotherapeutic drugs destroy the specific stem cells in marrow, which can reduce the number of mature and functional blood corpuscles in peripheral blood. The degree of reduction is related to the lifetime of cell components in peripheral blood, for instance, the lifetime of hematid is long, so the number of hematid in the peripheral does not change apparently; while the lifetimes of blood platelet and granular cell groups are shorter with 3 days and 67 hours respectively, so the numbers of peripheral blood platelet and granular cell groups reduce rapidly if the groups of megakaryocytic stem cells and granular cell groups are destroyed. After administering drugs, stem cells increase the time of division to make up for the amount in the process of restoration.

Most antineoplastics can result in the gastrointestinal mucosa reaction by inhibiting gastrointestinal mucosa epithelial cells.

Many kinds of antineoplastics can lead to renal toxic reaction and also affect the excretion of drugs through the kidney. It must be noticed that the damage of renal function can aggravate the general toxic symptoms or worsen the inhibition of marrow.

Many kinds of antineoplastics can damage liver in different degree and affect liver function.

Such serious geneal toxic reaction of chemotherapy can lead to nausea, vomit as well as anorexia, even being unable to take food. Consequently, the general anticancer ability declines obviously and the function of anticancer system of host cells is weakened apparently. The anticancer ability of organism and evolution of cancer are locked in a "zero-sum" game, which conduce to the further development of tumors.

4. Theoretic foundation of choosing chemotherapeutic drugs

Choosing chemotherapeutic is based on cell generation cycle and pathology and physiology of cancer, or accords to the principle of pharmacokinetics. The current chemotherapeutic scheme does not always accord with the theory of cell generation cycle. During the period of treatment (3~5d), cytotoxic drugs will inhibit cancer cells. After the treatment, these cancer cells continue to proliferate and divide. Currently, the use of chemotherapeutic drugs differs in different medical institution, in which some use the treatment of 5 days, others are 3 days; some of the used drugs aim at S stage and some are for M_1 stage. No matter the treatment is 3 to 5 days or 5 days, the effective period of cytotoxic drugs on cancer cells is less than 120 hours with cell generation cycle of 50 to 80 hours, so the treatment can only act on one and a half cell generation cycles. However, the proliferating cycle of cell mass continue for years, while the effect of chemotherapeutic drugs can only last from 3 to 5 days, so the effect of killing cancer cells can just happen at the stage of proliferating cycle when the drugs take effect, such as S stage, and then disappear. After the treatment of 3 or 5 days, cancer cells continue to proliferate and divide. As a result, tumors and the metastasized lymph nodes may shrink in volume, but they are likely to augment soon.

5. Failure to take actions to control cancer cells continuously and consolidate the effect at the interval of two times of chemotherapies

The treatment between two times of chemotherapies is blank, and the actions to continuous killing or control on cancer cells are not taken to consolidate the curative effect. What have been done is waiting the restoration of leucocytes and blood platelets to achieve the aim of stand chemotherapy next time. Actually, the treatment at the interval is very important, for cancer cells are out of control and proliferate and divide further positively and potentially at intervals due to the heavy decline in immune function. The more times of chemotherapies and the larger dosage of drugs, the more cytotoxic drugs will be used correspondently, so that the general immune function is worse and worse and the immunity of organism is less and less able to control the proliferation of oncocytes and prevent the metastasis leading to relapse and metastasize after continuous chemotherapies. Therefore, it is necessary to adopt immunological therapy or Chinese traditional medicine for regulating immunity to avoid relapse.

6. Theoretical foundation of postoperative auxiliary chemotherapy, the length of the intervals between two times of chemotherapies and the time of chemotherapy

The arrangements of chemotherapy differ in different locations and medical institutions, among which some use once a month or once every two months, some adopt six times in a row, or continuous four or eight times. The treatment is much blinder, especially postoperative auxiliary chemotherapy. The current arrangement of chemotherapeutic period is that only when leucocyte and blood platelet restore, can the next chemotherapy be taken. In fact, it is more helpless instead of meeting the pathological and physical demands (since the time of restoration is longer for some patients, when cancer cells have been in the process of division and proliferation continuously). What is the aim of auxiliary chemotherapy? How to achieve the aim? Are there any residual cancer cells in the body although the aim of chemotherapy is to kill cancer cells? Where do the cancer cells hide after surgeons, in the local of the surgeon, lymph nodes or in the blood? Taking gastrointestinal surgeon for instance, do the residual cancer cells hide in portal vein blood, or in celiac lymph nodes, or even in the local area of the surgeon? How long can the residual cancer cells lurk after surgeons before devastated by host cells? How to arrange the period of postoperative auxiliary chemotherapy? Knowing the location of cancer cells may be good for controlling the residual cancer cells in the area of surgeons and portal vein.

In a word, the current choice of postoperative auxiliary chemotherapy and the arrangement of chemotherapeutic period are very blind. It is essential to do further clinic research to ensure the indication, contraindication, medication and route of administration as well as a more uniform scheme so as to conclude analysis and evaluate.

7. Blindness of current chemotherapy

It may be helpful for some patients to take on chemotherapy blindly just according to experience, but it is harmful for a considerable number of patients. For instance, if some patient was resistant to this kind of drug, it would be harmful, rather than fruitless, for the cytotoxic drugs of chemotherapy can not act on cancer cells, instead of killing normal histiocyte, especially immunocyte, myeloid cell, which will lead to the prostration of immune function.

Drugsensitive test is a must to verify whether the patient is allergic to the used drugs. Only doing like this can ensure the accuracy of administering drugs. Currently, it is common that clinical administrate of drugs depends on experience blindly. Such blind administrate is potentially dangerous. If the drug is really sensitive to the patient's cancer cells, it will be effective (CR, PR). But if the drug is not sensitive to the cancer cells, it will only kill the normal cells and inhibit the marrow hematopiesis leading to the reduction in leucocyte and blood platelet as well as the decline in immune function without any damage on cancer cells, which will definitely promote the evolution of tumors and result in the prostration of immune function and hematopiesis. The decrease in immune function makes tumors be beyond the immune monitor and develop further, and then promote the relapse and metastasis. Therefore, it is necessary to take on individual drugsensitive test and drug resistant test.

8. Cure of cancer aims to kill tumors, reserve organism and regain health

The cure of cancer should always run through both strengthening health and wiping evil off, in which wiping evil off means inhibiting and killing cancer cells, clearing up lumps; strengthening health means protecting organismal ability to recognize dissidents, exciting the organismal positive factors of anti-cancer and improve the organismal ability to resist cancer. These two are dialectic and united. However, the current treatment on cancer only emphasizes killing cancer cells and ignores the protection of host cells, which damages the immune system and the system of marrow hematopiesis resulting in wiping both evil and health away. If tumors are drug resistant to this chemotherapeutic drug, it is likely to be harmful to health without wiping evil away. The treatment on cancer needs a scientific designed scheme, for cancer results from losing the balance between the organismal immune capacity of anti-cancer and the development of tumors, and from losing immune monitor, which leads to the further development of tumors. So it is necessary to try to restore the balance. Taking teeterboard in a children's playground for instance, tumor and the immunity of host cells represent the two ends of a teeterboard respectively. The comparison of the two parties' power decides the direction of tilt and the final result. Besides, the example of "scale" can be explained in the same way. However, chemotherapy does not emphasize the protection of host cells but promotes the diffuse and evolution of tumors.

9. Standards for the curative effects of chemotherapy should be good quality of life and prolonged lifetime

How to evaluate the curative effect of postoperative auxiliary chemotherapy? As the tumor has been ablated, it is unable to evaluate the effect in terms of its shrink.

Most patients only regard untoward reactions after chemotherapy, like decline in leucocyte and blood platelet, nausea and disgorge, anorexia, hypodynamia and abdominal distention as the curative effects, but they hardly realize that these symptoms are not the effects at all. It is unable to evaluate the postoperative curative effects until now. The current diagnostic methods are still laggard, as when tumors are detected, they have been very serious. Therefore, molecular biology is the only way to solve this problem.

Generally speaking, the standard for curative effects is remission. In terms of remission, the efficiency is defined as the shrink of the tumor, however, the quality of life is not improved and the lifetime is not prolonged, which is not the aim of handling diseases for the patients with cancer.

10. Anti-Carcinomatous drugs used currently can not always resist metastasis and relapse and the drugs for anti- carcinomatous metastasis and anti-cancer should be different

For many cases, postoperative auxiliary can not prevent relapse and metastasis, which relates to the fact that the current anti- carcinomatous drugs are not always able to resist metastasis and relapse besides other various possible factors mentioned above. Drugs for anti-metastasis should be different from anti-carcinomatous drugs as generally anti-cancer drugs have cytotoxicity and aim at killing cancer cells, destroying and inhibiting cell division and proliferation, whereas drugs for resisting metastasis are mainly used to resist the invasion of tumor cells, to antagonize the adherence of cancer cells inside the blood vessels, to inhibit the nascent micrangium and strengthen the organismal immunity to kill cancer cells. Most of anti- carcinomatous metastasis drugs have no cytotoxicity.

Research on anti-cancer drugs has stepped into a new stage. It is confronted with theoretical and technical renovations and the change in the train of thoughts when the field of research on anti-cancer drugs is not restricted to the traditional thoughts based on cytotoxic and the working method of cytotoxic drugs. New methods like inducement of differentiate, regulator of biological reaction, immunoregulation, genetherapy, combination of Chinese and western medicine, etc. have been taken into consideration in succession.

Although chemotherapy has been applied for sixty years, it is not satisfactory that many problems still exist reflected by the statistic, analysis and evaluation of applied information from a large number of clinical suffers. It is pitiful that cancer may metastasize and relapse after or during the process of chemotherapy.

In conclusion, the possible reasons that postoperative auxiliary chemotherapy is unable to prevent relapse and metastasis are, ①chemotherapeutant can promote the decline in immune function and inhibit hematopoiesis of marrow; ②failure to continue aftertreatment at the intervals of chemotherapies; ③chemotherapeutic drugs can not protect host cells; ④lumps may has drug resistance; ⑤chemotherapeutic drugs may be not sensitive; ⑥chemotherapeutic drugs for solid tumor may be not infiltrate into tumors; ⑦the arrangement of chemotherapeutic period is not reasonable; ⑧drugs may not act on the sensitive period of cell proliferation; ⑨it is difficult to restore immune function and hematopoiesis probably.

II. Main Contradictions in Traditional Chemotherapy

So far, the aim of chemotherapy has been still focusing on killing cancer cells. The majority of chemotherapeutic drugs are cytotoxic drugs without selectivity, so both cancer cells and normal ones will be damaged. Besides, chemotherapy has serious untoward reaction, suffers will have intensive feeling and have to give up the treatment at last. In the last ten years, the author has helped nearly ten thousand cancer cases in Wuchang Shuguang Tumorous Clinic, many of whom have tried chemotherapy. They came to anti-carcinomatous clinic for treatment as there were no curative effects after several periods of treatment. It can be implicated that auxiliary treatment does not prevent carcinomatous invasion, relapse and metastasis, and it also can not improve the quality of life and prolong lifetime obviously. Through the feedback of those cases, analysis, evaluation and reflection, the author have recognized that there are the following contradictions in traditional chemotherapy.

1. The contradiction between chemotherapeutic cytotoxic and the damage to host cells

The aim of curing tumor is to eliminate tumors and preserve the organism as well as regain health. However, currently the chemotherapeutic cytotoxic kills both cancer cells and the normal with internecine result of damaging host cells, which is the heavily unreasonable contradiction between cytotoxic and suffers (or host cells). What should be done is to try to eliminate or resist the effect of killing normal cells and to research positively on intelligent anti-carcinomatous drugs with selectivity.

2. The contradiction between succession and discontinuity

It means the contradiction between the continuous divisions of cancer cells and the discontinuous chemotherapeutic period of treatment. The division and proliferation of cancer cells are continuous according to cell cycle, but chemotherapeutic drugs can be used with intervals for they inhibit the hematopoiesis of marrow and the blood corpuscle in the peripheral, which results in the severe contradiction between continuous divisions and proliferation of cancer cells and the discontinuous chemotherapies. Cancer cells divide successively, whereas chemotherapies are of interval, so cancer cells continue to divide during the intervals. Even a large dosage of chemotherapeutic drugs can only kill limited number of cancer cells, but can not destroy the whole. Even the majority of the cancer cells can be killed during the 3 to 5 days with chemotherapeutic drugs, the residual tumorous stem cells will continue to divide, to proliferate, to clone, and then metastasize and relapse when the effects of medicine fade away after several days. Therefore, killing cancer cells simply does not accord with the biological traits and behavior of cancer cells.

3. The contradiction between increase and decrease in immunity

That chemotherapeutic drugs usually can reduce the immunity contradicts the fact that the treatment on cancer should improve the immunity. As chemotherapeutic drugs can weaken the immunity, the longer the period of treatment, the more decrease in immunity, which promotes the decline in immunity, and even leads to lose monitor and the further development of tumors. This unreasonable contradiction between chemotherapy and immunity can weaken the curative effects heavily and even lead to diffuse. Therefore, treatment on tumors must aim at improving immunity and restoring immune monitor so as to stabilize the cancer, to make it and regain health.

4. The contradiction between periods of treatment and curative effects

That chemotherapy can inhibit marrow forces the peripheral leucocytes and blood platelets decline, so it is necessary to design the time of administering with intervals, which means the next time of chemotherapy should be taken on after restoration. Currently the intervals are just for waiting, instead of taking any measure to control cell division. On one hand cancer cells proliferate successively, on the other hand the chemotherapy stops. Due to this contradiction, it is difficult to gain the curative effects though chemotherapy. The more times of chemotherapy, the more serious immune inhibition will be, the more actively cancer cells proliferate during intervals, which results in evolution and metastasis during the process of chemotherapy.

5. The contradiction between the period when drugs act and the cell cycle during the period of administer through intravenous drip

It is only effective when the time of administer meets the sensitive cycle of cancer cells. If not, it is of no effect. Chemotherapeutic administer aims at cell cycles. During the period of administer, the cell cycles of most cancer cells in the crowds are not simultaneous but much different from each other, for instance, administer via intravenous drip from 8 am to 10 am when some of the cancer cells are in S stage, others are in G_1 or M stage. Thus, if the drug aims at S stage, it is effective to the cancer cells in S stage, but the drug given at this period (8 am to 10 am) is of no effect to the cancer cells in other stages, that is to say the sensitivity of chemotherapeutic drugs to cancer cells in different stages are differential. So during the period of administer through intravenous drip, it is effective to some sensitive cancer cells but not to those in insensitive periods.

6. The contradiction between inhibition and protection of marrow

Chemotherapy is cytotoxic and can inhibit the hematopiesis of marrow where hematopoietic stem cells are stored. Inhibition of marrow is a common clinical toxic reaction, which is the kinetic effect of chemotherapeutic drugs on specific stem cells. Chemotherapeutic cytotoxic drugs can damage the specific crowd of stem cells in marrow and will definitely reduce the number of mature and functional blood corpuscles in the peripheral blood. The degree of reduction relates to the lifetime of the cell components in the peripheral blood, for instance, the lifetime of hematid is longer, so the degree of reduction in the amount of blood corpuscles in the peripheral blood and the number of blood corpuscles in the peripheral blood during the treatment do not change obviously. However, the lifetimes of blood platelet and granular leucocytes are shorter with 3 days and 67 hours respectively, so the numbers of peripheral blood platelet and granular leucocytes reduce rapidly if the groups of megakaryocytic stem cells and granular cell groups are destroyed. If the amount of leucocytes and blood platelets decline to a very low level, it is extremely easy to cause subsequent serious infection or haemorrhage. In some cases, using large amount of broadspectrum antibiotic to resist the serious infection may lead to double infection or mycotic ingection, even endangers the life.

To sum up, in order to solve the contradictions in the current chemotherapy, to ameliorate its disadvantages and make it better, the author thinks that it is necessary to update thoughts and to research on new drugs and new principles to resist cancer and metastasis as well as relapse, except improving chemotherapy further in traditional thoughts, only the changes in the opinions on curing cancer and the creativities and reforms of technologies can bring further development into the treatment of cancer.

Chapter 6 The reform and improvement Cancer surgery and chemotherapy

1. The reform objectives and methods of tumor surgical treatment

Surgical operation is a definite and effective cure for malignant tumor therapy. Even though today's cancer treatment has developed to the multi-discipline and multimodality treatment, surgical operation is still one of the most central and common means for malignant tumor therapy, and makes itself an integral part of multi-discipline and multimodality treatment.

In the 18ᵗʰ century, therapists held that the early cancer was a local disease, which could be cured by surgical treatment. In 1881, Bill-roth first carried out the surgical removal of tumor — subtotal gastrectomy. In 1890, Halsted actualized the radical resection of breast. He first elucidated the principle of en bloc resection, which meant resections of lymphatic vessel and lymph node in the chosen zone of primary tumor. This resection laid a good foundation for most modern surgical operations of tumors. The surgical technique of tumor resection has been developing along with surgery. After the middle of the 20ᵗʰ century, it gradually developed into an independent subject — tumor surgery. Since the 1950s, due to the improvement and development of surgical technique, preoperative (postoperative) care and operative supporting measures, such as blood transfusion, anesthesia, aseptic technique and antibiotics, the surgical risk, complications and fatality rate have reduced greatly; the range of tumor surgical technique tends to expand; a series of super radical operations arise, such as expansive radical mastectomy. But many years' practice proves that expanding the range of surgical resection cannot improve the survival time without tumor and total survival time of most tumors, such as lung cancer, liver cancer and pancreatic cancer.

Since the 1970s, people's understanding of tumor biology has changed a lot. At present, people hold that most tumors are not local diseases and may have been systemic diseases since the clinical examination. The hematogenous spread is common. When finally diagnosed, many patients may have suffered from micro-metastases. Whether obvious metastases have happened since the clinical examination, depends upon biological characteristics of tumor cells and interactions between tumors and hosts. Neither the more extensive regional surgery nor the share of surgery and radiotherapy can affect metastases.

1). Great Achievements in Surgical Removal of Tumor in 20th Century

In the 20th century, great achievements mainly focus on researching various methods of tumor surgical resections, operation procedures, preoperative (postoperative) care and cleaning range of lymph nodes; studying, understanding and getting familiar with regional anatomy and pathophysiology of bearing cancer organs, such as resection technique and organ reconstruction technique of liver cancer, pancreatic cancer, stomach cancer, esophageal cancer, colorectal cancer, lung cancer, breast cancer, cervical cancer, brain cancer and so on; taking measures to raise resection rate, reduce complications, lower operative mortality rate and improve perioperative care. In terms of esophageal cancer surgery, how to raise the resection rate? How to reduce anastomotic leakage? How to improve Esophagogastrostomy upon (down) Aortic Arch? How to carry out the cervical anastomosis? How to improve anastomose technique, such as scarf-type anastomosis? And in the case of liver cancer, how to perform regular or irregular hepatectomy? How to conduct (expanding) lobectomy of liver? How to carry out combined segmentum hepatis resection, second resection of intrahepatic recurrent cancer after resection, and liver cancer resection of special regions? How to retain residual liver functions? For the breast cancer, how to perform radical or super radical operation? Then how to conduct conservative operation procedures? In the case of stomach cancer, how to carry out D2 and D3 operations? How many groups of lymph nodes are needed to clear? For the operation procedure of rectal cancer, select Mile or Dixon procedure? Retain anus or not? Use anastomat or not? In terms of pancreatic cancer, select Whipple or Child procedure? How to conduct anastomose procedure of gall bladder and bowel? How to perform the resection of hepatic hilar cholangiocarcinoma? For the lung cancer, how to carry out the resection of pulmonary segments, lung lobes or the whole lung? In conclusion, researches are about how to resect the tumor en bloc and completely? How to increase operative resection rate? How to reduce or avoid complications? How to lower operative mortality rate? And how to help patients recover? By the 1990s, cancer resections of esophagus, stomach, bowel, liver, gall bladder, pancreas, lung, mammary gland and thyroid gland fully pass the test. All the operative routine techniques are already mature. Operative mortality rates have dropped to a very low level. Operations are basically safe. Many cancer radical operations have been widely diffused among county hospitals and basic hospitals. But how to prevent recurrence and metastasis has not yet generally attracted people's attention.

In some large hospitals, doctors have perceived that though operations are performed very thoroughly and canonically, postoperative recurrence and metastasis in the short (long) term still puzzle some specialists. Then in the 1990s, some experts have followed suit, announcing the study that disposes cast-off cells caused by operative wound. Chen Junqing in Shenyang has spent over ten years on researching and processing cast-off cells of stomach cancer, finally making brilliant achievements. The study conducted by South Hospital, which heats, washes and processes cast-off cells after the operation of rectum cancer, has got satisfactory efficacy. Yang Chuanyong at Tongji Hospital has always been devoting himself to exploring the pharmacokinetics of intraperitoneal chemotherapy of hepatic portal venous blood. At present, the technique of surgical excision of the tumor is basically successful, which is an honorable achievement in the 20th century. But these difficulties that cancer patients suffer from postoperative recurrences and metastases with no good countermeasure, and frequently come back to the clinic for further consultation, still bother vast numbers of medical workers.

2). The Objectives of Surgery in 21st Century Should Be the Study on Prevention and Control of Recurrence and Metastasis after Radical Operation of Carcinoma

In 1985, the writer himself made follow-up to more than 3,000 patients who had accepted surgical radical excisions of tumors. The results show that 2~3 years after the operation, most patients suffer from recurrences or metastases. While some patients even bear it after six months, less than a year or just over one year. These patients do not always come back to the previous surgery physician for further consultation but go to Tumor Hospital or Tumor Department for medical treatment. Once recurrences appear, however, only a few patients can accept the second operation. But most patients cannot receive effective therapies and soon pass away. It has made the writer more aware that though the operation at that time was successful and standard, the long-term follow-up result is dissatisfactory. That is, the late result is a failure (Certainly tens of patients can survive for 10, 20 or 30 years after the operation, but it is only a very few cases.). Therefore, the study must be done to prevent postoperative recurrence and metastasis. Follow-up results present an important problem that postoperative recurrence or metastasis is the key factor for long-term postoperative effectiveness. While researching method and measure of preventing postoperative recurrence or metastasis plays the key role in improving long-term effectiveness and lengthening survival time. Therefore, the clinical fundamental research must be done for preventing cancer recurrence and metastasis. If no breakthrough in the field of fundamental research, it will be hard to improve clinical effectiveness. Then the writer as well as his colleagues has established the Institute of Experimental Surgery, where they have carried out experimental tumor research, implemented transplantation of cancer cells to animals, constructed tumor animals' models. They have also developed a series of experimental tumor researches: ① Explore mechanism and rule of cancer recurrence and metastasis; ② Probe into the relationship between tumor and immunity, and that between tumor and immune organ; ③ Research into the method of arresting progressive atrophy of immune organs with the growth of tumor and the way of immunologic reconstitution; ④ Seek effective measures to adjust and control cancer invasion, recurrence and metastasis; ⑤ Conduct inhibition rates experiments of tumor-bearing animals to respectively filter 200 literature-approved traditional Chinese medicines which are commonly used for anti-cancer; ⑥ Carry out experimental researches to seek new drugs from natural drugs with resistances to cancer, recurrence and metastasis.

The writer has gone through a complete review of almost 54-year practical cases of clinical treatment and also made the follow-up. Then he analyzes and rethinks the lessons of success and failure, from which he comes to understand a truth. That is, conquering cancer needs to break with the conventional ideas and update the thought; conduct investigations, researches and analyses with patients; carry out self-reflection and self-evaluation. Renew ideas, innovate methods, look for an opening in urgent problems of tumor researches and weak links of modern medicine. The writer has also realized that techniques of surgical resections of tumors in the 20th century have made brilliant achievements. The next researching objective and task of surgeons are not only to have further studies on seeking for greater perfection of radical operation, but also to prevent postoperative recurrence and metastasis. Experiments and clinical researches on preventing recurrence and metastasis after cancer radical operation should be done to further improve postoperative long-term effectiveness. Because the operation is just a regional treatment, if the tumor is limited in a certain visceral organ, the surgical effect may be very good; but if the tumor is not just limited in this visceral organ but has invaded the serosa outside the organ, no matter how thorough the operation is, the possibility of recurrence and metastasis is still in existence. Especially for stomach cancer and rectum cancer, though lymph nodes are cleared completely, many cancer cells still remain in venous blood vessels. A lot of research materials have identified that clearance of lymph nodes is only to prevent lymphatic metastasis but that is just one side. The involved lymph nodes should be cleared, but excising lymph nodes cannot prevent hematogenous metastasis. Therefore, hepatic metastases rates in the short/long term are both high after operations of stomach cancer and intestinal cancer. At present, surgical excision of the tumor as well as regional lymphatic vessels and lymph nodes cannot prevent hematogenous metastasis and spread, implantation and dissemination of cast-off cells. Consequently, the next objective of tumor surgeons' research work should focus on experiments and clinical researches for preventing cancer recurrence and metastasis after radical operation. That is, in the early 20th century, researchers should make great achievements on studies of preventing cancer recurrence and metastasis. If postoperative recurrence and metastasis cannot be solved, short/long-term effectiveness of surgical cancer treatment will fail to get satisfactory result.

3). Design of Surgical Radical Operation of Tumor to be Further Studied and Perfected

Since recurrence and metastasis happens after the radical operation, it is necessary to analyze whether the radical operation itself has connection with postoperative recurrence and metastasis, and carry out retrospective analysis and reflection. Among the present radical operations, some have been used for over 100 years, such as the radical operation of breast cancer. Over a century, thousands of cancer patients have accepted different kinds of radical operations, the majority of which have got satisfied short-term effectiveness. But long-term recurrence and metastasis rates are still very high. As the name implies, "radical cure" means thorough or eradicating treatment; but if it is "radical operation", why the purpose of radical cure fails to achieve and the recurrence still happens? Now that lymph nodes have been cleared, why the metastasis still appears? The question is whether those recurrences and metastases are due to cast-off cells left by operation or operative techniques, related to procedure design, concept foundation of operative design or not entirely consistent with the present known Biological characteristics and biological behaviors of cancer cells. The present radical operation refers to the en bloc resection of primary tumor and regional lymph nodes. Logically, it is not the radical cure, and cannot approach the purpose of radical cure. That is because the malignant tumor has four routes of metastasis, which are lymphatic channel metastasis, hematogenous metastasis, implantation metastasis and direct spreading. While the surgical operation just completely clears lymph nodes and radically cures the route of lymphatic channel metastasis, it has no specific technical measure to prevent hematogenous metastasis, and also do nothing to bring forward definite and effective countermeasures to implantation of cast-off cancer cells as well as implantation and dissemination of chest and peritoneal cavity. Lymph nodes having been thoroughly cleared off cannot prevent hematogenous metastasis, and moreover, only the clearance of lymph nodes can't prevent peritoneal implantation and dissemination of peritoneal cavity by cast-off cancer cells, either. Surgical operation belongs to a regional treatment. Experts in tumor surgery hold that cancer develops in a local area of the body, invades the surrounding tissues and metastasizes to other areas through lymphatic vessels, etc. Accordingly, the main point of treatment is often put on the local area, controlling local growth and diffusion, especially lymph nodes metastasis, such as the clearance of lymph nodes. For years surgical treatment has been updating on the operation method and type, but its long-term effectiveness — 5-year survival rate still has no obvious improvement. The postoperative recurrence and metastasis seriously threaten patients' postoperative survival. Therefore, the present radical operation is just a relative one, which is on a quote. Young doctors should know that the present type design still has weak links, which need the further experimental and clinical studies to explore new techniques and methods to definitely and effectively prevent routes of metastases. Accordingly, in recent years the writer's laboratory has always been doing experimental exploration in this respect, such as experimental study of free-tumor technique in radical operation (Fig. 6-1), free-tumor technique study in radical operation of cancer-bearing animal models, counting of intraoperative cast-off cancer cells as well as detection and counting of cancer cells in venous angioma, experimental observation of dyeing tracking of gastric lymph nodes. Preventing postoperative cancer metastasis and recurrence must be started from the radical operation.

In order to study why cancer cells can dissociate and cast off from the tumor body, cast-off cancer cells still have the vitality and can implant to other areas, the writer's laboratory use electronic microscope to observe and study cancer cells' ultrastructural organization of cancer-bearing animal models (Fig.6-2, 6-3).

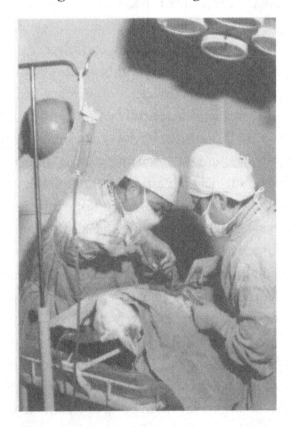

Fig. 6-1 Experimental study of free-tumor technique in radical operation

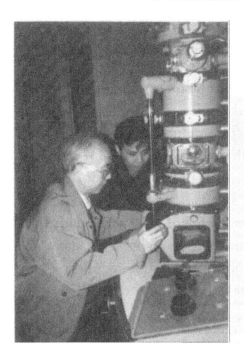
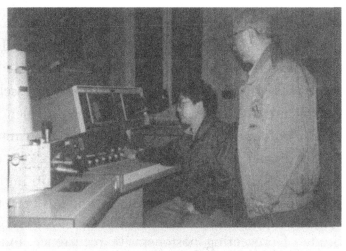

Fig. 6-2 Observation of ultrastructural organization of experimental model's cancer cells with electronic microscope

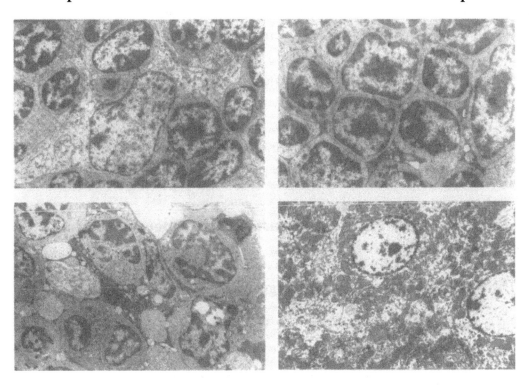

Fig. 6-3 Ultrastructural organization of hepatic cancer cells of cancer-bearing mouse H$_{22}$

4). Strengthening Fundamental and Clinical Study on Molecular Biology of Radical Operation of Recurrence and Metastasis after Operation

Inhibiting angiogenesis factors to induce the formation of blood vessels and preventing endothelial cells to construct new blood vessels are both new ways to explore preventions from recurrence and metastasis. In the experimental study of inhibiting actions of ethyl acetate extractives (TG) of traditional Chinese medicine — Common Threewingnut Root with different dosages on new blood vessels of transplanted tumor of mice peritoneum, the writer's laboratory observe influences of TG on the form and number of new-born micro-vessels in and around transplanted tumor of mice peritoneum, and on the diameter and flow rate of tumor arterioles and venules. They have made the preliminary confirmation that TG has certain inhibiting actions on new-born blood vessels of metastatic carcinoma focus and has been taken on clinical trials.

Study of preventing postoperative recurrence and metastasis of cancers must base on establishing animal models of recurrence and metastasis, and also proceed on levels of Molecular Biology and Gene. In the past decade and more, due to the rapid development of Molecular Biology, experts have found that the generation, progress, invasion, metastasis and recurrence of tumor are all in connection with cancer genes, cancer suppressor genes, metastatic genes and suppressor metastatic genes. To research related genes and seek control methods to prevent recurrence and metastasis as well as clinical measures of preventing recurrence, such as biological therapy, gene therapy, biological reaction control agent therapy, may be an important research aim in the future. In the 21st century, gene therapy will provide new efficient way for tumor therapy, and Molecular Biological Immunology will also stimulate the development of tumor therapy.

5). Prevention of Recurrence and Metastasis after Operation Should Be Established in Operation

(1) Surgical techniques of cancer surgery

Free-tumor technique is vitally important, which should prevent operation techniques from causing or actuating hematogenous metastasis of cancer cells.

Surgical principles of general surgery also applies to tumor surgery, such as operation techniques of aseptic operation, sufficient exposedness of operative location, the least intraoperative damage of normal tissues for the early-stage healing, etc. In addition, tumor surgery should take note of preventing the dissemination of cancer cells in the operation, in which the free-tumor technique is vitally important.

Ever since the end of the nineteenth century, people have realized that operation techniques may cause or actuate the dissemination of cancer cells. Therefore, the free-tumor technique of tumor surgery has been attracting more and more attention in recent years. For instance, intraoperative procedures of preserved skin, extrusion and anatomy can directly lead to the dissemination of tumor cells, stimulate formations of tumor embolism and metastasis which are near to or far away from blood vessels and lymphatic vessel. And tumor cells cast off and pollute surgical wounds, which results in local implantation recurrence, etc. Along with the development of Cell Pathology and inspection technology of tumor cells in blood stream, the phenomenon of tumor dissemination has been confirmed in clinical trials and animal experiments. For example, active cancer cells and cancer tissue masses can be found in vessel douche and surgical wounds douche of tumor operative specimen; cancer cells can be easier found in the output venous blood flow of tumor during the operation. Therefore, it is important that in the operation surgeons should first ligate and cut off output vena of tumor.

It should be noted in surgical operation that all the techniques are favorable toward preventing cancer cells' metastases. Do not stimulate or increase chances of cancer cells' metastases to cause iatrogenic metastasis and dissemination. For the surgical resection of tumor, all the operations must stress and observe free-tumor concept and technique, no matter big or small. Surgeons should give equal emphasis on free-tumor concept and aseptic concept, free-tumor technique and aseptic technique. The free-tumor technique is even stricter than aseptic technique. The surgical knife, scissors, needle and thread in the surgical operation, even every procedure is possible to cause metastasis of cancer cells. Such a possibility may increase with excessive extrusion, needle punching through the skin, knife cutting and other negative operative procedures by surgeons on tumor body or tissues. At present, applied molecular biology or immunohistochemistry method has proved that the operation technique itself can cause iatrogenic implantations, diffusions and metastases of cancer cells. Cancer cells can be found in surrounding blood circulations when many patients are undergoing the surgical operation; or cancer cells convert from the preoperative negative result to the postoperative positive result. The above evidences indicate that operation techniques are possible to induce the diffusion of cancer cells. It also suggests that some patients' postoperative recurrence and metastasis may be caused by improper operation techniques, such as the incision implantation.

Therefore, preventing postoperative recurrence and metastasis must start out from all the techniques in the surgical operation.

The route and type of tumor dissemination vary according to different pathologic types of tumor. Whether or not the metastasis can come into being is also related to the body's immune state. Consequently during the therapeutic process, the modern tumor surgeons should both prevent tumor dissemination and be careful to maintain the body's resistibility or immunity.

(2) Prevention from the dissemination of cancer cells

It is well-known but always overlooked that tumor's localized examination and operation techniques should be gentle and skillful to prevent the dissemination of cancer cells. Therefore, the following points should be noted: ① Preoperative tumor palpation should be gentle, and the number of times ought to be minimized. ② Preserved skin for operation should be gentle and skillful, or more cancer cells will invade small veins by the over friction. ③ operation techniques should be gentle and skillful, incision must be sufficient to expose, dissect and resect. Avoid pressing the tumor. ④ Adopt sharp dissection (dissecting knife or scissor); Strictly avoid blunt dissection to reduce dissemination. ⑤ Deal with the output vein before the artery. ⑥ Dispose the farther lymph nodes before the nearby lymph nodes to resect them wholly with the tumor.

(3) Prevention from the implantation of cancer cells

Cast-off cancer cells easily implant and grow on the traumatic tissue wounds, so: ① Use the gauze pad to protect cutting shoulder and wound surface. ② if the tumor is unwittingly incised or cracks, it should be covered and bound up with gauze pads. Replace timely polluted gloves and surgical instruments. ③ Adequate excision extent, involving enough normal tissues around the pathological changes. ④ Avoid the blood out-flowing from polluted wounds when anatomizing tissues near the tumor. Therefore, when two blood vessel forceps are used to clamp blood vessels, they should stick close to each other. Ligate immediately after being cut off. Replace timely gauze pads that are contaminated with blood.

Postoperative local recurrence (cover about 10%) of colon and rectum cancers often occurs in anastomotic stoma, incision of abdominal wall or outside of intestinal wall. This kind of recurrence is usually caused by the implantation of cancer cells. In recent years, a strip of cloth is used to ligate intestinal canals belonging to the upper and lower segment of tumor before the excision of intestinal loop, in order to stop cast-off cancer cells from continuing to diffuse along the intestinal cavity in the surgical operation. Use

1:500 corrosive sublimate or fluorouracil solution to douche intestinal cavities of both ends before the anastomosis, which can obviously improve the long-term effectiveness and may be relevant to the before-mentioned reduction of recurrence.

After all, to review significant achievements of 20-century techniques of surgical tumor excision; to preview glary prospects of 21-century tumor surgery study of prevention from recurrence and metastasis. In the coming period, the highlight of anti-cancer work should be anti-invasion, anti-metastasis and anti-recurrence. Anti-recurrence is the key of operative effectiveness; and anti-metastasis is the core question of cancer treatment. Cancer invasion and metastasis depend on specific potentials of two factors: biological characteristics of tumor cell itself and the host's influence on its restraining factors. To keep a balance is to control; to lose a balance is to progress.

2. Opinion on Improving and Perfecting Treatment of Cancer with Traditional Chemotherapy

I. On "gain" and "loss" after taking anti-cancer drugs

The treatment of cancer, no matter in early stage, mid stage or advanced stage, involves the comprehensive multi-discipline treatment.

The operation is a method of local treatment. The surgical oncology scientists hold that the cancer occurs locally at first, then encroaches the peripheral tissues and transfers to other places via lymphatic vessel and blood vessel, as a result, they stress on the local treatment, that is to say, the stress on control over the local growth and diffusion, especially when the cancer meets with metastasis via lymph, the lymph node is cleaned down by operation. For years, although the operative treatment has been improved continually in methodology, the long-term curative effects have not made remarkable progress as yet. The reoccurrence and metastasis after operation seriously threatens the prognosis of the patients, attracting high attention from the medical field, however, there has been no effective prescription up to now.

The radiotherapy is also a method of local treatment, which plays a role in killing off the cells from the local tumor per unit dosage. The radiotherapy effects are mostly affected by the factors including oxygenation of cells, type of tumor and restoration of cells and so on, all these characteristics determine that the radiotherapy is locally inferior to the surgical removal with respect to tumor.

The biological characteristics of cancer are invasion, reoccurrence and metastasis, which are the important reasons why the treatment with operation and radiotherapy fails.

In recent years, some one holds that cancer is a kind of generalized disease, so the generalized treatment should mainly depend on radiotherapy, however, it is a pity, in despite of the emerging new drugs and continually undated therapeutic methods and plans, the radiotherapy effects are not satisfactory. Since the cytotoxic drugs have no selectivity, they kill the cancer cells as well as the normal cells of the host, especially the immunological cells, in addition, they have severe side effects, inhibiting hematopiesis function of the bone marrow and reducing the immunity. Therefore, the traditional radiotherapy does not entirely conform to the well-known actual conditions of the biological behaviors of the cancer at present, for example, the invasion behaviors and metastasis of the cancer cells are of multi-link and multi-step. At present, people have cognized that the anti-tumor drugs do not always prevent the metastasis and reoccurrence.

In 1980s, the tumorous bioremediation emerged, such as immunological therapy, cytokine therapy and gene vaccination therapy. It was proven that some therapies could mediate the immunity of the patients, however, it has not proven that which immunological preparation or method could induce the extinction of tumor.

In the recent 20 years, so many reports on treatment of cancer with traditional Chinese medicine have been made and its outlook has been concerned by the people. Especially, with the further development of the study on medicine and immunology, people have realized that the disorder of the immune system of the organism is closely related to the occurrence and development of tumor and traditional Chinese medicine has its own characteristics and advantages in tumor treatment through mediating the immunologic function of the organism. The immunoregulation of traditional Chinese medicine and development of immunoregulator of traditional Chinese medicine will attract more attention and favor all over the world. With the assistance of operation, radiotherapy and chemotherapy, the traditional Chinese medicine can bring its immunoregulation into full play in the process of treatment and obviously prolong the survival time and improve the survival quality, in this way, the characteristics and advantages of the traditional Chinese medicine are fully embodied, however, it is disadvantageous in unremarkably improving the tumor.

Since the above-mentioned methods have different characteristics in action mechanism and effect with respect to treatment of cancer and different curative effects as well as their own disadvantages, so it is necessary to focus on the advantages and disadvantages of various therapies aiming at the "gain" and the "loss" of the paints, for example, what's the "advantage" and the "disadvantage" after taking the therapy, what's the "gain" and the "loss" of the patients? We should learn from the strong points of one therapy to offset the weakness of the other therapies and combine these therapies organically and reasonably to form the comprehensive therapeutic plans for cancer, only in this way, can the side effects from the drugs be obviously reduced, the survival quality of the patients be improved and the total survival time be prolonged. In the past 16 years, Tumor Specialized Clinic of Shuguang Tumor Research Institute has treated over 12000 cancer patients in mid and advanced stage with XZ-C immunoregulation therapy in practice and most of the patients have achieved the effects of improving the survival quality, stabilizing the lesion, controlling the metastasis, keeping survival with tumor and remarkably prolonging the survival time.

II. Actual conditions of chemotherapy in tumor: main cause affecting further improvement of curative effects of chemotherapy

The total effective rate of treatment with anti-tumor drug in clinic is only 14%, the factors impeding chemotherapy' better curative effects mainly include:

1. **Blindness of current chemotherapy**. Now it is unknown whether the chemical medicine used in the current therapeutic plan for chemotherapy is sensitive to the cancer cells of the patients just because most of the patients are not subject to the drugsensitive test to cancer cells. If the medicine is used by experience, it has blindness, that is to say, it may be beneficial to some patients while harmful to other patients. Based on the drugsensitive test results, remarkable curative effects have been made in treating the infectious diseases with antibiotics, as enlightens us on reasonably and jointly administrating drug through testing the sensitivity of the cancer cells of the patients to the cytotoxic drugs for chemotherapy so as to replace the blind chemotherapy with "individualized" chemotherapy. It is shown by the data that it can double the effective rate of chemotherapy.

2. **Drug resistance of chemotherapy**. Most of the solid tumor, such as stomach cancer, cancer of large intestine, is lowly sensitive or insensitive to the chemotherapy. Some tumor is remitted after chemotherapy, however, it meets with reoccurrence, resulting in ineffective chemotherapy, indicating that the cancer cells has the drug resistance to the chemotherapy drug. The reasons why the drug resistance appears include many factors such as drug transmission

disturbance of solid tumor, cell proliferation, difference in dynamics, immunity and metabolism and so on.

3. Selectivity toxicity of chemotherapy anti-cancer drug. The chemotherapy drug is the cytotoxic drug, killing the cancer cells as well as the normal histiocytes, without selectivity, especially the hemopoietic stem cells of the bone marrow with exuberant proliferation and immunological cells as well as stomach cells and intestinal cells. Compared with the volume of the normal tissue, since the cancerous protuberance only accounts for a minimal proportion, it is possible to "kill one hundred enemies while injuring three thousand soldiers on one's own side". The blindness of chemotherapy and the drug resistance of chemotherapy result in low curative effects, in case that it is expected to improve the curative effects by means of increasing the dosage, increasing the kinds of drugs and shortening the time, the toxic effects will be further aggravated, so the chemotherapy in cancer is still satisfactory in despite of great progress. The drugs shall be selected by testing the sensitivity and drug resistance of the chemotherapy drug so as to have a definite object in view. If the drugsensitive test is made on the chemotherapy patients so as to avoid the damage on the patients from the blind chemotherapy and benefit the chemotherapy patients, the epoch of chemotherapy will be opened up.

III. Suggestion on improving and perfecting the chemotherapy in cancer

Since nitrogen mustard drugs were reported by Gillman and Phillips in 1946 to treat the tumor in hematopiesis function, the chemotherapy has made great progress for 60 years and the great achievements have been made in therapeutics of the malignant tumor, for example, the chemotherapy has cured over 10 kinds of malignant tumor including chorionepithilioma, acute lymphocytic leukemia, Hodgkin disease, seminoma of testis, small-cell carcinoma of the lung and Wilms tumor and so on, and remitted the tumor including breast cancer, children' lymphadenoma, neuroblastoma and osteosarcoman and so on, resulting in prolonged survival time. Thus three principles of treatment including operation, chemotherapy and radiotherapy are established. Since the chemotherapy has made great achievements, especially in the recent 20 years, it has been widely used for various solid tumor, especially in the assistant treatment after operation, so the metastasis and dissemination in some patients has been restrained and improved, giving hope to treatment of solid tumor after operation. However, it is a pity that the reoccurrence and the metastasis happen again after several months and the patients still die of the cancer despite chemotherapy or intensive chemotherapy again.

According to the follow-up survey to over 12000 metastasis and reoccurrence patients and the analysis of and experience in treatment summarization in Tumor Specialized Clinic of Shuguang Tumor Research Institute, it is found neither metastasis nor the reoccurrence could not be restrained on thousands of patients receiving the assistant chemotherapy after operation, the survival time and the survival time without cancer are not obviously improved. At present, although the assistant chemotherapy after operation has been made all over the country, there has been no prospective and correlatable scientific data, the assistant chemotherapy after operation is still in study. Of course, there are lots of patients receiving assistant chemotherapy after operation who have been in good condition over 10 years even 20 years, however, due to lack of prospective and correlatable scientific data, what is the comparison result between chemotherapy and non-chemotherapy in the patients after operation? What is the long-term survival rate of the patients not subject to chemotherapy? How to prove the long-term survival results from the chemotherapy after operation? All of these issues shall be further studied. At present, the reports in China lack lots of prospective and correlatable follow-up survey analysis data as well as the prospective and correlatable evaluation data about the assistant chemotherapy after operation just because the case history is kept by the patient instead of the hospital, as a result, the doctors and the hospital cannot make the follow-up survey. Of course, the in-hospital case history is kept for study, however, the in-hospital case history just reflects the short-term curative effects, most of the effects reflected in the in-hospital case history are relatively good because if it is not so good, the patient is not allowed to leave hospital. However, most patients are in good condition temporarily, for example, after the incision heals up, the patient begins to take food again and takes case of itself, the short-term curative effects are good, but it is hardly realized that the cancer cells may be in metastasis and it cannot be tested at present, of course, some tumor markers can be dynamically observed, such as CEA and AFP and so on.

Then, how to make the further study? Start from the existing problems to settle the problems through experiments and clinical study. The treatment of cancer shall be people-oriented and aim at curing the sickness to save the patient.

1. Actively searching, studying and developing intelligent anti-cancer drugs. The main contradictions in chemotherapy have been mentioned above and now we should pay attention to how to study and perfect them. The main issue is: the chemotherapy is the cytotoxic drug, without selectivity, so it cannot selectively distinguish the cancer cells from the normal cells, killing off all of them, resulting in some side effects and contradictions. So we should update the thought and actively study, search and develop the "intelligent anti-cancer drug" that only selectively kills the cancer cells instead of the normal cells of the organism, especially the immunological cells. In June 2004, American Society of Clinical Oncology held the annual meeting in New Orleans, with over 20000 oncologists as the attendants and 3700 papers called. Among these 3700 papers, there were 30 papers greatly affecting the treatment of cancer, of which there were 9 papers discussing the intelligent anti-cancer drugs. The intelligent anti-cancer drugs only affect the specific molecules in the cancer cells. The research findings of intelligent anti-drugs come into the world, indicating the treatment of cancer would shift to the epoch of accurate administration with little side effects from the one of chemotherapy with very great side effects. In research and development of the intelligent anti-cancer drugs, the research and development personnel do not spread these drugs at present. I believe that in the coming future, with the wide use of these drugs, people would feel the great effects from them and the patients would benefit from them. **Among the 48 kinds of anti-cancer drugs with relatively good tumor-inhibiting rate screened by this lab from 200 kinds of natural vegetable drugs, there are 3 kinds of vegetable drugs that can entirely inhibit and kill the cancer cells entirely and has no effects on the cultured epithelial cells or fibrous cells in the culture in vitro experiment on cancer cells, including XZ-C1-A, XZ-C1-B and XZ-C1-C. In the in vivo tumor-inhibition experiment on tumor-bearing animals, their tumor-inhibiting rate is 85%-95%. They are a part of XZ-C1, XZ-C immunoregulation anti-cancer medicine.** This experiment takes chemotherapy drug CTX as the control group and CTX obviously inhibits the immunity and the bone marrow. XZ-C anti-cancer medicine has no effects on bone marrow.

2. Suggestion on immunologic chemotherapy. Namely immunological treatment + chemotherapy. The immunological drugs can be administered in peri-chemotherapy period so as to reduce the side effects from chemotherapy; after chemotherapy, the immunologic treatment should be continued for a period to enhance the curative effects. The immunological treatment is the most reasonable treatment, it is of 0 order kinetics, however, it ① has relatively small acting force, it acts on 10^{5-6} cancer cells strongly; beyond this range, it acts weakly. ②The immunological drug can improve the immunity of the organism and enhance the immunological surveillance in the organism. ③ It can be continually administered or taken orally. Because the cancer cells are continually divided and proliferated, the treatment shall be also continual. XZ-C immunoregulation medicine can protect the hematopiesis function of the bone marrow, protect the thymus, improve the immunity, improve the symptom and raise the life quality; the action is relatively slowly, little but durably. Since the biological characteristics of the cancer cells are the continual division and proliferation, our countermeasures must be also continual.

Chemotherapy and immunological treatment currently adopted should learn from other's strong points to offset one's weakness and be comprehensively applied so as to improve the curative effects. The chemotherapy is of intermittent administration while the immunoregulation treatment is of continual treatment. If both of them assist with each other, the curative effects will be improved undoubtedly. If the cancer patient has inferior immunologic function, the operation on cancer will bring down the immunologic function further. In operation, the cancer cells entering the blood circulation by extrusion increase. How to eliminate or control the cancer cells entering the blood circulation in operation? It is held by us that XZ-C medicine should be added before, in and after operation for immunological treatment. $XZ-C_4$ can protect the thymus and $XZ=C_8$ can protect the bone marrow. In this way, the central immune organ and immunologic function of the host can be protected, the curative effects of the chemotherapy can be strengthened and the side effects of the chemotherapy inhibiting the immunologic function can be reduced, as a result, it will reduce the opportunity of metastasis of cancer cells, therefore, the improvement of immunologic function of the patient in the peri-operation period or in the period of assistant chemotherapy after operation is an important link of comprehensive treatment.

3. Making sensitivity test of chemotherapy drugs and implementing "individualized" immunological chemotherapy. Now the chemotherapy in cancer has stepped into the stage of "individualized" chemotherapy in many hospitals. Previously, the different cancer patients are subject to the same chemotherapy plan, unavoidably resulting in blindness, not conforming to the actual conditions of the patients. It is shown by the study that even though the same kind of tumor with same type of tissue, even the different stages of the same cancer, has different sensitivities to the chemotherapy drugs, therefore, it is necessary to make the drugsensitive test on the individual cancer patients and it is urgent to select the sensitive drugs from various anti-cancer drugs. It is proven by the clinical experience in chemotherapy that the effective rate of administration by experience is very low (14%), if the drug can be selected according to the results measured by drugsensitive test, the effective rate can be raised to 28%-35%.

The effect of chemotherapy in the solid tumor is not as good as the one in malignant tumor in the blood system and the transmission hindrance of drug in the solid tumor is the upmost factor of drug resistance of solid tumor.

It is an important way and one of the current study hotspots to make the sensitive test on chemotherapy drug for tumor and carry out the individualized chemotherapy plan so as to improve the effects of chemotherapy in tumor and reduce the side effects.

Generally, the drugsensitive test on tumor can be made with the method of culture in vitro and culture in vivo, the former includes cell culture method and tissue culture method and the latter refers to the method of culture in vivo in animal. Among the test methods, the method of transplantation in vivo in the nude mice can obtain true and reliable results with respect to drug test or new drug screening, however, the process is long, the operation is complicated and the price is high. The method of cell culture is the most simple, convenient and feasible, however, since the kinetics is not entirely same to the tumor in vivo, the test results often differ from the drug reaction of the tumor in vivo, so it cannot be used to directly guide the administration of the different tumor patients.

Someone makes a study on 3D tissue culture method of tumor, namely Hoffman 3D tissue culture method, which directly uses the clinical samples, avoids the repeated digestion of tumor cells with enzyme or mechanically and features quickness and relatively high success ratio. This method would be helpful to guide the individualized chemotherapy, improve the chemotherapy effects and reduce the drug resistance.

(1) In vitro drugsensitive test: it is very important to establish the reliable anti-cancer in vitro drugsensitive test method so as to help the clinicians select the effective chemotherapy drugs, reasonably design the therapeutic method, improve the curative effects, avoid the side effects from the ineffective drugs and directly screen the new anti-cancer and anti-metastasis drugs with the fresh human tumor samples.

There are so many methods of in vitro sensitive test of anti-cancer drug and they have the common characteristics: simple method, high sensitivity, smaller dose than the in vivo method, quick judgment results, without too many animals; in addition, they also can screen the anti-cancer drugs and most of them are parallel to the in vivo method with respect to the procedures.

(2) in vivo chemotherapy drug sensitive test: at present, as to the chemotherapy drug sensitive test methods, the in vitro method prevails and it has the advantages of quickness, convenience and simple as well as good clinical correlation and good repeatability, however, it also has some disadvantages because it breaks away from the in vivo environment of the tumor and is not consistent with the human tumor in histology and cell kinetics, reducing the coincidence rate of the test results and the clinic.

Various drugs have different concentrations in the body fluid and are affected by the body weight, route of medication, liver and kidney function and so on, in this way, the in vitro method cannot represent the change in drug concentration. Some drugs should be activated and metabolized in vivo before playing a role in anti-cancer, such as CTX; some drugs acting on the cancer cells will bring into play through the immune system. The reaction of the cancer cells to these drugs cannot be tested with in vitro method.

The solid tumor are the spatial structure occupying a certain space. Besides the tumor cells in blood, breast and ascites are directly contact with the drugs, the solid tumor is not so simple. The drugs cannot reach up to the deep part easily; the anoxia caused by ischemia; the uneven blood flow in the tumor; the difference in PH value and osmotic pressure will affect the sensitivity of the solid tumor cells to the chemotherapy drugs.

It is necessary to select the optimal "individualized" joint chemotherapy plan through the drugsensitive test.

3. The mothed for Improving Measures for Assistant Chemotherapy after Operation on Cancer

In 1985, I made the follow-up survey of over 3000 patients after operation on cancer in general surgery and thoracic surgery, finding that most of the patients met with reoccurrence and metastasis within 2-3 years after operation, some even met with reoccurrence within several months, which made me realize that the operation was successful and standardized while the long-term curative effects were unsatisfactory or the long-term treatment was unsuccessful.

Since 1990s, in view that the reoccurrence and metastasis rate of cancer after operation was very high, in order to prevent the reoccurrence and metastasis after operation, a series of assistance chemotherapy after operation has been adopted, what's more, the chemotherapy was made before operation (for example, the breast cancer), however, the results had been not so satisfactory. Reoccurrence and metastasis take place in assistant chemotherapy after operation or in the period of treatment or the metastasis takes place synchronously in chemotherapy. It can be seen from so many patients in Wuhan Shuguang Tumor Special Clinic that neither reoccurrence nor metastasis cannot be prevented by the assistant chemotherapy after operation, even in some cases, the intensified chemotherapy promotes the adynamia of immunologic function. All these things should be seriously, calmly, practically and realistically thought and reflected by the clinicians: why the assistant chemotherapy after operation cannot prevent the reoccurrence? Why the assistant chemotherapy after operation cannot prevent the metastasis? Why the assistant chemotherapy after operation on some patients promotes the adynamia of immunologic function? What's the problem and disadvantage of the assistant chemotherapy after operation? What measures should be taken? How to further study and perfect it? How to reform and innovate in the assistant chemotherapy to improve the curative effects?

I. Why to make the assistant chemotherapy after operation on cancer or assistant chemotherapy in peri-operation period?

Currently, the treatment of cancer mainly depends on the operation, however, the reoccurrence and metastasis rate is still relatively high after operation.

1. The potential reason why the local reoccurrence and metastasis after radical operation on cancer takes place may be the following factors viewed from clinic:

(1) Insufficient attention has not been paid to the free-tumor technique, as a result, the operation such as exploration and touch causes the cancer cells on the serosa surface to fall into the intra-abdominal implantation.

(2) The tumor tissue is not thoroughly removed by the operation, as a result, the remained cancer cells are continually proliferating.

(3) The existing metastasis lesion is not found in operation and is not removed, for example, the lymph node in metastasis is not found or is removed incompletely.

(4) As to the clearing of lymph node in operation, traditionally, it adopts the passive separation, in this way, the apocoptic micro-lymphatic vessel may lead to the fluxion, dissemination, residual and transplantation of the cancer cells.

(5) The operation leads to the transplantation of the cancer cells, the cancer cells invading the esophagus, stomach serosa or colon, recta and serosa may easily fall into the abdominal cavity and form the transplantation lesion and the damaged peritoneum in the area of operation may easily meet with transplnation and reoccurrence. The reoccurrence of anastomotic stoma of the colon may be the intracavity exfoliation and transplantation of the enteral cancer cells in the operation.

(6) The metastasis of the lymph node in the patients in the late stage is relatively wide and syzygial, in this way, it is difficult to remove it with operation.

(7) In the operation on gastrointestinal tract cancer, the metastasis of cancer cells in the portal vein takes place, resulting in the metastasis of liver cancer cells after operation. However, it is unseenable in the operation by the naked eyes.

For example, when the "radical operation on gastric carcinoma" is made, the cancerous protuberance and the tumid lymph nodes of gastric carcinoma can be seen by us, however, whether the cancer cells exist in the vein and the blood of the portal vein is unknown? How many cancer cells exist? Where do these cancer cells in the vein go? Whether these cancer cells in cluster that can be touched and extruded into the venous blood in operation arrive at the portal vein? Or arrive at the branch of the portal vein in the liver? It is not impossible to touch the cancerous protuberance in exploration and excision of gastric cancerous protuberance and cleaning of lymph node, the operation necessarily makes a large number of cancer cells be extruded and fall down, then they flow into the portal venous blood, resulting in metastasis in liver after operation.

(8) The operation brings about the traumas to the organism, resulting in the inferior immunologic function, in this way, the organism losses the immunological surveillance or is weakened in immunological surveillance, leaving opportunity to the residual cancer cells or the cancer cells in dormancy for reoccurrence and metastasis.

(9) As to the cancer in the progressive stage, the metastasis of cancer cells may take place before operation while these cancer cells in metastasis cannot be seen by the physician in operation. However, it is reported in the pathological section report that the cancer embolus can be seen in the blood capillary and the lymphatic vessel.

Based on the above-mentioned, after the radical operation of the cancer, the residual cancer cells may still exist, resulting in reoccurrence and metastasis of the residual subclinical cancer lesion after operation.

Then, how to make up for the shortage of radical operation with residual cancer cells? Adopt the chemotherapy in peri-operation period to hunt the residual cancer cells in operation with the chemotherapy cytotoxic drug and remove the cancer cells falling off or remained or transplanted in the operation.

However, could the traditional assistant chemotherapy after operation hunt the residual cancer cells in operation? Could it remove the cancer cells falling off, remained or transplanted in operation?

2. Why the current assistant chemotherapy after operation cannot prevent the reoccurrence and metastasis? It shall be reviewed, analyzed and reflected:

(1) The route of administration of assistant chemotherapy after operation shall be further studied and reformed. At present, it mainly adopts the general intravenous chemotherapy after operation, the cytotoxic drug injected is generally distributed, acting on the histiocytes of the viscera in the whole body, in this way, the ones killed are mainly the proliferative cells, immunological cells and bone marrow cells of the normal tissue organs in the whole body. However, the field of operation accounts for a little ratio in the whole body, in this way, the dose obtained is very small, it is difficult to kill the local residual cancer cells or the cancer lesion in the field of operation or the residual cancer lesion of the cancer cells falling off in the operation, therefore, the route of administration shall be reformed.

(2) The assistant chemotherapy after operation is blinded and the drug administered is not subject to the drugsensitive test. Since the drugsensitive test on the cancer histiocytes of patient is not carried out, the drug is administered by experience, so it is unknown whether the drug is sensitive. If the drug administered is insensitive or drug resistant, it is not only fruitless, without any action on the residual cancer cells, but also kills the proliferative cells, the immunological cells and the bone marrow cells of the normal tissues in the whole body, while these normal tissues in the whole body do not need the cytotoxic drug, resulting in the remarkable side effect, damaging the patient and making the patient suffer from the pain of the side effect. Thus, although the chemotherapy has been made for several times, the expected curative effects cannot be realized, in addition, the cytotoxic drug injected intravenously in the wholly body covers the whole body, kills the general immunological cells and the hematopoietic cells of the bone marrow and makes the immunologic functions of the patient further descend. Actually, the cancer patient is inferior in immunologic function, while the radical operation further brings down the immunologic function, plus the assistant chemotherapy of the cytotoxic drug after operation, the immunological function of the patient is further reduced, like one disaster after another, resulting in metastasis while in chemotherapy. Therefore, as for the assistant chemotherapy after operation, if the drugsensitive test is not made and the drug is administered in form of individualization, the chemotherapy would benefit some patients while damage some patients.

(3) Assistant chemotherapy after operation. **Since the tumor is removed and the lymph clearing is made, the drug administration plan and the dosage should differ from the ones for the patients without removal by operation,** the dosage in the assistant chemotherapy period after operation would differ from the one before operation, before removal of the tumor, the dosage is calculated as per the body surface area so as to realize the goal of remission and shrinkage, however, after the radical operation, the tumor is removed, so it shall target the potentially residual cancer cells or the micro-metastasis in operation instead of the remission and shrinkage, since both targets differs from each other, in order to remit and shrink the tumor of the patient without operation, the drug must have a certain lethality, as a result, the drug administration plans shall be combined and the dosage shall be up to the one the patient can bear, in this way, the curative effect of remission and shrinkage can be realized. Meanwhile, the assistant chemotherapy after operation, depends on radical operation primarily and the chemotherapy secondarily, only targeted for removal of the potentially residual cancer cells or the cancer cells falling off in the operation or the cancer cells in metastasis to make some subsidiary treatment to prevent the reoccurrence and metastasis. Therefore, its drug administration plan and dose shall differ from the former and the dosage of the cytotoxic drug shall be greatly reduced.

(4) What determines the indications and the contraindications of the assistant chemotherapy after operation? At present, the indications of assistant chemotherapy after operation are discordant, for example, do the residual cancer cells exist in the patient after this operation on earth? Where? How many? To what extent? All those things should be taken into account and estimated, however, most of the patients receive the "radical operation on cancer" in the general surgery or the specialized surgery, after operation, they come back to the local hospitals or the tumor clinic, the chemotherapy after operation is the general intravenous chemotherapy, the plans selected differ from each other in each place, each hospital by each physician, namely there is no uniform plan, these physicians or nurses responsible for general intravenous injection for the assistant chemotherapy after operation are not always aware of the patient's condition, pathological analysis, the range and the extent of cancer invasion seen in the operation as well as the estimation of the potential residual cancer lesion in operation, the extent of the radical operation and so on. They should know TNM stage and the immunity chemotherapy and estimate the potential residual cancer cells. Who knows it clearly? Only the operation doctor because he can see the range and extent of the cancer invasion through exploration in operation. Therefore, what determines the selection of chemotherapy or radiotherapy after

operation? The operation physician shall determine the indications and the contraindications of the assistant chemotherapy after operation as well as the chemotherapy plan, times, dosage and so on to satisfy the actual conditions of the patient.

(5) How to assess the curative effects of the assistant chemotherapy after operation? At present, there is no uniform understanding or standard. The objective curative effects of the chemotherapy on the solid tumor before removal of the tumor shall be assessed according to the area of tumor and the remission of the tumor recognized in the world. However, since the tumor is removed, it shall be assessed according to the improvement of the symptom and the condition instead of area of tumor. At present, what role does the assistant chemotherapy after operation play? Does it kill the cancer cells? How many? Do the residual cancer cells exist in the patient's body? What is the effect? All these things are kept unknown. However, it is well known that it kills the normal cells, the immunological cells and the hematopoietic cells of the bone marrow because the white blood cells fall down, the blood platelets fall down too, but it is the extent of the side effect rather than the effect. As to the tumor sign, it is difficult to determine the definite standard at present and it is necessary to make the fundamental study and clinical study.

II. How to Do well in Assistant Chemotherapy after Operation on Cancer or Assistant Chemotherapy in Peri-operation Period?

XU ZE made a suggestion of reforming and developing the assistant chemotherapy after operation on cancer in abdomen (the malignant tumor such as liver cancer, gallbladder cancer, pancreatic cancer, gastric cancer, intestinal cancer and abdominal cancer) as follows:

1. Reform the route of administration and change the general intravenous chemotherapy into the chemotherapy through intravascular administration in target organ. All of the operations on cancer in abdomen, no matter the radical operation or palliative excision, or the operation only for exploration instead of removal, shall adopt the built-in pump in ductus venosus in stomach omentum, or built-in pump in portal vein, or arterial pump, or built-in pump in vein of mesentery as much as possible. Why is the chemotherapy pump built in portal system? Firstly, it is necessary to know where the cancer cells after operation on cancer exist. The administration must be targeted for the cancer cell group and the cancer cells of liver cancer, gallbladder cancer, pancreatic cancer, gastric

cancer and intestinal cancer are in the tuberiferous veins, which flow towards the portal vein and gather at the portal vein, then flow towards hepatic vein via sinus hepaticus and into the lungs via the right atrium. Therefore, the portal system adopts the targeted intravascular administration targeted through the chemotherapy pump, so it is the direct target and it is reasonable and scientific. It can make the residual cancer cells prowling in the portal vein after operation directly contact the chemotherapy drug to produce the curative effect.

2. Reform the dosage of administration: since the built-pump in portal vein is directly targeted for the cancer cell group in the blood of the portal vein and the chemotherapy drug needed is greatly reduced by contrast with the dosage of general intravenous administration. Since the drug is administered through the target organ of the portal vein, the dosage can be greatly reduced. Because the radical operation on cancer has been made, the cancerous protuberance has been removed and the next thing to be done is to remove the potentially residual cancer cells, generally, the immunological cells in the human body can remove these cancer cells, however, since the immunologic function of the cancer patient comes down, the assistant chemotherapy after operation is used to assist in removal, so only a small quantity of dosage is needed, it shall strive for killing 10^{5-6} cancer cells without damage to the normal cells as much as possible. The rest 10^{5-6} cancer cells will be removed by the immunological cells of the organism. However, as to the tracking and hunting of the potential cancer cells in metastasis in the portal system, although the targeted administration reduces the dosage greatly, the drug concentration in the portal vein will be greatly increased out of question, resulting in the improvement of the curative effect. **Since the dosage is greatly reduced, it will necessarily reduce even eliminate the side effect of the chemotherapy greatly. The elimination of the side effect of the chemotherapy, will benefit millions of cancer patients. Over the past half century, millions of cancer patients have deeply suffered from the pain of the side effect from the chemotherapy and the radiotherapy all over the world, what's more, the lives of some patients have been endangered. Since the side effect of chemotherapy is eliminated, so many cancer patients are secured. The cancer seriously endangers the health of the human beings and makes the medical expenses rapidly increase as well. The direct expenses for cancer treatment in China are approximately RMB one hundred billion Yuan, bringing a heavy economic burden to the patients even the whole society. Now Professor Xu Ze holds: the intravascular administration in the specific target organ, reduces the dose, improves the curative effects, eliminates the side reaction, necessarily leading to great reduction of medical charge,**

saving billions of medical charges and expenditures (in RMB Yuan) for the state and the patients and being advantageous for settling the problems of being difficult and expensive in taking medical treatment.

3. Reform the blindness of the drug administered for assistant chemotherapy after operation. The drug for chemotherapy after operation shall be subject to the drugsensitive test together with the histiocytes of the cancer tissue of the patients for the individualized chemotherapy. All operations on cancer, no matter the radical operations or the palliative operations or the exploratory operations, shall try to obtain the specimen of the cancer tissue, the cancer tissue will be cut up into two halves in aseptic manipulation, one for cultivation of cancer tissue and drugsensitive test and another for pathological section and chemotherapy of immunity group for definite pathological diagnosis.

Why the specimen of cancer tissue is selected for cultivation of cancer cells and the drugsensitive test? Since the detection of sensitivity and drug resistance of tumor chemotherapy is the foundation of "individualized" chemotherapy. To this day, the tumor chemotherapy has stridden forward to the "individualized" chemotherapy. In the past days, the different tumor patients receive the same chemotherapy mode (plan), resulting in blindness inevitably. It is shown by the study that the same kind of tumor with the same tissue, even the same tumor in different stages has the incompletely consistent sensitivity to the chemotherapy drug. Therefore, it is necessary to make the drugsensitive test on the tumor patient to select the sensitive drug. Especially, with the increase of the anti-tumor drug at present, it is more urgent. It is proven by the clinical experience in tumor chemotherapy that the effective rate of drug administered by experience is very low (14%) while it will be increased to 28%-35% if the results measured with the existing drugsensitive test method is used to guide the selection of the drug, which is a great fruit.

The detection of the sensitivity and drug resistance of tumor chemotherapy offers an important basis to the foreseeable chemotherapy to reasonably use the anti-tumor drug to reduce the blindness and improve the pertinence, which would undoubtedly improve the level of tumor chemotherapy greatly.

4. The key is to manage and disposal the pump after operation: the drug pump for portal system is in-built in the operation. After operation, it is necessary to continually adopt the long-term light (trace) nontoxic chemotherapy drug and inject the heparin to prevent the embolism, prevent the cancer embolus and prevent the cancer cell group. Where are the cancer cells in the peri-operation

period? The cancerous protuberance of liver, gallbladder, pancreas, spleen, stomach and intestine will be carried off by the blood separately after flowing into the blood of the portal vein or many cancer cells meet with homoplasmic adhesion or heterogenetic adhesion with other cells to form the cancer cell group, which floats with the blood and forms the cancer embolus in the blood vessel, then the deciduous cancer cell embolus moves along the direction of the blood of the venous system. The cancer cells continually enter the blood circulation and transfer along the normal direction of the blood. Most of the cancer cells entering the blood circulation will be eliminated by the host and only a few of the cancer cells survive. Within several days after operation, a large number of cancer cells flow over into the portal system via tumorigenic vein in virtue of operation technique and exploratory extrusion. The surviving cancer cells are adhered to the endothelial cells of the wall of the target organ and then enter the target organ after passing through the wall and form the minute metastasis lesion. The cancer cells from gstrointestinal tract can flow into the liver along the portal vein and the liver is the end point of the blood of the portal vein, therefore, the cancer of gastrointestinal tract often transfers to the liver, forms the cancer cells of the metastasis lesion of the metastasis liver cancer and invades the central vein via the minute branch of the portal vein. The cancer cells can enter the hepatic vein and then flow back to the right atrium via the lower caval vein, then to the lung via the pulmonary artery and form the metastasis lesion of lung.

It can be often seen that the cancer embolus exists in the portal vein branch in the pathological report or the cancer embolus forms in the portal vein branch in CT or MRI report. The cancer embolus is the main factor in the formation of the metastasis lesion. The cancer cells, the fibrin and the blood platelet constitute the embolus and then it is carried to other parts, passes through the wall and forms the secondary tumor around the blood vessel. The formation of cancer embolus is related to the following factors: ① the inherent adhesion and aggregation of the cancer cells; ② the action of Thrombo-Pletinlike substances; ③ action of blood platelet; ④combined action of fibrin.

It is important to do well in management and application of pump after operation. Someone is inbuilt with chemotherapy pump and does not pay a return visit or use the pump after leaving hospital. After operation, the regular return visit shall be paid and the heparin shall be injected via the pump to prevent the blockade and the cancer embolus. A few of chemotherapy drugs shall be injected to hunt the floating cancer cells remaining in the the blood circulation of portal vein.

The surgeons and the nurses shall be responsible for the arrangement, follow-up survey, registration, filling, consultation answer, statistics and summary of the assistant chemotherapy after operation.

5. Reform the single goal of killing cancer cells into the immunological mediation and control therapy in an all-round way. Abandon the goal of only killing the cancer cells, attach importance to the resistance of the organism, reform it into the immunological mediation and control therapy in an all-round way and give attention to both of them, thus, the curative effect will be improved. XZ-C medicine shall be orally taken in the period of assistant chemotherapy after operation and after the treatment course of the assistant chemotherapy to carry out the immunological chemotherapy (immunity + chemotherapy) or immunological chemotherapy radiotherapy (immunity + radiotherapy) so as to reform the unilateral therapeutic outlook of singly killing the cancer cells into an all-round therapeutic outlook of killing the cancer cells as well as improving the immunity of the organism.

III. Why the Assistant Chemotherapy after Operation Cannot Achieve the Expectation

In the past 10 years, the assistant chemotherapy after operation has been widely adopted all over the country, however, most of the assistant chemotherapy after operation is made by experience, the treatment plans differ from each other in different hospitals; the chemotherapy drugs selected differ from each other; the same to the departments and doctors in the same hospital due to the difference experience. The days and the interval of chemotherapy drugs administered differ a little from each other in different hospitals in different places: once per month for someone, once per two months for someone, once per week for someone, 4 times continually for someone, 6 times continually for someone and even 8-10 times continually for someone. The treatment courses are arranged with a certain blindness and differ from each other, without uniform or consistent standard. Because most of the hospitals have not made the drugsensitive test, so the "individualized" chemotherapy cannot be made.

At present, the plans for assistant chemotherapy after operation adopted in different places are basically similar to the ordinary chemotherapy plans, however, the goal or target of the ordinary tumor chemotherapy aims at the primary cancer lesion or the metastasis cancer lesion and the goal of treatment is to shrink, eliminate or remit the primary cancerous protuberance or metastasis cancerous protuberance or the tumid lymph node. These solid cancerous protuberances occupy a relatively large area, so, in order to shrink the cancerous protuberance, it is necessary to take the combined chemotherapy drugs with a relatively large quantity, otherwise, it is difficult to shrink the cancerous protuberance.

However, the assistant chemotherapy after operation is entirely different from this because the radical operation removes and cleans down the primary cancerous protuberance and the tumid lymph node around it, in this way, there is no solid cancerous protuberance. Since the cancerous protuberance is removed, the assistant chemotherapy after operation aims at the potentially residual cancer cells after operation, the potentially remnant micro-metastasis cancer cells or the cancer cells in metastasis and it is targeted for the remnant cancer cells or the potentially metastasis cancer cells instead of the solid cancerous protuberance, so the dosage shall be relatively small, without damage to the immunological cells of the host or with a little damage to the host. So how to assess the curative effect of the assistant chemotherapy after operation shall be measured according to the assessment standard including the improvement of immunity, the improvement of the survival quality, the improvement of the symptom, the elevation of the immunity indexes, the descent of the tumor sign and good mental state and appetite instead of the shrinkage of the tumor.

How to do well in assistant chemotherapy after operation? It is held by us that attention shall be paid to the following:

1. As to the patients receiving the radical operation on the cancerous protuberance, the fresh tumor specimen shall be selected for the chemotherapy drug sensitive test so as to individualize the assistant chemotherapy after operation to avoid the blindness of drug administration.

2. How to judge or estimate whether the remnant cancer cells exist in the body after radical operation so as to determine the indication of the assistant chemotherapy after operation, in this way, the immunity indexes and the tumor signs shall be detected.

3. How to judge the curative effect of the assistant chemotherapy after operation? Are the cancer cells killed or not? Since the tumor is removed, the curative effect cannot be judged as per the existence of the tumor of the volume of the tumor. The immunity indexes, the cytokines and the tumor signs shall be detected to judge the possibility of the reoccurrence and metastasis after operation.

4. The drug administered for the assistant chemotherapy after operation shall differ from the one for primary tumor or the metastasis cancer lesion because

the goals are different: the former is to eliminate the primary cancer lesion and the latter is to eliminate the residual cancer cells, as a result, the dosage shall be different and it shall be greatly reduced.

5. The patient receiving the radical operation on cancer is very weak in the body condition and inferior in immunologic function, so the assistant chemotherapy after operation must be accompanied with the immunological mediation and control therapy, namely the immunological therapy + chemotherapy, called immunological chemotherapy. As above-mentioned, the elimination of the cancer cells in metastasis or the cancer cells or the cancer cell group in the blood circulation after operation mainly depends on the immunological cells in the organism of the host. It is shown by the experimental study that the immunological cells in the organism can eliminate 10^5 cancer cells, so the dosage for the assistant chemotheray after operation shall not be too large under the precondition of not damaging or slihgtly damaging the immunological cells because it is very important to carry out the immunological mediation and control therapy and improve the immunity of the organism to eliminate the cancer cells in metastasis. We deeply realize that in the past 16 years, Wuhan Shuguang Tumor Special Clinic under Wuhan Research Institute of Anti-cancerometastasis and Anti-reoccurrence has diagnosed so many patients like this, some of them are of valetudinarianism or accompanied with other diseases, resulting in failure to chemotherapy and radiotherapy; some of them fail to the chemotherapy again due to the severe response after 1-2 chemotherapy after operation; some of them refuse the chemotherapy after operation; most of the patients meet with the cancer invading serosa and are accompanied by metastasis of lymph node, so they take XZ-C medicine for treatment in the new mode of XU ZE new concept of anti-cancerometastasis treatment and orally take XZ-C medicine for a long term, resulting in a relatively good curative effect.

6. Although the assistant chemotherapy after operation has been widely popularized all over the country at present, there are short of the forward-looking, comparable and appreciable reports on the assistant chemotherapy after operation. According to the report on 5-year's follow-up survey of the assistant chemotherapy or radiotherapy after operation on the patients suffering from the stomach cancer by American Stomach Cancer Group, it was reported by Lence (1994, 3, 3, 1390) that the total survival rate was still low in the patients suffering from the stomach cancer even the patients with the cancer removed through operation, therefore, the people hope to improve the prognosis through the assistant chemotherapy and radiotherapy for the patients with low tumor

load after operation. It was shown by the results of the assistant treatment with mitomycin and fluorouracil on the first group of the patients in 1976 by British Stomach Cancer Organization that it had no benefit to the patients after operation, for this reason, the study on the assistant treatment of another group of patients had been made.

The forward-looking, random and contrapositive grouping study had been made on 430 patients suffering from the gastric gland cancer in Stage II and III after operation, accompanied with radiotherapy or the combined chemotherapy of mitomycin, adriamycin and fluorouracil (MAF) plan over 5 years, among which 372 patients died, 7 of which died of the surgical complication and 327 of which died of the reoccurrence of tumor. In the random grouping study, 145 cases only adopted the operation therapy; 153 cases accepted the assistant chemotherapy with the rang of irradiation including hilum of spleen and porta hepatic with the dosage of 4500cGy and the increase in dosage of 500cGy in operative field area; another 138 cases accepted the combined chemotherapy (MPA Plan) with mitomycin 4mg/m^2, adriamycin 30mg/m^2 and fluorouracil 600 mg/m^2, intravenously injected, 3 weeks as a cycle, totaling 6 cycles. The total two-year's survival rate of this group of patients was 33% and the total five-year's survival rate was 17% (13%~21%), compared with the patients with the single operation therapy, as to the patients accepting the assistant chemotherapy, the survival rate was not raised: the five-year's survival rate of the patients with single operation therapy was 20% and the one of the patients accepting the operation plus radiotherapy was 19%.

Therefore, operation is still the standard therapeutic method of the stomach cancer and the assistant therapeutic measures shall be restricted within a certain scope of study.

To sum up, it is held by the author: some large hospitals or medical centers in China should make the forward-looking comparable grouping study to obtain a large number of appreciable scientific data in China. At present, the assistant chemotherapy after operation is still restricted within a certain scope of study.

4. The basic Model and Specific Scheme of Anti-cancerometastasis Treatment

Traditional chemotherapy against metastasis mainly aims to kill cancer cells. No matter it is the primary carcinoma, metastatic carcinoma, the postoperative adjuvant chemotherapy preventing reoccurrence and metastasis or when metastasis of lymph nodes is found, intravenous chemotherapy drugs are adopted in all cases. However, because chemotherapy drugs are of no selectivity and kill both cancer cells and normal cells (especially the immunological cells), they act as a double-edged sword. The author holds that various schemes for intravenous chemotherapy are mainly the different combinations of cytotoxic drugs, which are not certainly in line with the multi-link and multi-step biological characteristics of the cancerometastasis process.

I. The basic model of anti-cancerometastasis treatment

Among the innumerable patients in this clinical practice, it is not uncommon to see that some of them are not free from metastasis after the postoperative adjuvant chemotherapy. What is worse is that some of them suffered a simultaneous metastasis in chemotherapy or suffered from the metastasis again after chemotherapy again. All these phenomena make us deeply think about the reason behind the failure to prevent metastasis. Is it the traditional chemotherapy not in line with the biological characteristics of cancerometastasis process? Whether it is necessary to update our knowledge and thinking, or to change our conceptions and treatment model on anti-canceromestasis? Xu Ze's design concept of anti-cancerometastasis countermeasures is just an innovation of the concepts, thinking, methods and models of the traditional anti-metastasis treatment.

Anti-metastasis drugs tend to interfere or blockade a certain link or step of the metastasis process of cancer cells or the cancer cell clusters so as to inhibit the formation of metastasis focus. Although the chemotherapeutic cytotoxic drugs can kill tumor cells, suspend the growth of primary carcinoma and delay the occurrence time of metastasis, they fail to inhibit the process of invasion and metastasis. At present, the ideal drugs killing the primary carcinoma and inhibiting invasion and metastasis are unavailable. Thus, it is necessary to study the strategy of interdiction, prevention and treatment aiming at the development steps and mechanism of the cancerometastasis summarized as "eight steps and three stages".

The invasion and metastasis of carcinoma is a complicated process of many steps and the metastasis process could be generalized as following: proliferation of primary cancerous protuberance→ the formation and growth of newly born micrangium of tumor→ invading and breaking through basement membrance→ cancer cells breaking away from parent tumor and breaking through basement membrance and then perforating micrangiums or micro lymphatic vessels→ the survival and floating of invading blood in the circulatory system→ formation of small cancer embolus from cancer cells clusters wrapped by blood platelet and delivery to remote target organs together with blood stream→ the detention in the micrangium of target organs→ the attachment or adherence of cancer embolus to the wall of micrangium→ breaking through blood vessels and forming micro metastasis focus→formation of newly born micrangium of tumor as the metastasis focus→ the proliferation of the metastasis focus. If we could find the way to blockade one or several links or steps, it is possible to control metastasis, as is the context in which Xu Ze's new model of anti-cancerometastasis treatment is formed and developed.

II. The specific plan of anti-cancerometastasis treatment

According to biological behaviors of modern oncology on cancerometastasis and theory of reoccurrence and metastasis, this libratory has been always searching for new anti-metastasis drugs among traditional Chinese herbs extracted from natural herbs for years. Through experimental study on of tumor-bearing animal bodies with traditional Chinese medicine as well as the combination of traditional Chinese medicine and western medicine, we interfere, obstruct and intercept all the links of the metastasis, and develop an anti-metastasis scheme and countermeasure with XZ-C medicine, including XZ-C-TG against the formation of micrangium, XZ-C-AS dissolving cancer embolus, XZ-C-MD against invading into and breaking through blood vessels, XZ-C-LM with antigenicity, XZ-C-Ind against PGE2; VA and XZ-C-CA as calcium channel blocking drugs against invasion, XZ-C-GB against adherence, XZ-C-TIMP against the resistance to drugs, XZ-C$_1$ inhibiting cancer cells rather than normal cells; XZ-C$_4$ protecting thymus and improving immunity; XZ-C$_8$ protecting bone marrow and improving hematogenesis function and Emulsion of Brucea Javanica into lymph nodes. The comprehensive measures of the above-mentioned treatment schemes have achieved sound curative effects in the clinical practice by our anti-cancer cooperative group.

Because cancerometastasis is a complicated process of multi-step and multi-link, it is necessary to adopt the comprehensive measures in an all-round way to treat the cancerometastasis instead of a certain drug or measure. Thus aiming at the steps of metastasis, we scientifically design and adopt different treatment schemes and countermeasures shown in the following table. Those treatment schemes and countermeasures aiming at the steps of metastasis are to achieve the same goal of anti-metastasis.

The new model of anti-cancerometastasis treatment of Xu Ze's new concept (treatment schemes and countermeasures for the steps of canceromestasis)

Metastasis step	Treatment countermeasures	XZ-C medicine and its role
Proliferation of primary cancerous	Operation, chemotherapy	$XZ-C_1$ inhibiting cancer cells
		$XZ-C_4$ protecting thymus and improving immunity
		$XZ-C_8$ protecting bone marrow and improving hematogenesis function
Growth of newly born micrangium of tumor	Inhibiting the formation of micrangium	XZ-C-TG against formation of micrangium
		XZ-C-CA against adherence
Invasion into basement membrance	Anti-adhesion, anti-kinesalgia and inhibiting the activity of hydrolase	XZ-C-K(LWF) against adhesion
		Ind against PGE2
		XZ-C-MD against kinesalgia
Breaking through blood vessels or lymphatic vessels	Anti-adhesion, anti-kinesalgia and inhibiting the activity of hydrolase	XZ-C-MD against invasion into blood vessels
		XZ-C-K (LWF)
		$XZ-C_{1+4}$ mediating immunity
In the blood of circulatory system	Inhibiting the aggregation and coagulation of blood platelet. Biological response modification (BRM)	XZ-C-N (CZR) against the aggregation of blood platelet
		XZ-C-LM
		XZ-C-ASP dissolving cancer embolus
		$XZ-C_{1+4}$ mediating immunity
The formation of cancer embolus	Promoting blood circulation and removing stasis and resisting thrombus	XZ-C-K (NSR) against cancer embolus
		XZ-C-N (CZR) against aggregation of blood platelet
The breaking out of cancer embolus from blood vessels	Resisting adhesion, kinesalgia, and the activity of hydrolase	XZ-C-MD against the breaking out of cancer embolus
The formation of metastasis focus	Operation, radiotherapy, chemotherapy	$XZ-C_{1+4}$ mediating immunity
		XZ-C-TG inhibiting the growth of blood vessels
The metastasis of lymph nodes	Liposoluble drugs	The Emulsion of Brucea Javanica as the carrier of lipa entering into the lymph nodes

The correlative factors of the invasion of cancer cells are adherence, enzymatic secretion and kinesalgia. The inhibition of adhesion, kinesalgia and enzymatic secretion is also helpful to inhibit the exfoliation of cancer cells from parent tumor, its break into matrix and the formation of the newly born blood vessels of the tumor besides its contribution to prevent the invasion of primary carcinoma. For years the researches on inhibitors inhibiting the growth of newly born blood vessels are seen in reports. Meanwhile, it is also discovered in the tumor-bearing animal experiment screening the anti-cancerometastasis drugs by this libratory that traditional Chinese medicine TG is of sound inhibiting effects on newly born blood vessels. Tumor cells are in weakest condition to resist the host environment when entering into the blood of the circulatory system and can be easily eliminated by the immunological cells of the host.

It is proved by some literature that a vast majority of cancer cells entering into the circulatory system are killed by immunological cells and only a number of approximately 0.01% thereof could survive and possibly become the focus of metastasis. Except the mechanical damage factors, the cancer cells in blood stream are mainly eliminated by the damaging effects of the immunological function of the hosts against tumor cells. Tumor-bearing patients usually suffer low immunological function inhibited by tumor and chemotherapy. Therefore, it is necessary to adopt immunotherapy, biotherapy and biological response modification and traditional Chinese medicine for immunological mediation to protect the function of immune organs so as to improve the immunity of the host. It is found that XZ-C medicine can protect bone marrow and improve hemogenesis function, protect hemogenesis function of bone marrow as well as stem cells, improve immunologic function and inhibit the metastasis of tumor. According to the clinical application on the innumerable patients in the clinic of Anti-cancer Cooperative Group of Traditional Chinese Medicine Combined with Western Medicine over ten years, XZ-C medicine against cancer and metastasis has achieved significant curative effects.

III. The important role of immunotherapy in anti-cancerometastasis treatment

Among all the current therapeutic methods, operation and radiotherapy are both local therapy while chemotherapy, immunotherapy, biological therapy, therapy with traditional Chinese medicine are systematic therapy. At present, the chemotherapy mainly targets the focus of primary cancer or metastasis focus and the criterion to judge the curative effects is to alleviate and shrink the tumor. In order to fulfill of the above criterion, a significant dose of chemotherapeutic cytotoxic drugs are in need to shrink the lump. Additionally in view of the cell cycle, medicines are necessarily combined in order to achieve a certain level of lethality. If it is a 1cm×1cm^2 lump, it would contain a number of 10^{12} cancer cells and this, requires a considerable dose of chemotherapeutic drugs to shrink it into half. However, it only needs a slight dose if cancer cells are eliminated in the process of metastasis by chemotherapy, because the amount of cancer cells in metastasis process only accounts to 10^7 to 10^8 and most of them could be eliminated. The problem happens as a large amount of immunological cells in blood circulation are destroyed by chemotherapeutic cytotoxic drugs whereas the anti-metastasis mainly depends on the system against cancer cells of the organism itself. Thus it would be a great loss to patients. Chemotherapy could only be conducted with intermission during which time a large amount of cancer cells and immunological cells would be both eliminated. However there still exist a handful of escaped cancer cells during this period which continually split and proliferate or are even more active.

More than that, the destroyed immunological cells, decreased immunity and weakened immune surveillance would also lead or contribute to the development and metastasis of cancer cells.

Therefore, the chemotherapeutic drugs should not be overdosed in the anti-metastasis treatment and should not impair a large amount of immunological cells. Meanwhile, chemotherapy should be accompanied by Immunotherapy, Biotherapy, Biological Response Modification (BRM), XZ-C medicine and tonic traditional Chinese medicine so as to give play to each other's advantages and make up each other's imperfections. Because a properly protected and activated immune system of the body could eliminate 10^6 cancer cells and additional chemotherapeutic drugs could destroy most cancer cells in the process of metastasis, it is possible to hold up and cut off the metastasis path and put the diffusion and metastasis under further control.

Xu Ze's new concept of anti-metastasis treatment promotes the application of immunochemotherapy, namely the combination of immunotherapy and chemotherapy. To be specific, immune drugs would be used in the peri-chemotheraputic period, in other words, at the week before the chemotherapy to be implemented, and would not be ceased in the chemotherapy period unless in case of serious chemotherapy response. The immunotherapy will continue for 6 to 9 months after chemotherapy and during intermission for the maintenance of a certain level of immunity and the consolidation of the curative effects. All these above are proved to be reasonable. For 16 years the Dawn Specialist Out-patient of our anti-metastasis laboratory uses XZ-C anti-cancer traditional Chinese medicine for immunological mediation to coordinate chemotherapy, which usually causes less chemotherapy response. Most of the postoperative in our out-patients suffer the liver, gallbladder, pancreas, stomach, intestine, lung and breast cancer. Some suffer a multi-part lymphatic metastasis after radical operations but then meet with serious response after chemotherapy thus come to our out-patient for treatment. Some fail the exploratory operation and some are under palliative operations. Therefore, the author, through combining the small-dosed chemotherapy with XZ-C medicine, usually finds less response and hemogram variation. Because of different conditions of the patients and the absence of comparability, it is impossible to conduct the comparative observation of perspective random allocation. Therefore, the perspective clinical study is conducted by comparatively observing the curative effects of the immunotherapy group and the chemotherapy group with immune indexes (IFN, IL-2 and TNF), the level of tumor marker, the quality of life and the survival time as the evaluative criteria of the two groups.

The immune drugs used in the above-mentioned immunochemotherapy shall increase the immunity indexes of the body. Actually not all traditional Chinese medicine that support healthy energy and eliminate evil are able to improve immunity because some are of bidirectional regulating function, which would improve immunity at a certain dosage range but lower immunity at another dosage range. For example, the glossy privet fruit could significantly increase the spleen and thymus indexes; the bupleurum roots lead to the atrophy of the mice thymus; and the liquid made from the pilose antlers of a young stag could improve the weight of the spleen and thymus of the mice if it is poured into their stomach. Additionally, barrenwort polysaccharide would lead to the atrophy of the thymus but a long-term oral administration turns to increase the weight of thymus. $XZ\text{-}C_{1+4+8}$ medicine is proved to be able to increase cytokines like IFN, IL-2, TNF etc and to decrease the level of tumor markers of many terms by many animal experiments and long-term clinical observation. To be specific, $XZ\text{-}C_4$ could protect bone marrow and thymus and improve hematopoiesis functions and immunity thus raises the overall immune level. The test by cultivating cancer cells in vitro reveals that the series of XZ-C1 medicine, including $XZ\text{-}C_1\text{-}A$, $XZ\text{-}C_1\text{-}B$ and $XZ\text{-}C_1\text{-}C$, are the three pharmaceutics that 100% kill cancer cells, 100% cause no harm to normal cells and achieve an 85% to 95% tumor-inhibiting rate in tumor-inhibiting experiments on the body of tumor-bearing animals. Cyclophosphane (CTX) as the control group only achieves a tumor-inhibiting rate of 45% and also significantly decreases the immunity.

The removal of focus of primary cancer and metastasis focus depends on local surgical removal or radiation exposure. The focus of primary cancer should be removed by surgical removal if possible and in case of impossibility, it would be helpful to turn to interventional therapy, radiotherapy, radio frequency, focused ultrasound or the injection of absolute ethyl alcohol so as to control the local focus.

The metastasis of tumor is an essential expression of malignancy. The reason why cancer treatment is failed is that the treatment isn't proper and the immunity of the patients isn't sufficiently strong to kill all the cancer cells. Literatures show that a marginally small tumor (1 to 8g) could release millions or even thousand millions of cancer cells in 24 hours into blood. However, a vast majority of these cancel cells would be eliminated by the human body's immune system and only 1% of them are possibly able to survive and evolve into metastasis tumor. The test data of our libratory reveals that the immunity of mice is capable of killing 100,000 cancer cells. The amount could be increased to more than 1,000,000 if $XZ\text{-}C_1$ medicine is used. The question is what destroys them? It is the immunological cells of the body itself. Thus Xu Ze's new concept holds that the immunological cells of body should be protected and not be damaged by any treatments. It is necessary to find ways to protect and activate the immunological function of the host. It would be beneficial for the patients if the immunotherapy and a small-dosed chemotherapy are combined as immunochemotherapy, learning from each other's strong points and offsetting each other's weakness.

5. New Mothed of Cancer Treatment

I. Strengthening of immunological therapy and improving side effects from chemotherapy

1. Side effects of traditional chemotherapy: when chemotherapy is made on cancer, it usually inhibits immunologic function and hematopoiesis function of the bone marrow, descends WBC and PLT and damages liver and kidney function as well as gastroenteric function, leading to the side effects such as nausea, emesis, abdominal distension, anorexia and so on.

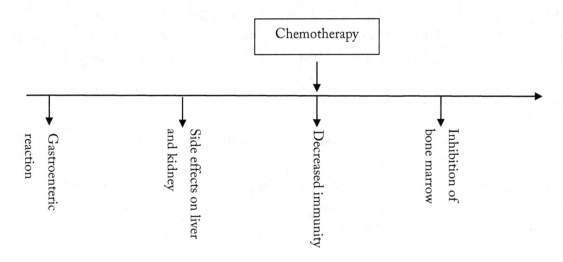

Fig. 1 Side effects of traditional chemotherapy

2. The countermeasures of Xu Ze's new concept: the method to improve the side effects of chemotherapy is to strengthen the supporting therapy and take effective measures to protect the host. Among the traditional Chinese medicine for immunological mediation, XZ-C$_4$ can protect thymus thus and improve immunity; XZ-C$_8$ can protect hematopoiesis function of the bone marrow and generate more stem cells; XZ-C medicine for immunity mediation can strengthen physical strength of cancerous patients. See Fig. 2.

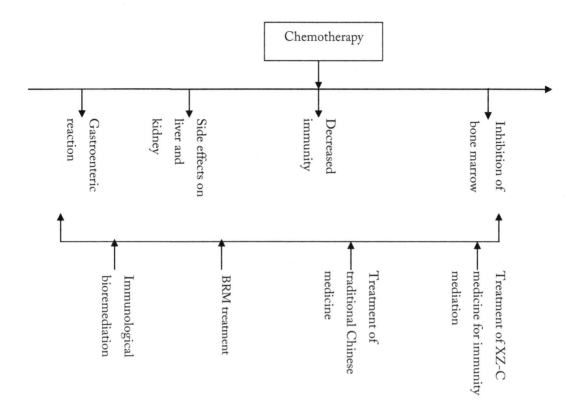

Fig. 2 Countermeasures for side effects of chemotherapy

II. Changing intermittent treatment into continual treatment

1. Traditional intravenous chemotherapy is an intermittent therapy, that is to say, after the drug for chemotherapy is applied for 3-5 days, it is necessary to apply the chemotherapeutic drug for the second course of treatment when WBC and PLT return to normal after 3-4 weeks. The drug for chemotherapy shall not be continually applied during the intermission between the first and the second course of treatment, whereas the cancel cells are still continually and uninterruptedly proliferated and divided in the intermission and increase at the speed of geometrical progression. In addition, because of the inhibition of immunologic function caused by chemotherapeutic drug, the cancel cells escape from or are free of the immunological surveillance, their proliferation and division are quickened during the intermission between these two courses, in other words, the longer the course of treatment of chemotherapeutic drug, the more the combined drug and the more the dose, the more serious of the attack against immunity of the human body, resulting in lack of immunological surveillance, and even resulting in reoccurrence and metastasis in chemotherapy, and shrinkage of tumor firstly before continual enlargement later (see Fig. 3). These cases occur commonly, how to treat

them? It is held by us that the following model should be adopted for a continuous immunological therapy in the intermission between two courses of treatment.

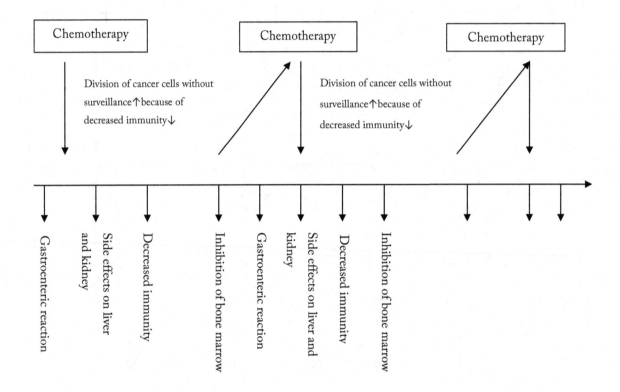

Fig.3 Easy reoccurrence of tumor without treatment in the intermission

2. Xu Ze's new concept and model of cancer treatment is a continuous treatment. It adopts traditional Chinese medicine for immunological mediation, namely $XZ-C_1$ + $XZ-C_4$, or BRM for treatment during the intermission. $XZ-C_1$ was screened through the experimental study on tumor-bearing animals over 7 years and has been proven by a sixteen-year clinical verification that it has only inhibited the cancel cells rather than normal ones and that it can benefit spleen and stomach. $XZ-C_4$ can protect thymus from atrophy, prevent immunity from decreasing and make it better. Continual treatment in the intermittence with XZ-C medicine can control proliferation of caner cells and also protect the function of immune organs such as thymus.

The combination of chemotherapeutic drug and XZ-C medicine can decrease teh side effects from chemotherapy and strengthen chemotherapy effects against the loss of immunological surveillance as well meanwhile. See Fig. 4.

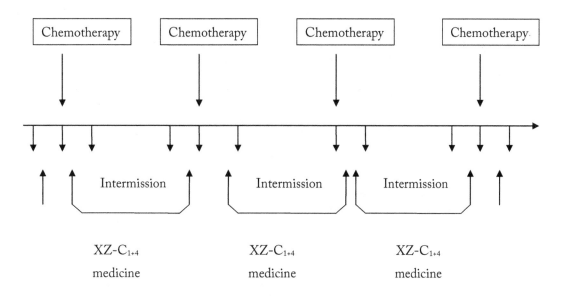

Fig. 4 Continual treatment in the intermission

III. Therapy of protecting the host instead of damaging the host

1. Traditional chemotherapy tends to damage the hosts: chemotherapeutic drugs are the x drugs and function as a double-edged sword, killing both cancer cells and normal ones for the lack of selectivity, inhibiting bone marrow and decreasing peripheral WBC and PLT. See Fig. 5.

2. Xu Ze' new concept and model of cancer treatment tends to protect the hosts: the new-type anticancer drugs only inhibit cancer cells, have no effects on normal cells, protect thymus, improve immunity and protect bone marrow. Among XZ-C medicine, $XZ-C_1$ only inhibits the cancel cells and have no effects on normal cells; $XZ-C_4$ protects thymus from atrophy and improves immunity; $XZ-C_8$ protects bone marrow and produces blood, all of which have been screened through the experiments on tumor-bearing animals over 7 years and have been proven by the clinical data of nearly 10000 cases in the cooperative anti-cancer clinic over 10 years. See Fig. 6.

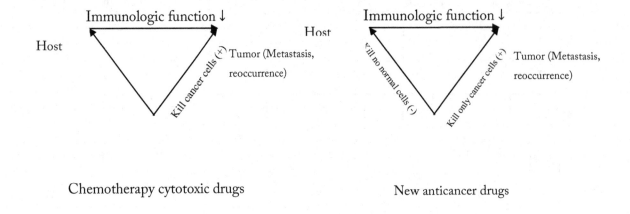

Fig. 5 Effects of traditional chemotherapy

Fig. 6 Effects of Xu Ze's new model of cancer treatment

IV. Rebalancing the unbalance between the host and tumor

It has been proven by the abovementioned findings from the experimental study that the positive relationship exists between the occurrence and development of tumor and the structure and immunologic function of immune organs of the host such as thymus and marrow. Enlightened by the seesaws in children's park and the weighing scale in the laboratory, the author took a tumble: if immunologic function was too inferior, tumor would grow up, meanwhile, when the former was improved to a certain level, then the later would be controlled in a stable or improvement condition (Fig. 7). However, the fluctuation of the level depends on further experimental observation and test.

Thus, the occurrence and development of tumor depends on the relationship between immunologic function of the host and the intrinsic biological characteristics of tumor. Similarly, the invasion and metastasis of cancer also rests with the relationship, namely, carcinoma would be put under control in case of the balance between biological characteristics of tumor cells and impacts of the host on the inhibition factors; otherwise, the cancer would grow up.

Traditional radiotherapy and chemotherapy are inclined to weakening immunologic function and lead to a worse unbalance between both of them.

Xu Ze's new model of cancer treatment aims to improve the immunity of patients as much as possible, level off the decreased *immunity* (Fig. 8) and thus inhibit tumor growth and strengthen immunological surveillance.

Immune system is the one composed of immune organs, immunological cell and molecules executing immunologic function, mainly including central lymphatic tissue, peripheral lymphatic tissue and immunological cells. Central lymphatic tissue, the home to immune cells for their occurrence, differentiation and maturation, includes thymus and bone marrow. Peripheral lymphatic tissue includes lymph nodes, spleens and stomachs, in which T cells and B cells settle and these cells make their immune response after the identification of foreign antigen.

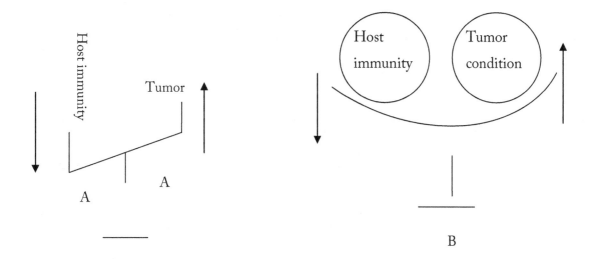

Fig. 7 Schematics of "seesaw" and "weighing scale"

A. tumor grows up in unbalance; B. stabled improvement conditions in balance

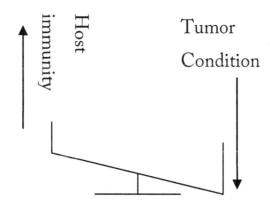

Fig. 8 Improved immunity and controlled tumor

V. Protecting central immune organs instead of damaging it

1. Traditional chemotherapy inhibits immunologic function: when cancer happens, thymus has been inhibited by "cancer-inhibiting thymic factor" and atrophied. Meanwhile, chemotherapy inhibits immunity and bone marrow, damages hemopoietic system and finally lead to the adynamia of the central immune organs as a whole.

In case of cancerometastasis, a large number of cancer cells are swarming into lymph nodes and destroy their immunologic function. As to the spleen, it could inhibit or destroy cancer cells intruding in the spleen along the blood and provide nowhere for the existence of free cancer cells due to its intrinsic structures and functions. Thus there is generally no primary or secondary malignant tumor in the spleen. However, it is shown by the experiments that the immunologic function of the spleen to tumor is bidirectional, namely, it effectively inhibits tumor in the early stage of cancer but fails in the late stage.

2. Xu Ze's new model of cancer treatment can protect thymus and bone marrow and prevent the immunologic function of the host from damage. According to anatomic experiments on more than 2,000 tumor-bearing animal models, it was found that the growth of tumor is accompanied with the thymus atrophy in form of simultaneously direct proportion. In addition, the death of mice is also proportional to the tumor growth and thymus atrophy. Conclusively, it is necessary to protect thymus and improve immunity. As well as that, in studying the reason why cancer leads to death on thousands of late tumor-bearing animal models, it is found by us that the thymuses apparently atrophied among all grouped dead animals in the final stage of carcinoma, their central immune organ met with atrophy and malfunction. It may be one important reason why the cancer patients died of cancer. It is a common fact that most cancer patients die of cancer in clinic. But further careful analysis and profound consideration would reveal the close relationship between infection bleeding, the failure of organ function and adynamia of immunologic function, which enlightens us to try to prevent or inhibit the thymus atrophy of tumor-bearing animal models in the late stage of tumor. We just aim to find the way to prevent or alleviate thymus atrophy, no matter what measure is taken. After a long-term experimental research, it is found by us that XZ-C_4 and XZ-C_8 screened from the natural herbs, the former can protect thymus and improve immunologic function and the later can protect bone marrow and produce the blood.

XZ-C_4 can protect thymus from atrophy and increase lymphocyte and T cells.

XZ-C_8 can protect hematopoiesis function of the bone marrow, rebuild erythrocyte and leucocyte system and correct anemia.

VI. Non-damage therapy instead of damage therapy

1. For half a century, the traditional anti-cancer therapies have been always the operation, the radiotherapy and the chemotherapy, the first two are the local therapy and the last one is the systematic therapy, all of which would damage the patients to a certain extent. To be specific, operations would attack the ability of the patients to resist disease at a certain level and also cause an implantation, dissemination or residue of exfoliated and free cancer cells, thus resulting in reoccurrence or metastasis after operation. Radiotherapy would cause radioactive inflammatory pathological changes. Chemotherapy has great systemic side effects on the human body. Although currently the traditional therapies have been gradually improved as regional selective local therapy with intubation or catheter on target organs, which aims to increase local concentration and narrow down the damage range of cytotoxic drug, the whole body would still under the effects of medicine disseminated systemically and be subject to obviously toxic effects such as decreased immunity, inhibition of bone marrow, gastroenteric reaction, hair shedding, renal and hepatic injuries and so on. In addition, radioactive rays and chemotherapeutic drugs are two carcinogenic factors despite of the ability of radiotherapy and chemotherapy to kill cancer cells, thus they would be obviously harmful to the patients.

2. The characteristics of the effects of the new non-damage therapy and Xu Ze's new model of cancer treatment: so many new therapies such as biotherapy, immunotherapy, differentiation and induction therapy, gene therapy, Chinese medicine treatment, combined therapy of traditional Chinese and western medicine and so on, have been emerging in the past 10 years, most of which devote to improving immunity, protecting the host, simulating and inducing the anticancer cell clusters within the anticancer system of the host (including NK cell clusters, K cell clusters, LAK cell clusters, macrophage cell clusters and TK cell clusters) as well as the factor system of anticancer cells (including IFN, IL-2, TNF, LT), regulating and controlling neurohumor system and endocrine system, strengthening the immunologic function and antineoplastic ability of the host and maintaining a balance and sustainability for the host. Z-C medicine was screened from natural herbs on tumor-bearing experimental animals, got a remarkable curative effect by a ten-year follow-up clinical verification with data of approximate 10,000 clinical cases and categorized as non-damage medicine, which could actually constitutes a non damage therapy.

The effects of burgeoning non-damage therapy could be summarized as follows: ① directly improve the anti-tumor ability of the host; ② indirectly improve the anti-cancer ability of the host by diminishing inhibition mechanism; ③ improve the resistance power of the host against oncotherapy; ④ enhance the immunogenicity of tumors.

No matter the traditional therapy or the new concept therapy, operation is the preferred method to treat solid tumor. Radical surgery to resect tumor is the currently best therapeutic method in the range of indication. In 1960s, the author resected huge abdominal tumor more than 6kg for 4 patients, one of which was a female patient, aged 50, with a hysteroma over 18kg. Such a huge solid tumor can't be removed by chemotherapy, immunity, traditional Chinese medicine or BRM. The strategy for treatment of cancerous protuberance is to adopt different methods to eliminate the number of cancer cells to a certain order of magnitude (Someone fixes the order of magnitude at 10^6 mice cells or corresponding 3.5×10^9 human cells and describes it as a spherical nodule with a diameter of 1.5cm) and remediate the human body under this condition. $Z-C_{1+4}$ are verified by the experiments from this laboratory that they could put 10^5 cancer cells under control. Thus if XZ-C medicine is applied in adjuvant therapy after the tumors resection surgery of patients, the body resistance could be strengthened so as to eliminate pathogenic factors and diminish reoccurrence and metastasis.

Chapter 7 Preliminary Establishment of XZ-C Immuno-modulatory Cancer Therapy System

1. The new understanding and new concepts of cancer etiology and pathology

1). The cause of cancer and pathogenesis

One of the etiology and pathogenesis of cancer may be thymic atrophy and decrease of immune function (by the new investigation: this is the first time in the world.). In our laboratory from the experimental study it was found that : in tumor bearing mice thymus was progressive atrophy and volume reduction, cell proliferation blocked, mature cells decreased. In the tumor late stage the thymus is extremely atrophic, hard texture, may be thymic atrophy, central immune organ dysfunction, immune function decrease and immune surveillance capabilities decrease and immune escape.

2). Cancer forms in the human body

(1) There are two forms of expressionin traditional concept of cancer therapy that:

The first form of expression - the primary foci;

The second form of expression --- metastasis foci.

Traditional cancer therapeutics target or "target" is for these two forms,

first, for the first form of expression - the primary cancer foci;

The second is for the second form of expression --- metastasis foci.

This traditional concept of treatment is used more than a hundred years and this treatment goal or "target" is for these two forms of expression - the primary tumor foci or metastasis, but ignore the cancer cells on the way of metastasis. As we all know, metastasis is the biological characteristics and biological behavior of malignant tumors.

The difference between benign tumor and malignant tumor is that the former does not metastasis and the latter metastasis so that anti-metastasis is the key to cancer treatment. If there is no blockage for the cancer cells on the way of metastasis, you cannot control the metastasis of cancer cells, and thus it is difficult to obtain the possibility of cancer treatment heal.

(2) In Xu Ze new concept there are three forms of cancer in the human body and there are three forms of performance:

The first form of expression - the primary foci;
The second form of expression --- metastasis foci;
The third form of expression - is in the process of metastasis of cancer cells, cancer cell clusters and micro-tumor thrombus metastasis.

The goal or target of treatment are also against these three forms:

One for the first form of expression - the primary cancer foci;
Second, for the second form of expression --- metastasis foci;
Three for the third form of expression is being transferred on the way of the cancer cell population.

This new concept is that cancer in the human body exists for the performance of three forms, which is more complete and more comprehensive and clarifies the dynamics, causality and affiliation relationship among the three forms, is a complete and new concept of cancer treatment and a comprehensive explanation of the whole process of cancer development and how to control the whole process of cancer cell metastasis. This new doctrine will bring about the dawn of the fight against cancer.

3). The new concept of cancer metastasis --- "two points on the line"

New understanding: the whole process of cancer development, "two lines." About the treatment of cancer, both at home and abroad in the past and now it only knows and pays attention to the two points and ignores the line. In fact, the treatment of cancer not only should pay attention to two points, but also should pay attention to the front line. To cut off the line is the key to anti-cancer metastasis.

What is the two points and a line? Two points is the starting point of metastasis, the primary foci; and the end point of metastasis, metastatic foci. Line is a route between two points of the primary foci and metastasis foci which a cancer cell in the foci travels a long distance to distant organs (see Figure 7-1)

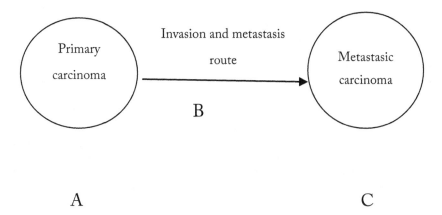

Fig. 1 Sketch Map of Two Points and One Line of Carcinoma Development

Note: A. Primary carcinoma, the starting point of metastasis; B. Invasion and metastasis route; C. Metastasic carcinoma, the end point of metastasis

Traditional cancer treatment often only pays attention to "two", but ignores the "frontline."

XUZE new concept of cancer treatment, both should pay attention to "two points", but also to cut off the front.

In summary we can see, XUZE new concept of cancer not only attach importance to the primary tumor and metastatic foci of surgical resection and radiotherapy, chemotherapy, should pay attention to the transfer of cancer cells on the way to intercept and kill. This is called "two points and a line" of the new theory, its significance is reflected :

The emphasis on anti-metastasis should not only pay attention to "two points", should pay attention to "line." Only to cut off the transfer of cancer cells can improve cancer curative effect.

2. The new concept of cancer therapy

1). The principle of cancer treatment

1)). The cure should be controlled rather than killing

(1) Traditional Therapeutics: cancer is the continuous division of cancer cells, proliferation, so the treatment goal is to kill cancer cells.

(2) The new concept that cure should be through the control rather than kill, the final step in the treatment of cancer is to mobilize the host control role in the reproduction, rather than killing the final cancer cells. Therefore, the medication period (to a certain dose) may kill cancer cells, to obtain temporary relief, but can not kill all and the remnants of cancer cells are still split and proliferation, cancer will relapse.

(3) The basis of the new concept: the experimental study found a new revelation, that is, must be to prevent thymic atrophy, promote thymic hyperplasia, protection of bone marrow producing blood function, improve immune surveillance, control of malignant cell immune escape.

2)). Protection of thymus and increase the immune function(to protect the thymus, increased immune), protect the marrow producing blood (to protect the bone marrow hematopoietic stem cells).

3)) The establishment of a comprehensive treatment concept: the goal of cancer treatment or target, must also target both the tumor and the host, the establishment of a comprehensive treatment concept. In the current country including inside and outside the hospital, chemotherapy is a single kill cancer cells, we believe that this is a one-sided treatment concept, not only does not protect the patient's immune, but also kills a large number of the main immune cells and bone marrow hematopoietic cells, resulting in the more chemotherapy the lower the immune function; resulting in while the side of the chemotherapy is used, the side of the metastasis happens.

4)). Cancer treatment model --- the establishment of multi-disciplinary comprehensive treatment program

The current domestic and foreign hospitals for cancer treatment is to put radiotherapy chemotherapy as the main body, the results still did not prevent recurrence and metastasis.

We propose: full treatment for the spindle: the main surgery + biological therapy, immunomodulatory treatment, integrated traditional Chinese and Western medicine treatment, immune regulation and treatment.

Short-term treatment, supplemented by axis: to put chemotherapy and radiotherapy which cannot be a long course of treatment, not excessive.

2). The principle of cancer metastasis therapy

1)). The key of cancer treatment is anti-metastasis: metastasis is the main cause of cancer deaths, so the transfer is the key to cancer treatment.

The original traditional therapy failed to reduce the long-term high mortality rate, the failure of the main reason is not arming for the metastasis and for controlling transfer.

How to control the transfer? To kill cancer cells in the body should rely on two forces: First, surgery, radiotherapy, chemotherapy, external forces;Internal forces of immune system. The drugs, surgery and all of the treatment technology are important for the patients, but the body's own immune system is more important.

Many problems must be solved by the patient's own strength because the body has a complete set of anti-cancer system.

2)). The third field of anti-cancer metastasis treatment

What is the third area of anti-cancer metastasis treatment? All aim at the third form of cancer in the existing human body --- is cancer cells treatment on the way of the metastasis.

How to kill the metastasis cancer cells on the way of the transfer?

Cancer patients usually have low immune function, especially with the cancer development cellular immune function is becoming increasingly low, but many research results show that, although the tumor-bearing host may have systemic immune deficiency, but in general have a normal T cell response. In animal experiments and clinical research it can stimulate an effective anti-cancer response. The key is how to break the tumor inhibition of the immune system to stimulate the effective, especially in T cell-based immune response.

How to effectively regulate the host immune function and to improve the local immune microenvironment, in order to facilitate the host to play the anti-cancer effect to prevent cancer metastasis and the elimination of residual cancer cells is an important and effective measures for comprehensive treatment of cancer which is an important part.

The circulatory system has a large number of immune surveillance cells.

Cancer cells in the blood circulation are blocked, captured and swallowed by immune cells. Therefore, it can be said that the blood circulation is the main battlefield to destroy the transfer of cancer cells, the immune cells are the effective strength to kill cancer cells.

The circulatory system has a large number of immune surveillance cells can kill and phagocytosis the original cancer cells with heterosexual resistance; combined with the impact of blood flow and shear force, a single crucian cancer cells is difficult to survive; in order to avoid the immune cell chase and kill the cancer cells adhere platelets and attach to the inner wall of blood vessels, endothelial cells in the blood vessels, do amoeba movement, through the microvascular outside settled in the new organs, and gradually form a new metastasis.

3). cancer metastasis therapy "three steps"

How should anti-metastasis be done? The metastasis steps should be understood so that the goal of treatment can become more specific. For these extremely complex, dynamic, continuous multi-step, and multi factor in the process of cancer cell metastasis, the book will summarize the process of cancer metastasis as "eight steps" theory.

In order to get the scientific design, to block the transfer step and to break down each step, based on the molecular mechanism of the "eight steps" and "three-stage" on the transfer of cancer cells, the author designed and formulated measures for various stages of prevention and treatment, known as anti-cancer metastasis therapy "three steps."

In the first step of anti-cancer metastasis the control objectives: to prevent cancer cells into the blood vessels, to reach the purpose "enemy outside the door of the country".

In the second step of anti-cancer metastasis the control objectives: to activate immune cells, to protect thymus tissue function, enhance immune, protect the marrow blood, to promote blood circulation.

The cancer cells in the circulation are captured by the immune cell population, swallowed, surrounded by annihilation.

In the third step of anti-cancer metastasis the control objectives: to improve the local micro-environment tissue immune so that cancer cells are not easy implantation, inhibition of angiogenic factors, inhibition neovascularization-based intervention, suppression measures.

Why? The above-mentioned anti-cancer metastasis therapy "three steps" locate the treatment of cancer metastasis treatment of space in the blood circulation; time locates in three different stages; focuses on enhancing the host immune, regulating local microenvironment.

The important point is to enhance the host immune system, the specific summary can be summarized as Table 7-1 and Figure 7-2.

Table 1 Xu Ze Three Steps of Therapy of Carcinoma Metastasis

Metastasis stage of cancer cell	Metastasis process	Prevention and cure countermeasures
The stage before the cancer cell intrudes the circulation First step of anti metastasis	Separating the cancer cell from the primary cancer→degrading ECM→adherence and de-adherence→movement→before entering the blood vessel.	● anti-adherence ● anti-degradation ● anti-movement ● anti stroma metal protease
Transportation stage of cancer cell in blood circulation Second step of anti-metastasis	The cancer cell group and micro cancer embolus float in the blood circulation and are damaged due to being phagocytized and captured by the immunological cell and be subject to the shearing force of the blood.	● enhancing and activating various immunological cells in circulation, improving the immunologic function as the main battlefield of killing off the cancer cells in the routing of the metastasis ● anti-adherence ● anti-aggregation of blood platelet
The stage in which Cancer cell escapes the blood circulation and anchors "target" organ Third step of anti metastasis	After cancer cell escapes from the blood vessel, it anchors the organ for nidation, forms the new blood vessel and forms the metastatic lesion.	● anti cancer embolus ● TG ● Inhibiting angiogenesis factor ● Inhibiting angiogenesis ● Improving immunological regulation ● Improving the immunity of local microenvironment.

Before the circulation(From the primary tumor to shedding off of tumor cells to adhere to degradation of ECM to movement)

In the circulation(Tumor cells go into the blood vessel to the single cell to tumor groups to tumor thrombus with platelet cells)

↓

After the circulation (move out of the vessel to tumor cell get together to the metastasis foci)

Fig 2 Three stages of anti-cancer metastasis

4). The new concept and method of cancer metastasis of research process are outlined in Figure 3.

New Concept and Way of Treatment of Carcinoma (3)

In 1985, the author surveyed more than 3000 cases of thoracic and abdominal surgeries made by him and found that relapse and metastasis are the key factors that affect postoperative curative effects.

↓

It is necessary to do basic clinical research to prevent relapse and metastasis

↓

The author built a laboratory foe animal experiments

↓

Made cancer-bearing animal model

↓

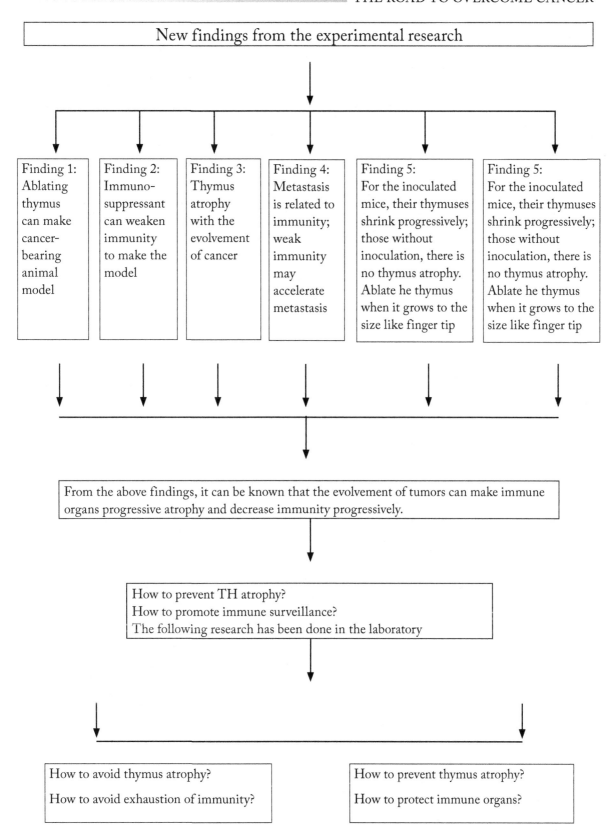

New findings from the experimental research

Finding 1:
Ablating thymus can make cancer-bearing animal model

Finding 2:
Immuno-suppressant can weaken immunity to make the model

Finding 3:
Thymus atrophy with the evolvement of cancer

Finding 4:
Metastasis is related to immunity; weak immunity may accelerate metastasis

Finding 5:
For the inoculated mice, their thymuses shrink progressively; those without inoculation, there is no thymus atrophy. Ablate he thymus when it grows to the size like finger tip

Finding 5:
For the inoculated mice, their thymuses shrink progressively; those without inoculation, there is no thymus atrophy. Ablate he thymus when it grows to the size like finger tip

From the above findings, it can be known that the evolvement of tumors can make immune organs progressive atrophy and decrease immunity progressively.

How to prevent TH atrophy?
How to promote immune surveillance?
The following research has been done in the laboratory

How to avoid thymus atrophy?
How to avoid exhaustion of immunity?

How to prevent thymus atrophy?
How to protect immune organs?

Immunologic reconstitution by adoptive immunity through transplantation of fetal liver, thymus and spleen cell

Look for the medicament that can prevent thymus atrophy and strengthen immunity.

The experimental results indicate that in the group of combined transplantation of S, T, L cells, the complete regression rate in near future is 40% and that of forward future is 46.67%. Those with regression can survive for a long time with good curative effects.

Screen 200 kinds of traditional Chinese medicines by experiments to find out the medicine that can protect thymus and strengthen immunity, promote hematopiesis and resist relapse and metastasis.

Experimental articles can not be published

The experiments for screening in the laboratory: ①screening experiment by the rate of inhibiting tumors in vitro; ②screening experiment by the rate of inhibiting tumors in vivo of cancer-bearing animal model

Screen and look for natural medicament from traditional Chinese herbs through animal experiment.

From a series of experimental research on tumors with cancer-bearing animals over 7 years, there is a deeply-felt that it is necessary to persist in research on resisting cancerometastasis with Chinese characteristics, namely the combination of experimental research and clinical verification. It is essential to do experimental research on tumors, or it is difficult to improve clinical curative effects.

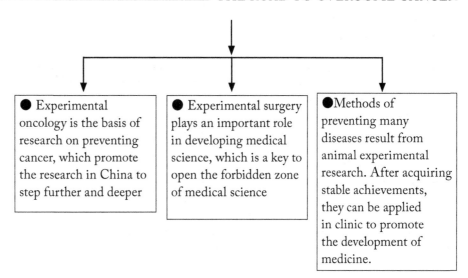

Chapter 8 Series of XZ-C anti-cancer immune regulation drugs

1. Overview

1). The prospect of Immunomodulatory drugs is gratifying and promising

No matter how complex the mechanism behind cancer, immune suppression is a key cancer progression. Removal of immunosuppressive factors and restoration of recognition system cells to cancer cells can effectively resist cancer. More and more evidence shows that by regulating the body's immune system, it is possible to achieve the purpose of controlling cancer. Many researchers in the field are currently excited by activating the body's anti-tumor immune system to treat cancer. The next major breakthrough in cancer is likely to come from this.

In order to investigate cancer etiology, pathogenesis, pathophysiology, we conducted a series of animal studies, the experimental results from the analysis, access to new discoveries and new revelation: thymus atrophy and immune dysfunction is one of the cause of cancer and pathogenesis, therefore Ze (Xu Ze) professor proposed causes of cancer at international conferences, one of the mechanisms that may be thymus atrophy, central immune sensory dysfunction, immune dysfunction, decreased immune surveillance and immune escape ability.

As a result of experimental studies real laboratory findings: in cancer-bearing mice thymus showed progressive atrophy, central immune sensory dysfunction, decreased immune function, immune surveillance decrease so that its treatment principle must be to prevent atrophy of the thymus, to promote thymic hyperplasia and protect bone marrow function improve immune surveillance, which provides an experimental evidence and theoretical basis for the immune regulation treatment of cancer.

Based on the above revelation about cancer etiology, pathogenesis of experimental results, is put forward a new concept and new methods of xz immunomodulatory therapy. After 16 years of oncology clinics in more than 12,000 cases, clinical validation of Advanced cancer patients, confirming that protection of thymus and increase immune function treatment principle is reasonable, the efficacy is satisfactory.

Application of immune regulation medicine has achieved good results, improving the quality of life and prolong the survival.

Professor Xu Ze immune regulation law is that XZ-C(XU ZE-China) first proposed in 2006 in his monograph << new concepts and new methods of treatment of cancer metastasis>> which he believes under normal circumstances the body's defenses and cancer are in a dynamic equilibrium and the cancer is caused by the dynamic balance disorders. If the state has adjusted to normal levels, it can control cancer growth and make it subside.

As we all know, the incidence of cancer development and prognosis, depending on the comparison of two factors, namely, the biological characteristics of cancer cells and the host defense against the body's own cancer-dimensional constraint cells, such as the balance between these two, the cancer can be controlled, if the two of those are imbalances, then the cancer develops.

Under normal circumstances, the host organism itself has a certain capacity constraints against cancer cells, but in cancer patients, these constraints are subject to different levels of defense suppression and damage, leading to the loss of the immune surveillance of cancer cells, immune escape occurred so as to lead to the further development of cancer cells and metastasis.

Through Basic experimental study of investigated the recurrence and metastasis mechanism by more than four years, and after three years of the inherent natural medicine herbal experiment in vivo anti-tumor cancer-bearing mice, herbs selected from a group of traditional Chinese medicine which have better inhibition rate are composed of anti-cancer immune regulation medication $XZ-C_{1-10}$.

2). China's traditional anticancer drug market is developing rapidly

The following excerpts «reference news» column "science and technology frontier" September 10, 2015 published an article, you can see the efficacy of traditional Chinese medicine anticancer and its market prospects.

Bloomberg News reported on Sept. 9:

For years, China, the world's leading cancer powerhouse, has been one of the fastest-growing anticancer drug markets, and now another two-fold increase in the market for antitumor drugs: traditional Chinese medicine.

Traditional Chinese anticancer drugs usually contain some strange ingredients, such as toad skin and shells, etc. According to market research in the Chinese medicine and Pharmaceutical Information (Group) Co., Ltd. estimates that sales of traditional Chinese anti-cancer drugs soared 35% last year, approaching 17 billion Yuan Chinese yuan, an annual growth rate of 17 per cent for the Chinese market with a size of 65 billion yuan, said Richard Yeh, an analyst at Citibank Group.

In 2014, only Livzon Pharmaceutical Group Co., Ltd. production of Shenqi injection which is an anti-tumor and improve the tolerance of chemotherapy drugs, sold 1.3 billion yuan.

China now has become a pioneer in the comprehensive treatment of cancer, even the largest cancer medical centers in the United States are receiving this therapy last week, the Chinese scientific research Personnel confirmed that Shenqi Fuzheng can improve the effectiveness of radiotherapy and reduce side effects in lung cancer patients.

"Traditional Chinese medicine is more used for adjuvant therapy," says Zhao Yingjie, president of the Singapore Chinese Medicine Association and cancer expert. "Clinical practice shows that Chinese medicine can help patients with chemotherapy or radiotherapy go much more smoothly."

Researchers in other countries are eager to test their efficacy, although randomized controlled clinical trials to assess the efficacy and safety of Chinese herbal medicines are being conducted less frequently.

To tap the anti-cancer effects of traditional Chinese medicine, the National Cancer Institute funded numerous research projects, covering the natural ingredients of traditional Chinese medicine, acupuncture and qigong this combination of action, meditation and martial arts of traditional Chinese fitness methods.

In June, researchers at the University of Texas MD Anderson Cancer Center conducted an experiment that showed that hot water extracts from the skin glands of some toads used to treat solid tumors in China can treat non-Hodgkin's lymphoma.

Zheng YQ, a professor of pharmacology at Yale University School of Medicine in New Haven, Connecticut, is conducting a clinical study of herbal formula called PHY906, which was published in March and showed that the formula enhances anti-cancer Effect of Sorafenib, a cancer drug.

Zheng Yongqi said that they are studying that the drug contains a variety of plant ingredients, the effect is more comprehensive, not a single molecule treatment of a specific disease.

3). A series of anti-cancer drug research and clinical verification profile

XZ-C immunomodulatory anticancer medicine are from traditional Chinese herbal medicines which are selected 48 kinds of anti-tumor Chinese herbal medicine with better inhibitory rate. After made up into the composition of the compound, and then tested by inhibiting cancer-bearing mice tumor experiments in cancer-bearing mice experiments, the compound inhibitory rate inhibition rate is much greater than single herbs. $XZ-C_1$, $XZ-C_4$ God grass, agrimony, Shu Yang Quan etc 28 Chinese herbal medicines, of which $XZ-_{C1-A}$, $XZ-C_{1-B}$ 100% inhibit cancer, 100 percent don't kill normal cells, with righting improvment of the role of the body's immune function. From our experiments XZ-C pharmacodynamics, s tudy results show: they has a good inhibitory rate on Ehrlich ascites carcinoma, S_{182}, H_{22} hepatocellular carcinoma; there are obvious synergy and toxicity attenuation; experiments also demonstrated that the immune XZ-C the regulation of traditional Chinese medications have significantly improved immune function.

After the acute toxicity test in mice, no obvious toxicity, no significant side effects for long-term oral clinical taking (2--6 years). XZ-C can significantly reduce the toxicity of chemotherapy while oral immune regulation medications are used with chemotherapy. Oral XZ-C drugs can increase the white blood cells, hemoglobin increased during the Chemotherapy Intermittent periods. Advanced cancer patients mostly have weakness, fatigue, loss of appetite, after taking XZ-C immunomodulatory anticancer medicine 4-8-12 weeks, the patient have more significantly improved appetite and sleep, relieve pain, gradually recuperate see Figure 8-1.

The author has done the following experimental research on the rate of tumor inhibition of traditional Chinese herbs

1. Cultivate cancer cells in vitro to do screen test on the rate of traditional Chinese herbs' inhibition of tumors

(1) screen test on inhibiting tumors in vitro: Cultivate cancer cells in vitro and observe the direct damage of cancer cells by drugs

(2) Screen test inside a test tube: Cultivate cancer cells inside test tubes and add crude drugs (500μg/ml); observe the inhibition of cancer cells

(2) Screen test inside a test tube: Cultivate cancer cells inside test tubes and add crude drugs (500μg/ml); observe the inhibition of cancer cells

Take screen tests on the 200 kinds of traditional Chinese herbs that are thought to have anti-cancer effects by traditional Chinese medicine one by one

Take screen tests on the 200 kinds of traditional Chinese herbs that are thought to have anti-cancer effects by traditional Chinese medicine one by one

Cultivate and test cancer cells with fibrous cell for comparison under the same condition

(3) Experimental results:
1. 48 kinds of traditional Chinese herbs with high rate of tumor –inhibition, other 152 kinds (that are thought to have good anti-cancer effects traditionally) have no effects on inhibiting tumors

Take a further step to make cancer-bearing animal model to do screen test on the rate of inhibiting tumors in vivo

Make the model with cancer-bearing animals inoculated with EAC or S-180 or H22 cancer cells to do screen test on the rate of traditional Chinese herbs' inhibiting tumors in vivo

(1) Screen test on inhibition of tumor in vivo: Make animal model, namely inoculate mice with EAC or S-180 or H22 caner cells

(2) Grouping:
Divide 240 mice into 8 groups in each experiment with 30 mice in a group; the 7th group is for blank control and the 8th group is used as control group with fluorouracil or cyclophosphane

After 24 hours from inoculation, feed the mice with specific dose of rough medical powder in a long period and observe the lifetime and untoward reactions; calculate the percentage of those whose lifetimes are prolonged and the rate of inhibiting tumors

(3) Experimental results:
48 kinds of traditional Chinese herbs do have certain rate of inhibiting tumors and 26 of them have better effects of inhibiting tumors

Optimize and regroup those 48 kinds of traditional Chinese herbs with high rate of inhibiting tumors

Repeat the above experiment and the experiment on immunity

Develop Xu Ze China$_1$~ Xu Ze China$_{10}$ pharmaceutics of traditional anti-cancer Chinese medicine for immunologic regulation and control with Chinese characteristics (XZ-C$_1$~XZ-C$_{10}$)

Figure 8-1 The brief introduction of the research of Z-C immune regulation of anti-cancer medications

① target: to find and to screen anti-cancer, anti-metastatic Chinese herbal medicine from the Chinese medicine;② Objective: To screen out the drug-resistant, high selectivity, non-toxic side effects, long-term oral administration of the "smart anti-cancer drugs"; ③ line: From experimental research to clinical validation, based on the success of animal experiments applied to clinical practice; ④ method: To this end, we had done the Animal Experimental Research of screening new anti-cancer, anti-metastatic drugs that traditional Chinese medicine has 200 kinds of anti-cancer effect of Chinese herbal medicine

1). The research of medication experiments

The author has done the following experimental research on the rate of tumor inhibition of traditional Chinese herbs

1. Cultivate cancer cells in vitro to do screen test on the rate of traditional Chinese herbs' inhibition of tumors

1>> Experimental studies

Our laboratory conducted the following new cancer screening experiment study from traditional Chinese medicine, anti-metastatic drugs:

1. **In vitro screening test:** the use of cancer cells in vitro was observed for cancer drugs directly damage cancer cells. Cultured cancer cells in a test tube, were placed raw meal drug products (500ug / ml) to observe whether there is inhibition and inhibition rate of cancer cells.

2. **In vivo antitumor screening test:** manufacture cancer-bearing animal model for the screening of Chinese herbs for cancer-bearing animal experiments suppressor rate, batch experiments with 240 mice were divided into eight experimental groups, each group 30, para. 7 group was the control group, Group 8 with 5-Fu or CTX as the control group. The whole group of mice were inoculated with EAC or S180 or H22 cancer cells inoculated 24h, the crude product by oral feeding crude drug powder, long-term feeding the herbs screened each mouse was observed survival inhibition rate was calculated.

Our experimental study for four consecutive years, with more than 1000 per year tumor-bearing animal models, four years made a total of two tumor-bearing animal models, mice each were carried out after the death of the liver, spleen, lung, thymus, 'kidney pathological anatomy, in the 20000 times slices.

3. Results: In our laboratory animal experiments after screening 200 kinds of Chinese herbal medicine, the selected 48 kinds indeed carry, even excellent inhibition of cancer cells, the inhibition rate of more than 75-90%. The group of animal experiments made screening test 152 had no significant anti-cancer effect.

2>> Clinical Vertification:

On the basis of successful experiments on animals to clinical validation

1. Methods: built oncology clinics and combination Research Group of anti-cancer, anti-metastasis and anti-recurrence, keeping the medical records, built perfect follow-up and observation system to observe the long-term efficacy and clinical validation. From experimental study to clinical verification means the clinical application on the basis of successful experimental study. Then new problems are found during the clinical application, which need fundamental experimental studies. Afterwards new experimental results are applied to clinical verification. Experiments → clinic → experiments once more → clinic once more, recurrent ascent continuously; through eight-year clinical practical experiences, knowledge also continues to improve. Summation, analysis, reflection and evaluation ascend to theory, putting forward new knowledge, new concept, new thought, new strategy and new therapeutic route and scheme.

Clinical criteria are: good quality of life, longer survival.

Results: XZ-C immunomodulatory anticancer Chinese medicines have significant treatment effect after applying through a lot in advanced cancer patients treated with observation,

2. Clinical information

(1) Hubei Branch of China Anti-cancer Research Cooperation of Chinese Traditional Medicine and Western Medicine, Anti Carcinoma Metastasis and Recurrence Research Office and Shuguang Tumor Specialized Outpatient Department had treated 4, 698 carcinoma patients in Stage III and IV or in metastasis and recurrence with Z-C medicine combined with western medicine from 1994 to Nov. 2002, among which there were 3, 051 men patients and 1,647 women patients. The youngest one was 11

years old and the oldest one was 86 years old, the high invasion age was 40~69 years. All groups of the patients were entirely subject to the diagnosis of pathological histology or definitive diagnosis with ultrasonic B, CT and MRI iconography. According to the staging standard of UICC, all the cases were entirely the patients in medium and advanced stage over Stage III. In this group, there were 1,021 hepatic carcinoma patients, among which there were 694 primary lesion hepatic carcinoma patients and 327 metastatic hepatic carcinoma patients; there were 752 patients suffering from carcinoma of lung, among which there were 699 patients suffering from the primary carcinoma of lung and 53 patients suffering from the metastatic carcinoma of lung; there were 668 gastric carcinoma patients, 624 patients suffering from esophagus cardia carcinoma, 328 patients suffering from rectum carcinoma of anal canal, 442 patients suffering from carcinoma of colon, 368 patients suffering from breast carcinoma, 74 patients suffering from adenocarcinoma of pancreas, 30 patients suffering from carcinoma of bile duct, 43 patients suffering from retroperitoneal tumor, 38 patients suffering from oophoroma, 9 patients suffering from cervical carcinoma, 11 patients suffering from cerebroma, 34 patients suffering from thyroid carcinoma, 38 patients suffering from nasopharyngeal carcinoma, 9 patients suffering from melanoma, 27 patients suffering from kidney carcinoma, 48 patients suffering from carcinoma of urinary bladder, 13 patients suffering from leukemia, 47 patients suffering from metastasis of supraclavicular lymph nodes, 35 patients suffering various fleshy tumors and 39 patients suffering from other malignancies.

3. Medicine and medication: the treatment aims to protect thymus and increase immune system, protect bone marrow so that improve the immune surveillance and to control cancer cells escape. From traditional Chinese medicine the treatment aims are to support healthy energy to eliminate evils, soften and resolve the hard mass and supplement qi and blood. $XZ-C_1$, $XZ-C_2$, $XZ-C_3$, $XZ-C_4$, $XZ-C$ $XZ-C_6$, $XZ-C_7$, $XZ-C_8$, ...$XZ-C_{10}$, according to different kinds of cancers, disease conditions, metastasis situations and according to disease syndrome, choose the above medications. According to the analysis and differentiation of the diseases, anti-cancer powder shall be taken orally and the anti-cancer apocatastasis paste shall be applied externally for the solid tumor or the metastatic tumor. In case of being in pain, anti-cancer aponic paste shall be applied externally. Icterus removal soup or dropsy removal soup shall be taken orally for the patients suffering from icterrus and the ascites.

4. Curative results : The symptom was improved, the quality of life was improved, the survival time was prolonged.

2. The Name and Application of XZ-C Series Anti - cancer Traditional Chinese Medicine

1). First, a series of traditional Chinese medicine name

XZ-C$_1$, also known as: smart talent anti-cancer

XZ-C$_2$, also known as: increasing immune blood anti-cancer

XZ-C$_3$, also known as cancer pain scattered

XZ-C$_4$, also known as: cancer Kang San

XZ-C$_5$, also known as liver cancer scattered

XZ-C$_6$, also known as bladder cancer powder

XZ-C$_7$, also known as lung cancer powder

XZ-C$_8$, also known as: marrow care blood scattered

XZ-C$_9$, also known as: prostate cancer powder

XZ-C$_{10}$, also known as: brain tumor scattered

2). XZ-C Prescription Principles

XZ-C immunomodulatory anticancer medicine XZ-C$_1$, XZ-C$_4$, are compound as a powder, or capsules, the compound is a mixture and multi-flavored powder rather than chemical, so each herb's active ingredients, pharmacological effects is alone and each herb can be individually separated.

XZ-C compound and traditional Chinese medicine or is completely different, after the traditional compound in A, B, C, D boiling component is completely changed, like eating "pot", the original pharmacological effect ofevery taste will lose after every taste boiled together and the original pharmacological effects will lose each flavor, after cooking it is difficult to know what the active ingredient is and to know what the pharmacological effects. Extract the active ingredient compound of boiling after work difficult is very complex technology. And XZ-C drugs are completely different, not boiling, every individual taste was fine grind level, and then mixed in different amounts together (do not have chemical reaction), the pharmacological effects of each herb and its active ingredient completely do not change while retaining all herbs and pharmacological effects of the active ingredient. This is a traditional Chinese medicine formulations reform and innovation.

Why do we use compound rather than single herb because the role of power is not enough, more herbs together have bigger role, such as A = a + b + c + d... then there must be A> a, A> a + b, A> a + b + c, etc., such as its single flavor inhibition rate of 20%, another 30% flavor, taste and then another 31%, and that this inhibition rate of three mixes may be 20 + 30 + 31. That may reach 81%. For improving the immune system, such as the first flavor is 19%, the second flavor 40%, the third flavor 24%, then mixed together of three flavors may be increased to 83%. Holding constant every individual taste is the most important, independent of each herb plays its role in anti-cancer and increase the role of immunity.

Furthermore, xz-c Prescription principles also was set up and selected by the biological characteristics of cancer and cancer metastasis multi-link, multi-step characteristics so that over the years we have achieved remarkable results with long-term taking xz-c immunomodulatory anti-cancer, anti-recurrence and metastasis medications in our anti-cancer specialist outpatient Integrative surgery center while we treat various patients after radiotherapy and after surgery. Many patients with advanced inoperable, or no tolerance through chemotherapy can achieve stable disease, control metastatic spread, improve quality of life significantly prolong survival with long-term taking xz-c immune regulation medicine. Because every herb of xz- C immunomodulatory anticancer medicine has been twice screening for solid tumor-bearing mice in vivo anti-tumor screening, for the first time as a single flavor screened to find out the better inhibition rate, and the second is for selecting the Prescription compound and the selected indicators are three: 1, it has a good anti-tumor effect; 2, without killing the normal cells or the body's toxic side effects; 3, increase immune function. If there is a high inhibition rate, but reduced immune function, it cannot be chosen. In the recently published book "the new concept and new methods of cancer treatment," which specifically for 16 years in our laboratory experiments work in cancer research it confirmed that tumorigenesis, development and recurrence, metastasis have certainly clear relationship with the level of host immune organ function and immune function abilities, may protect the immune organs, enhancing immune medications are more important than the inhibiting or killing cancer drugs. Currently we have recognized that the traditional anti-cancer drugs are not necessarily anti-metastatic and anti-metastasis drugs are not necessarily anti-tumor.

The experimental research and clinical validation observations of XZ-C anti-tumor immune regulation medication show that:

1. There is significant anti-tumor effect with a higher inhibition rate;

2. Have better roles of improving the body's immune function and the experiments showed it can make cancer mouse incomplete atrophy of the thymus and improve immune function;

3. Protect the hematopoietic system and the outer periphery white blood cells, platelets, red blood cells have been significantly improved after chemotherapy drugs inhibit the bone marrow

4. Have a good effect for advanced cancer patients; can significantly change the patient's appetite, sleep, physical and mental state, can significantly improve symptoms, improve quality of life;

5. Have a role in reducing the toxicity in advanced cancer patients with chemotherapy drugs. Its efficacy is superior to the treatment of chemotherapy drugs;

6. In animal experiments there is no toxic side effects. In clinics for 16 years on 16000 patients, especially in many cases of advanced cancer patients the medication were used for a long-term 3--5 years, and some patients even served 8--10 years, it showed no toxic side effects. If the patients have long-term medication adherence, their spirit, appetite, physical strength are good, significantly prolonged survival.

3). Clinical application of several commonly used drugs

(A) XZ-C1 "Smart talent cancer"

[Composition] Long grass, Shu Yangquan etc 8 flavor.

[Indications] Esophageal cancer, stomach cancer, colorectal cancer, lung cancer, breast cancer, liver cancer, cholangiocarcinoma, pancreatic cancer, thyroid cancer, nasopharyngeal cancer, Bladder cancer, ovarian cancer, cervical cancer, a variety of sarcoma and various metastases, recurrent cancer.

[Usage] After Z-C1 continuous service 1-3 months the patient can feel effect and can be long-term use, after serving three years it can be used every other day; after serving for 5 years it can be used 2 twice / week so that immune function, long-term cytokines can maintain stability in a certain level.

2. XZ-C2, also known as: increasing immune and blood anti-cancer drug

[Composition]

[Indications] leukemia, upper gastrointestinal cancer, tongue cancer, laryngeal cancer, nasopharyngeal cancer, esophageal cancer, cervical cancer, bone metastasis, esophageal cancer or gastric cancer after anastomosis recurrent stenosis (no longer surgery); have the effect of acute lymphoblastic leukemia in general, in other types of leukemia have a significant effect; On the control of bone metastases, a more significant effect.

[Usage] generally 1 capsule Qid or 2 capsules tid

Leukemia 3 capsules tid after meal, 7 days for a course of treatment.

3. XZ-C3, also known as: cancer pain scattered

[Composition] Shanai, turmeric and other 14 flavor.

[Anti-Cancer Pharmacology]

1). Qingrejiedu, anti-inflammatory analgesic, qi Sanjie pain;

2). Activating blood stasis, swelling and analgesia, played a total of Qingrejiedu, swelling and pain, and above the most prominent analgesic effect.

3). for acupoint application, simply apply pain which can better play the efficacy and achieve the purpose of rapid analgesic.

[Attending] liver cancer, lung cancer pain, pancreatic cancer back pain, bone pain points, neck, supraclavicular lymph node metastases.

[Usage] a total of research to take bees close amount, mix, stir evenly into a paste spare. For lung cancer spread in the milk root point (nipple straight 5, 6 intercostal); for liver cancer putting on (6 to 7 intercostal spaces), dressing with gauze covered, tape fixed, severe pain for 6h/change dressing, the lesser pain for 12h replacing 1, continuous use until the pain relief or disappear.

4. XZ-C4, also known as: cancer Kang San

[Composition] ginseng, Ganoderma lucidum and other 12 flavor.

[Indications] a variety of cancer, sarcoma, a variety of advanced cancer, metastasis, recurrence of cancer, adjuvant radiotherapy, chemotherapy, postoperative patients, especially dizziness, fatigue, fatigue, lazy words, less gas, spontaneous perspiration, palpitations, insomnia, qi and blood deficiency are more applicable.

[Usage] starting to take medications during preoperative time and after taking the medications every 4 weeks to do a clinical and laboratory tests, for 20 weeks.

Check items: conscious and objective total cholesterol, electrolyte, ALT, AST blood routine and platelet, lymphocyte count, T cells and B cells,

Globulin, urinary protein.

Treatment results: the number of lymphocytes increased, the role of inhibition of leukopenia; ② no effect on liver function; ③ to protect the kidneys, No kidney damage; ④ can significantly reduce the chemotherapy and radiotherapy caused by rash, stomatitis, etc.; ⑤ can have physical recovery effect after surgery, chemotherapy and radiotherapy; can increase appetite, improve body fatigue and increase body weight.

Z-C4 can reduce side effects from the radiotherapy and chemotherapy and improve the overall state of patients after surgery, is a necessary rehabilitation medicine.

4). A variety of cancer using XZ-C immune regulation of anti-cancer series of traditional Chinese medicine formulations

1. A variety of cancers XZ_{C1+4}:[Love with the most]: XZ-C immune regulation of Chinese medicine series

2. lung cancer: XZ-C1 + XZ-C4 + XZ-C7

3. breast cancer: XZ-C1 + XZ-C4 + Mushroom

4. esophageal cancer: XZ-C1 + XZ-C4 + XZ-C2

5. gastric cancer: XZ-C1 + XZ-C4 or + XZ-C5

6. H liver cancer: XZ-C1 + XZ-C4 + XZ-C5 + Scrophulariaceae + red ginseng

7. gallbladder cancer: XZ-C1 + XZ-C4 + XZ-C5 + capillaris

8. pancreatic cancer: XZ-C1 + XZ-C4 + XZ-C5 + XZ-C9

9. knots, rectal cancer: XZ-C1 + XZ-C4 + XZ-C5

10. renal and bladder cancer: XZ-C1 + XZ-C4 + XZ-C6

11. cervical and ovarian cancer: XZ-C1 + XZ-C4 + XZ-C5 + Lms + MDS

12. Lymphoma XZ-C1 + XZ-C4 + XZ-C2 + Dai

13. Leukemia XZ-C1 + XZ-C4 + XZ-C2 + XZ-C8 + Artemisia

14. Prostate cancer: XZ-C1 + XZ-C4 + XZ-C6

XZ-C1: 100% kill cancer cells, do not kill the normal cells; XZ-C4: a "protection of thymus and increased immune function "role, to promote thymic hyperplasia, enhance immune; XZ-C8: "marrow care"

Can ↑ T cell to anti-metastatic. In dawn cancer clinical out-patient clinics all of them have been validated for 18 years, 12,000 cases of advanced cancer, the clinical application can improve the symptoms, good spirits, good appetite, significantly improve the quality of life of cancer patients, prolong survival.

5). Several Chinese medications for cancer complications in out-patient center of cancer treatment:

1. Anticancer eliminate water soup for pleural effusion and ascites

2. Drop yellow soup for liver cirrhosis and jaundice

3. Anticancer soup after surgery for postoperative recovery

4. Starvation soup for cancer loss of appetite

5. Through Quiet soup for anastomotic stenosis

6. Adhesiolysis soup for adhesions after surgery for cancer

3. Mechanism and Application of XZ-C Anticancer Drugs

1). The Action Mechanism

With the deepening of traditional Chinese medicine research, it is known to produce a lot of traditional Chinese medicine and biological activity of cytokines and other immune molecules having a regulatory role, this time to clarify XZ-C from the molecular level immunomodulatory anticancer Chinese medication immunological mechanisms very important.

1. XZ-C immunomodulatory anticancer Chinese medication can protect immune organs, increasing the weight of the spleen and chest pay attention.

2. XZ-C immunomodulatory anticancer Chinese medication for hematopoietic function of bone marrow cell proliferation and significant role in promoting.

3. XZ-C immunomodulatory anticancer Chinese medication on T cell immune function enhancement effect on T cells significantly promote proliferation.

4. XZ-C immunomodulatory anticancer Chinese medication for human IL-2 production has significantly enhanced role.

5. XZ-C immunomodulatory anticancer Chinese medication activation of NK cell activity and enhance the role, NK cells with a broad spectrum of anticancer effect, can anti-xenograft tumor cells.

6. XZ-C immunomodulatory anticancer Chinese medication for LAK cell activity can enhance the effect, LAK cells are capable of killing of NK cell sensitive and non-sensitive solid tumor cells, with broad-spectrum anti-tumor effect.

7. XZ-C immunomodulatory anticancer Chinese medication to induce interferon and pro-inducing effect, IFN has a broad-spectrum anti-tumor effect Wo immunomodulatory effects, IFN can inhibit tumor cell proliferation, IFN can activate the skin to kill cancer cells and OIL cells.

8. XZ-C immunomodulatory anticancer Chinese medication for colony stimulating factor can promote credit enhancement, CSF not only involved in hematopoietic cell proliferation, differentiation, and in a host of anti-tumor immunity plays an important role

9. XZ-C immunomodulatory anticancer Chinese medication can promote tumor necrosis factor (TNF) role, TNF is a class can directly cause tumor cell death factor, its main biological role is to kill or inhibit tumor cells.

2). Principles of clinical application

BRM and BRM-like Z-C immunoregulatory anti-cancer Chinese medicine can enhance the immune response of the body, can strengthen the body's tumor immune surveillance, when the cell mutation or tumor is very small when the effect is good. Through surgery or radiotherapy, Drug treatment can minimize the tumor to the smallest and the best effects.

To have lost the opportunity to surgery, poor physical fitness, can not tolerate radiotherapy, chemotherapy, immunotherapy which the medications have a certain effect, can reduce symptoms and prolong survival time.

After radical resection of the tumor, in order to reduce the recurrence and metastasis, it is feasible to treat Z-C immunoregulation with traditional Chinese medicine. After surgical resection of large tumors, it may be feasible to eliminate possible residual cancer cells and distant cancer cells with Immune regulation of traditional Chinese medicine treatment.

If the tumor can not be removed, it can be treated with radiotherapy or chemotherapy, a large number of tumor cells to kill, so that after the body reduces the tumor load Z-C immune regulation of traditional Chinese medicine treatment can be used.

3). The scope of adaptation

1>> Anti-cancer postoperative metastasis: recover and improve postoperative immune function, improve postoperative quality of life, to kill residual cancer cells after surgery to prevent metastasis, inhibit cancer cell proliferation, prevent recurrence, consolidation and enhance long-term efficacy.

The adaptation: ① a variety of cancer after radical surgery; ② a variety of cancer palliative resection; ③ exploration cannot have resection of advanced cancer surgery; ④ only have gastrointestinal anastomosis or colostomy; ⑤ late cancer cannot have Resection, loss of surgical indications; ⑥ tumor resection + catheter pump after surgery.

2>> to improve the overall quality of life of patients with advanced cancer, prolong survival, inhibition of cancer cell mitosis, control of cancer cell proliferation, improve the overall immune function, mainly against the wide range of the metastasis.

The application scope ① various cancer postoperative short or long term recurrence; ② a variety of advanced cancer, liver metastasis, lung metastasis, brain metastasis, or a cancerous pleural effusion, cancerous ascites.

3>> to alleviate cancer pain: oral or topical Z-C drug treatment of various advanced refractory cancer pain and softening, reducing the body surface metastasis.

4>> with interventional therapy or intubation drug pump treatment, protection of liver, kidney, bone marrow hematopoietic system and thymus and other immune organs, improve immune function and improve the overall immune status after drug treatment, maintenance, consolidation and enhance intermittent and long-term effect to prevent the spread, to prevent the recurrence of a comprehensive improvement and improve liver cancer patients after intervention or intubation treatment quality of life and prolong survival.

5>> with radiotherapy and chemotherapy it can reduce toxicity, enhance treatment and protection of liver, kidney, bone marrow hematopoietic system and immune organs, improve immune function, or white blood cells.

6>> Z-C immune regulation of Chinese medicine and Chinese medicine decoction combination: such as the combination of anti-cancer Shugan Xiaoshui Decoction can be used for the treatment of cancer with ascites or peritoneal metastases of ascites; for the treatment of liver cancer with jaundice; for treatment of liver cancer with high transaminase and HbsAg positive and is used with Shengxue Tang for chemotherapy-induced leukopenia.

4). The application time

Cancer patients are mostly immune dysfunction because after diagnosis the patient is treated by surgery, radiotherapy, chemotherapy, three treatment may further reduce the patient's immune function, the results will reduce the patient's surgery or chemotherapy, radiotherapy endurance, and to reduce the immune surveillance of immune system in patients. Therefore, it should start Z-C immune regulation of traditional Chinese medicine in the operation or in radiotherapy, chemotherapy. Immunotherapy are oral drugs, as long as the patient can eat, oral Z-C Chinese medicine can be used. After 1 to 2 weeks of surgery it can the start. Before radiotherapy, chemotherapy, or post chemotherapy and radiotherapy, and in the gap of chemotherapy and the completion of radiotherapy and chemotherapy Z-C immune regulation of Chinese medicine can be used for a period of time and may be conducive to reduce or control the recurrence and metastasis. This will help reduce the side effects from chemotherapy on ; prevent chemotherapy to reduce immune function and increase the immune function ; promote the bone marrow function, bone marrow production of blood; activate the body's immune system and immune cell system, improve immune surveillance, help to prevent recurrence and metastasis.

Chapter 9 Z-C anti-cancer medicine active ingredients and molecular structural formula

1. Immune Function in Molecular Level of Anti - cancer Traditional Chinese Medicine

With more and deeper researches on traditional Chinese medicine, it has been proved that many kinds of traditional Chinese medicine can regulate and control the production and biological activity of cytokine and other immune molecules, which is meaningful to explain the immunological mechanism of XZ-C traditional Chinese anti-carcinoma medicine for immunologic regulation and control from the level of molecule.

I. Protecting Immune Organs and Increasing the Weight of Thymus and Spleen

That XZ-C traditional Chinese medicine can protect immune organs resulting from the following active principles.

1. XZ-C-T (EBM): Using its 15g/kg and 30g/kg extracting solution (equivalent to 1g original medicine) along with 12.5mg/kg, 25mg/kg ferulic acid suspension to feed the mice for seven days in a raw can increase the weight of thymus and spleen obviously, especially the effects of the group with high dose are more apparent. Intraperitoneal injection of EBM polysaccharide can also alleviate thymus and spleen atrophy obviously caused by perdnisolone.

2. XZ-C-O (PMT) Extract PM-2, feed the mice with 6g/(kg·d) PMT decoction for successive seven days which can increase the weight of thymus and celiac lymph nodes and antagonize the reduction in the weight of immune organs caused by perdnisolone. Drenching the mouse of 15 months old with 6g/kg decoction (with the concentration of 0.5g/ml) for 14 days can increase the weight and volume of thymus, thicken the cortex and raise cellular density apparently. The combined use of PM and astragalus root can promote non-lymphocyte hyperplasia and benefit the micro environment of thymus.

3. XZ-C-W (SCB) SCB polysaccharide can gain weight of thymus and spleen of a normal mouse. Lavage with it enables cyclophosphane to control the gain in the weight of thymus and spleen.

4. XZ-C-M (LLA) Drench a mouse with LLA decoction for seven days resulting in increasing the weight of thymus and spleen.

5. XZ-C-L For a 15-month old mouse, its thymus degenerates obviously. Astragalus injectio can enlarge the thymus significantly. The cortex under microscope is thickened and the cellular density increase obviously.

II. Effects on Proliferation, Differentiation and Hematopiesis of Marrow Cells

The following active principles of XZ-C traditional Chinese medicine have effects on hematopiesis of marrow cells.

1. XZ-C-O(PMT) extract(PM-2)and

2. XZ-C-Q (LBP) (1)Effects on the proliferation of hematopoietic stem cell (CFU-S) of a normal mouse: inject PM-2 with the dose of 50mg/(kg·d)×3d or 10mg/(kg·d)×3d LBP into the experimental mice respectively by venoclysis and kill them in the ninth day. It can be found that the number of spleen CFU-S in the group with administration increases obviously. The number of CFU-S in group PM-2 is 121% higher than that of the control group and it is 136% in the group with LBP.(2)Effects on colony forming unit of granulocytes and macrophages (CFU-GM): the experimental results indicate that LBP with the dose of 5~30mg/(kg·d)×3d can increase the number of CFU-GM and PM-2 can also strengthen the effect of CFU-GM with the effective dose of 12.5~50mg/(kg·d)×3d. In the early stage of cultivation, most CFU-GMs are units of granulocytes and then units of macrophages increase gradually. In the anaphase units of macrophages take over the dominance.

From the above experiment, it can be found that PM-2 and LBP can promote hematopiesis of normal mice obviously. The experiment proves that during the process of restoring hematopiesis damaged by cyclophosphamide, PM-2 and LBP stimulate the proliferation of granulocytes at first, and then marrow karyocytes multiply; at last these two promote the restoration of peripheral granulocytes.

3. XZ-C-D (TSPG) Ginsenoside, which is the active principle of ginseng to promote hematopiesis, can bring the recovery of erythrocyte in peripheral blood, haemoglobin and myeloid cell of thighbone in the mice of marrow-inhibited type, increase the index of myeloid cellular division and stimulate the proliferation of myeloid hematopoietic cell in vitro so as to make it into cell cycle with active proliferation ($S+G_2/M$ stage). TSPG can promote the proliferation and differentiation of polyenergetic hematopoietic cells and induce the formation of hemopoietic growth factor (HGF).

4. XZ-C-H (RCL) Steamed Chinese Foxglove can promote the recovery of erythrocyte and haemoglobin for animals with blood deficiency and accelerate the proliferation and differentiation of myeloid hematopoietic cell (CFU-S) with the effect of predominance and hematosis significantly. Peritoneal injection of rehmannia polysaccharides for successive six days can promote the proliferation and differentiation of myeloid hematopoietic cells and progenitor cells as well as increasing the number of leucocytes in peripheral blood.

5. XZ-C-J (ASD) ASD polysaccharide has no effects on erythrocytes and leucocytes of normal mice, but for those damaged by radiation, injection of ASD polysaccharide can influence the proliferation and differentiation of both polyenergetic hematopoietic stem cells (CPU-S) and hemopoietic progenitor cells. But its decoction has no obvious effects.

6. XZ-C-E (PEW) Poria cocos (micromolecule chemical compound extracted from Tuckahoe polysaccharide) is the active principle that can strengthen the production of colony stimulating factor (CSF) and improve the level of leucocytes in peripheral blood inside the mouse's body. It can also prevent the decline in leucocytes caused by cyclophosphamide and accelerate the recovery with the effects better than sodium ferulic which is used to increase leucocytes.

7. XZ-C-Y (PAR) Its polysaccharide can obviously resist the decline in leucocytes caused by cyclophosphamide and increase the number of myeloid cells to promote the proliferation of myeloid induced by CSF as well as the recovery and reconstitution of hematopiesis for the mice irradiated by X ray. It can also increase the number of hematopoietic stem cells and myeloid cells along with leucocytes.

III. Enhancing Immunologic Function of T Cells By Z-C immune regulation medications

The active principles of XZ-C traditional Chinese medicine and their effects are following.

1. XZ-C-L (LBP) It can raise the percentage of lymphocytes in peripheral blood obviously. The LBP in small dose (5~10mg/kg) can cause the proliferation of lymphocytes, indicating that LBP can promote the proliferation of T cells apparently. 50mg/(kg·d)×7d is the best dose in that it will have no effects if lower than the level and it will bring the effects down if higher than the level. Oral administration of LBP can raise the conversion rate of lymphocytes for the sufferers who are weak and with fewer leucocytes.

2. XZ-C$_4$ It can regulate immune system and active T cells of aggregated lymphatic follicles, as well as stimulate the secretion of hemopoietic growth factor in T cells. Among the crude drugs of XZ-C$_4$, the extract from the hot water of atractylodes lancea rhizome can obviously stimulate the cells of aggregated lymphatic follicles, which is regarded as the base of XZ-C$_4$ immunoloregulation.

IV. Activating and Enhancing NK Cell Activity By Z-C immune regulation medications

Natural killer cell, NK cell is another kind of killer cell in lymphocytes for human beings and mice, which needs neither antigenic stimulation, nor the participation of antibodies to kill some cells. It plays an important role in immunity, especially in the function of immune surveillance as NK cell is the first line of defense against tumors and has broad spectrum anti-tumor effects.

NK cell is broad-spectrum and able to kill sygeneous, homogenous and heterogenous tumor cells with special effects on lymjphoma and leucocytes.

NK cell is an important kind of cells for immunoloregulation, which can regulate T cells, B cells and stem cells, etc. It can also regulate immunity by releasing cytokines like IFN-α, IFN-γ, IL-2, TNF, etc.

The active principles in XZ-C traditional Chinese medicine and their effects are following.

1. XZ-C-X (SDS)

Divaricate Saposhniovia Root can strengthen the activity of NK cells of experimental mice. When combined with IL-2, it can make the activity of NK cell higher, indicating that its polysaccharide can give a hand to IL-2 to activate NK cells and improve the activity.

LBP can strengthen T cell mediated immune reaction and the activity of NK cells for normal mice and those dealt by cyclophosphamide. Peritoneal injection of LBP can improve the proliferation of spleen T lymphocytes and strengthen the lethality of CTL increasing the specific lethal rate from 33% to 67%.

2. XZ-C-G (GUF)

Glycyrrhizin can induce the production of IFN in the blood of animals and human beings and strengthen NK cell activity at the same time. Clinical tests made by Abe show that after intravenous injection of 80mg GL, the raise of NK cell activity reaches 75% among 21 sufferers. Peritoneal injection of 0.5mg/kg GL on mice can strengthen the activity of NK cells in liver.

3. XZ-C-L (AMB)

Its bath fluid can promote NK cell activity of mice both in vivo and in vitro, and can also induce IFN-γ to deal with effector cells under the certain concentration of 0.1mg/ml. Cordyceps sinensis extract can strengthen NK cells activity of the mouse both in vivo and in vitro. Fluids with the concentrations of 0.5g/kg, 1g/kg and 5g/kg can strengthen NK cell activity of mice.

V. Effects on LAK Cell Activity By Z-C immune regulation medications

Lymphokine activated killer cell, namely LAK cell can be induced by IL-2 cytokine. LAK cells can kill the solid tumors that are both sensitive and insensitive to NK cells with broad anti-tumor effects.

The active principles in XZ-C anti-carcinoma traditional Chinese medicine and their effects are following.

1. XZ-C-L (AMB)

Its polysaccharide can strengthen LAK cell activity within a certain range of dose with 0.01mg/ml being the most effective, which is three times better than the damage effects of LAK cells. The concentrations of both higher and lower than this level can not achieve the effects.

2. XZ-C-U (PUF)

It can significantly strengthen the spleen LAK cell activity of killing tumor cells and improve the activity of erythrocyte C3b liquid. PUF and IL-2 are synergistic that can be used as regulator for biological reaction in tumor biological therapy based on LAK/Ril-2.

3. XZ-C-V

ABB polysaccharide can also raise LAK cell activity for the mouse and inhibit tumors remarkably. Its anti-tumorous mechanism relates to its strengthening immunity and changing cell membrane features.

VI. Effects on Iterleukin-2 (IL-2) By Z-C immune regulation medications

The active principles in XZ-C anti-carcinoma traditional Chinese medicine and their effects are following.

1. XZ-C-T

EBM polysaccharide can enhance obviously the production of IL-2 for human beings when the concentration is 100ug/ml. At higher concentration (2500ug/ml and 5000ug/ml), it will lead to inhibition. Hypodermic injection of barrenwort polysaccharide for seven days in a row can significantly improve the ability of thymus and spleen of the mouse induced by ConA to produce IL-2.

2. XZ-C-Y

PAR polysaccharide has strong immune activity and is able to promote the production of IL-2. For the mouse bearing S-180 tumor, it can raise the ability of spleen cells to produce IL-2 obviously。

3. XZ-C-D

Ginseng polysaccharide has great promotion on IL-2 induced by peripheral monocytes for both healthy people and sufferers with kidney troubles. The effects are relevant to the dose positively.

VII. Function of Inducing Interferon and Promoting Inducement of Interferon By Z-C immune regulation medications

IFN are broad-spectrum in resisting tumors and can regulate immunity. It can also inhibit the proliferation of tumor cells and activate NK cells and CTL to kill tumor cells. Meanwhile, IFN can cooperate with TNF, IL-1 and IL-2 to enforce anti-tumorous ability.

The active principles in XZ-C anti-carcinoma traditional Chinese medicine and their effects are following.

1. XZ-C-Z

250mg/kg or 500mg/kg CVQ polysaccharide can improve significantly the level of IFN-γ produced by mouse spleen cells.

2. XZ-C-D

Ginsenoside (GS) and panaxitriol ginsenoside (PTGS) can induce whole blood cells and monocytes of human beings to produce IFN-αand IFN-γ. It can also recover the low level of IFN-γand IL-2 to the normal.

The IFN potency of ASH polysaccharide on S-180 cell line of acute lymphoblastic leukemia and S_{7811} cell line of acute myelomonocytic leukemia produced after acanthopanax polysaccharide stimulation is 5~10 times more than that of normal control group.

3. XZ-C-E

Hydroxymethyl Poria cocos mushroom polysaccharide has many kinds of physical activity like immunoloregulation, promoting to induce IPN, resisting virus indirectly and alleviating adverse reaction resulting from radiation. Do IFN inducement dynamic experiment on S-180leukaemia cell line by using 50mg/ml Hydroxymethyl Poria cocos mushroom polysaccharide. The results indicate that its potency to induce interferon at all stages is better than that of normal inducement.

4. XZ-C-G (GL)

It can induce IFN activity. Make peritoneal injection of 330mg/kg GL on mice. IFN activity reaches the peak after 20 hours.

VIII. Function of Promoting and Increasing Colony Stimulating Factor By Z-C immune regulation medications

Colony stimulation factor, namely CSF is a kind of glucoprotein with low molecular weight that can stimulate the proliferation and differentiation of marrow hematopoietic stem cells as well as other mature blood cells. Cells that can produce CSF include mononuclear macrophages, T cells, endothelial cells and desmocytes. CSF not only take part in the proliferation and differentiation of hematopoietic stem cells and regulating mature cells, but also play an important role in anti- tumorous immunity of host cells.

The active principles in XZ-C anti-carcinoma traditional Chinese medicine and their effects are following.

1. XZ-C-Q

PAR polysaccharide is able to promote to produce CSF by spleen cells of experimental mice. 100~500ug/ml PAP-II can encourage spleen cells to produce CSF depending on the dose and time with the fittest dose of 100ug/ml and best time of 5d. Moreover, lentinan can also increase the amount of CSF.

2. XZ-C-Q

Injection of LBP can facilitate the secretion of CSF by mouse spleen T cells and improve the activity of CSF in serum.

3. XZ-C-T

EBM icariin can promote the proliferation of mouse spleen lymphocytes induced by ConA and bring CSF activity.

IX. Function of Promoting TNF By Z-C immune regulation medications

Tumor necrosis factor, namely TNF is a kind of cytokine that can kill tumor cells directly. Its main effect is to kill or inhibit tumor cells, which can kill some tumor cells or inhibit the proliferation both in vivo and in vitro.

The active principles in XZ-C anti-carcinoma traditional Chinese medicine and their effects are following.

1. XZ-C-Y (PEP)

It can induce the production of TNF, so as PEP-1. Inject 80~160mg/kg PEP-1, once every four days. Collect peritoneal macrophages (PM), add 10ug LPS into culture medium to cultivate PM. Take the supernatant to determine TNF and IL-1. It can be found that PEP-1 can parallelly increase the auxiliary production of TNF and IL-1. The time of TNF inducement reaches the peak on the 8th day after the second intraperitoneal injection. Compared with the known startup potion BCG, the inducement of TNF has no difference.

2. XZ-C-E

Carboxymethyl-pachymaran (CMP) is the principle essential component distilled from traditional Chinese medicine Tuckahoe. It can not only strengthen the ability of mouse spleen to create IL-2 and macrophages and promote the activity of T cells, B cells, NK cells and LAK cells; but also encourage the production of TNF. The experiment proves that CMP is an effective potion to promote and induce cytokines.]

3. XZ-C-V

ABB polysaccharide can promote the production of TNF-b in mouse cells induced by ConA. It can also induce the synthesis of peritoneal macrophages and secrete 20ug/ml TNF-αachyranthes bidentata polysaccharides. The time of TNF-α to reach its peak is 2~6 hours after effects. Peritoneal injection of 100mg/kg achyranthes bidentata polysaccharides can accelerate the production of TNF-α, whose intensity of effects is comparable to that of BCG.

X. Effects on Cell Adhesion Molecule By Z-C immune regulation medications

Most adhesion molecules are glycoproteid and are distributed on cellular surface and extracellular matrix. Adhesion molecules take effect in the corresponding form of ligand-acceptor, resulting in the adhesion between cells, or between cell and stroma, or the adhesion of cell-stroma-cell. These molecules take part in a set of physical pathologic processes, like cellular conduction and activation of information, cellular stretch and movement, formation of thrombus as well as tumor metastasis, etc. Intercellular adhesion molecule-1, namely ICAM-1 is one kind of adhesion molecules in the super family of immune globulins.

The effect of Z-C immune regulation on ICAh4-1

The effective ingredients of Z-C immune regulation: The effect of corn stigma as an active principle in XZ-C traditional Chinese anti-carcinoma medicine:

Hobtemariam has proved that alcohol extract from corn stigma has significant inhibition on the adhesion of endothelial cells to inhibit effectively the expression of ICAM-1 and the adhesive activity with TNF, LPS as agents. The main pharmacological effects (see Table 9-1)

Table 9-1 Summary table of the main pharmacological effects of Z-C immune regulation anticancer Chinese herbal medicine (anti-cancer and increasing immune)

	Increased white blood cells	Enhanced phagocytosis	Enhance cellular immune	Enhance humoral immune	Enhanced hematopoietic function	Improve gastrointestinal function	(subtotal)	Enhance the weight of the thymus	Promote bone marrow cell proliferation	Enhanced T cell function	Enhanced NK cell activity	Enhanced LAK cell activity	Enhanced IL-2 activity levels	Enhance the level of interferon IFN activity	Enhanced TNF activity levels	Enhanced CSF colony stimulating factor	Antagonistic WCBYC ↓	Inhibition of platelet coagulation and antithrombosis	(subtotal)	Antitumor	Anti-metastasis	Antiviral	Anti-cirrhosis	Liver protection	Eliminate free radicals	Protein synthesis	Anti-HIV	(total)
Z-C-A-APL																				+	+							
Z-C-B-SLT																				+	+							
Z-C-C-SNL																				+	+							
Z-C-D-PGS	+	+	+	+	+	+	6	+	+	+	+			+	+	+	+	+	9	+	+	+			+	+		20
Z-C-E-PCW		+	+				2	+	+				+	+	+	+	+		7	+	+	+						12
Z-C-F-AMK		+	+	+	+	+	5				+			+		+			3	+		+		+				11
Z-C-G-GUF		+	+	+		+	4				+			+			+		3	+		+		+		+		11
Z-C-H-RGL	+	+		+			3		+	+				+	+		+		5	+					+			10
Z-C-I-PLP	+	+	+	+	+	+	6		+	+							+		3	+		+				+		12
Z-C-J-ASD	+	+	+	+	+		5	+	+	+				+	+	+	+	+	8	+				+				15
Z-C-K-LWF		+	+				2								+			+	2	+	+							5
Z-C-L-AMB	+	+	+	+	+		5	+	+	+	+	+	+	+					7	+		+			+			5
Z-C-M LLA	+	+	+	+			4	+		+									2	+					+			5
Z-C-N-CZR		+					1									+		+	2	+	+							5
Z-C-O-PMT	+	+	+	+	+	+	6	+	+	+							+		4	+		+	+	+	+	+		16
Z-C-P-STG							0												0	+								1

Z-C-Q-LBP	+	+	+	+	+	5		+	+	+	+	+		+	+	+	8	+	+				4		16
Z-C-R-NSR		+				1	+			+							+	3	+	+		+	+			8
Z-C-S-GLK	+	+	+	+	+	5			+		+	+	+	+		+		6	+	+			+		+	+	16
Z-C-T-EDM	+	+	+	+	+	5	+		+			+	+		+	+		6	+		+			+		14
Z-C-U-PUF		+	+	+		3		+	+	+								3	+			+				8
Z-C-V-ABB						1		+	+	+			+					4	+							6
Z-C-W-SCB	+					1	+									+		2	+			+	+			5
Z-C-X-SDS						0			+	+	+							3	+							4
Z-C-Y-PAR						0			+	+	+		+	+				5	+							6
Z-C-Z-CVQ						0					+							1	+							2

2. The Study on the Structure and Anti-tumor Effect of Z-C Anti-Cancer Traditional Chinese Medicine

The Study on the Antitumor Composition and Function of Z-C Anti - cancer Traditional Chinese Medicine

Z-C1 - A ApL

Anti-tumor components: agrimonniin

Effective parts: the whole plant for the plants.

Anti-tumor effect: Okucla other scholars isolated out agrimonniin from ApL grass which has proven to be the main component. Before and after inoculation MM2 breast cancer cells, 10mg /kg of this product is given by ip, the results were all tumor are rejected. No matter how it was given by P.O. or I.P., it can prolong survival time in tumor-bearing animals. Agrimonniin can inhibit MH 134 liver cancer and sarcoma Meth-A cellulose growth. With or without calf serum medium, MM2 breast cancer cells and agrimonniin together for 2h, then for 48h at 37 humidified CO_2 incubator, and found time without calf serum, agrimonnii on breast cancer cells showed MM2 strong cytotoxicity, and its IC50 is 2.66ug / ml, but adding fetal calf serum in the culture medium, then weakened to around 4% of the original, namely an IC50 of 62.5% ug / ml, after intraperitoneal injection of agrimonniin 4d, the absorption of H3-thymine on MM2 breast cancer and MH134 hepatoma cells was obviously inhibited.

These results indicate that agrimonniin is a potent anti-tumor acid and its anti-tumor effect may be due to the drug action on tumor cells and enhance the immune re ApL grass produces 1: 1, PH6.5 (1g crude drug / ml) solution by water extraction method to inhibit $_{S180}$, cervix U_{14}, brain tumors B_{22}, Ehrlich EAC, melanoma B_{10}, rats W_{256}

cancer. The results show that for more than transplanted tumors better inhibition, the inhibition rates were between 36.2 -6.59%, $P<0.05$, there is a significant difference.

ApL grass water extract has a strong inhibitory effect on human JTC-26 canein vitro and inhibition rate reaches 100% and meanwhile it promotes the growth 100%. While 30mg / kg ApL grass phenol was injected daily in intraperitoneal cavity, it has a significant therapeutic effect on rat sarcoma S_{37} and cervical cancer U_{14}. The inhibition rates on tumor growth were 47.0% and 38.7%. The inhibition was 47.4% on sarcoma S_{180} mice with 0.625g / day and was 52.6% on liver cancer.

Fluid extracted from liver cancer ascites was diluted with sterile physiological water 1-2x10⁷/ml, then inoculated into mice, each mouse by intraperitoneal injection 0.2ml, the next day were randomly divided into treatment group and control group 30mg / ApL grass phenol was injected in intraperitoneal cavity once daily for 7 days, saline was injected in control group, then observed 30 days to calculate life span. Results: the mean survival day was 26.2 disabilities 0.9 in 24 animals treatment group; the average rival was 17.5 + 1.3day in control group. Life span prolonged above 49.6%. ApL grass phenol has significantly prolong life in animal liver cancer ascites carcinoma.

Z-Cl - B SLT

Anti-tumor components: p-SoIamarine
Structure:

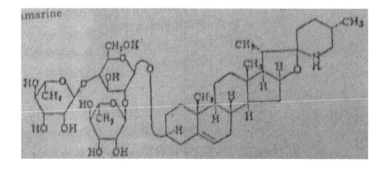

Effective parts: the SLT whole plant.

Anti-tumor effect: the whole plant has anti-tumor effect, in many countries for a long time as a folk medicine to cure cancer, p-Solamarine its active ingredient, at 30mg / kg on S_{180} mice the tumor weight from control group 1285 mg reduced to 274mg, the Inhibition rate was 78.6%.

The whole plant has anti-cancer effects on human lung cancer.

The studies have reported recently, extracted from the SLT anti-tumor active ingredient o health foods, it has given anti-tumor effect and almost no toxicity. SLT also contain solanine Australia which has inhibitory activity on S_{180} mice.

Recently it has been reported: an effective anti-tumor ingredient was extracted from SLT through water or an organic solvent or a mixture of water capacitive solvent, then be made into oral or parenteral medication: the oral dose serving as 1g /d; the parenteral drug as 60mg / d. The drug can inhibit a variety of tumors, such as S_{180} neck cancer with its low toxicity. Murakami Kotaro etc isolated two different body sugar from SLT, each with some anti-tumor effect.

SIT can inhibit S_{180}, cervical cancer U_{14} and Ehrlich ascites carcinoma. In vitro the product of hot water extract can has inhibition rate 100% on human cervical cancer JTC-26 system. And there was no effect on normal cells; in vivo experiments on mice S_{180} inhibition rate was 14.57%. This product contains an effective anti-cancer ingredient β-bitter solanine which significantly inhibited mice S_{180} and W256 mouse cancer.

Z-C1-C SNL
Antitumor Ingredient A: Vitamin A
Structure:

Existing parts: the whole plant for an amount of 9666 IU%.

Anti-tumor effects: vitamin A(Va) has anti-tumor activity. Wald had conducted a survey in 1975-1979, indicating Va having anti-tumor effect in vivo; Bontwell found that Va can stop cell membrane mucopolysaccharides aggregate effect induced by tumor promoters and block the receptor which bindstumor promoters. A new method for cancer treatment: normal sugar plus LETS (large cells are transferred outside sensitive protein from), two of which are affected Va material synthesis, which shows Va is important in cancer treatment. Meanwhile, Va and their derivatives can reverse cancerous cells inducedv by chemical carcinogens, viruses, and ionizing radiation.

Antitumor Component B: Vitamin C(Vc)
Structure:

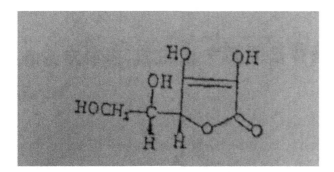

Existing parts: the whole plant for the plant, its content is 20mg%

Anti-tumor effects: Vc is antioxidants in anti-tumor effects in blocking nitrite and primary amine to synthesize carcinogenicity compounds in vivo. Cameron will use 10g / day Vc to hundred cancer patients from long-term, 42 times of higher efficacy than control group and has better effect in gastrointestinal cancer. Murata use Vc high-dose to treat cervical cancer and its effect is 5.7 times higher than the effect of small doses. Malistratos induced sarcoma growth with benzo, then treat them with lots of Vc. Vc inhibited sarcoma growth and occurrence. For bladder cancer and skin cancer, it has the preventive effect. In epidemiology cancer occurrence is also related with the intake of Vc.

Vc with various anticancer drugs in combination can increase the efficacy of the drug. As with Vincristine (VCR) it has a synergistic effect and V + CCNu have higher treatment efficacy than single CCNu in leukemia. The survival time extencle: twice, but also alleviate the condition of patients with advanced cancer. Cisplatin anticancer drugs, because of its toxicity and the larger application subject to certain restrictions, if Vc their combination, can reduce toxicity. New Jersey now Englehard company Hollis developed a cisplatin and Vc mixture composition which has better efficacy.

The whole plant contains Solasonine and solanine which also have activity against S_{180} sarcoma. Nigrum extract of dried green fruit of total alkali Solanum nigrum can inhibit animals transplanted tumor system by 40- 50%. In tissue culture 50-500mcg/ml 24h total alkali Solanum nigrum inhibit meningioma cells growth. Alkali component isolated from total alkali Solanum nigrum has the strongest antitumor activity and there are significant cytotoxicity. 10mcg / ml 15h concentration causes cells to collapse. A total extract also has inhibition effect on mice ascites sarcoma S_{180}. Solamine also be used as hematopoietic system stimulant, increasing leukocyte. barbata and comfrey it was used to treat malignant mole and the result is good. With surgery, chemotherapy, radiation it was used to treat uterine choriocarcinoma, -_in cancer, liver cancer and had effectiveness.

This product can inhibit cervical cancer U_{14} and S_{180}, Ehrlich ascites carcinoma and -hosarcoma, Ehrlich ascites carcinoma, L_{615} lymphatic leukemia, S_{180}, gastric cancer cells and leukemia in mice, etc

SNL has anti-cancer effect on nuclear division. Extract of SNL has inhibition rate of -50% on animal transplanted tumor. In tissue culture 50-50Oug/ ml 24 hr total SNL can inhibit brain tumor cell growth.

Z-C-D PGS
Anti-tumor components A: β-Elemene
Structure:

Existing parts: the root of the volatile oil and flowers of about 10%.

Anti-tumor effects: The product has significant anti-tumor effect on ECA and ARS etc transplanted animal ascites and S_{180} ascites.

Anti-tumor component B: PGS total polysaccharides:

Anti-tumor effects: animal experiments show: PGS total polysaccharides have a stimulating effect on immune function. It inhibit mice transplanted tumor S_{180} to a certain extent and significantly inhibited Ehrlich ascites tumor cells in mice at 400-800mg / kg. PGS polysaccharide doesn't directly kill many tumor cells; its anti-tumor effect may be due to the adjustment of the body's immune function so that =or-bearing hosts enhance antitumor capacity. There are also reports: PGS total - polysaccharide is administered at 460.620mg / kg / d in S_{180} abdomen the inhibition of tumor weight was76.81% (P <0 001.).

Another report, PGS total polysaccharides have some anti-tumor activity, its system may be induced tumor necrosis factor: PGS total polysaccharides on normal mice d tumor-bearing mice can enhance immune function and activation, PGS total polysaccharides also inhibit cancer cell growth.

Anti-tumor components C: PGS saponin Ginsenoside
Formula formula :

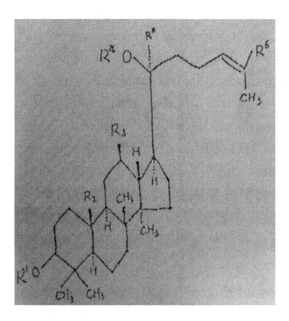

Anti-tumor effects:

On mouse sarcoma S_{180} it had significant inhibition at 120mg / kg/d x7 and the inhibition rate of its tumor weight was 60.48%; on Ehrlich ascites carcinoma (ECS) at a dose of I00mg / kg / d x70, its inhibition rate was 36.40%; on S_{180} at a dose of 100 mg / kg / dx10 its inhibition rate was 41-61% (P <0.05); large doses on U_{14} also have some anti-tumor effect.

With chemotherapy drugs CXT used in conjunction, it can enhance the anti-tumor effects of chemotherapy drugs.

Its anti-tumor effect is more complex; one, it can act directly with the cancer cell- -that the cancer cell growth was inhibited or be reversal. Second, it can also regulate the body metabolism and the immune function to resist diseases so that the tumor growth was inhibited. National and international clinical trials have proved: it has therapeutic effect on gastric cancer, not only reduces tumor; but also increases appetite, improves immunity and prolongs patients' survival time.

PGS soap component as a human anti-tumor agents, adapt to a wide range, almost no side effects. The application ranges: gastric cancer, colorectal cancer, breast cancer, uterine cancer, mouth, esophagus, gallbladder cancer, kidney cancer, lung cancer, brain cancer, liver cancer, skin cancer, etc., are valid for almost all tumors. The mode of administration: it can be taken orally at 100-300mg/day x2-3 doses. It can also used 1-10% of hydrophilic or hydrophobic ointment topically.

Korea Atomic Energy Research Institute Nguyen and other reports: Application -- carcinogens in laboratory animals treated, serving long red ginseng can reduce the incidence of cancer and inhibit tumor growth. Small Tajima and other reports: cultured hepatoma cell PGS soap can change the cancer cell structures indicating PGS can induce cancer cells to be reversed. Hiroko Abe and other reports: PGS saponin induced reversal to hepatic cancer cells. Li xianggao believes: PGS soap can inhibit 3-O- methyl glucose through the cell membrane and overflow on liver cancer cells so presumably the inhibition of membrane transporters of PGS saponin may non-specific.

In addition to the relevant ginseng root soap antitumor activity studies, ginseng flower total inhibition has also been reported: Yuyongli and other scholars studied, the effect of a total ginseng flower soap on NKC-IFN-IL-2 regulatory network

and inhibition of tumor Effect. The results showed that: PGS total promote natural killer activity in vitro mouse spleen, and in the presence of Con-A induces the production of Y-IFN and IL-2, indicating the total soap flower PGS has regulation -KC-IFN-IL-2 network to regulate the immune function by this adjustment extensive network.

Liang Zhongpei etc applied PGS to study how dimethyl buttery yellow sugar induced rat liver cancer. The results showed that: PGS can increase the percentage of ANAE e lymphocyte cells, reduce the incidence of liver cancer, the tumor is smaller, a degree of differentiation of cancer cells, the longitudinal fibers hyperplasia and cute infiltration around tumor tissue, indicating that PGS should be able to promote immune function so that it has prevention or control action to the chemical carcinogen-induced liver cancer.

Ginseng inhibits variety of experimental animals. Ginseng had reduced tumor incidence nor growth inhibition after rats and mice were fed with ginseng long-term for aflatoxin-induced rat lung adenomas, urethane-induced lung cancer in mice. Its main anti-tumor ingredient is Ginseng saponin of which ginseng saponin Rg3 can - inhibit tumor formation of new organs, inhibit tumor recurrence, proliferation and metastasis in mouse melanoma and S_{180} tumor. The inhibition rate was 60% and on a variety of animal and human tumor lung metastasis, liver metastasis the inhibition ached 60% -70%. Ginseng saponin Rg3 is promising as anti-metastatic drugs.

Z-C-E PCW
Antitumor points A, Adenine
Structure:

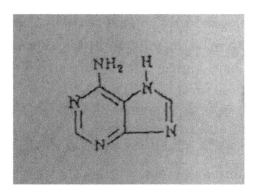

The presence of areas: plant sclerotia.

Anti-tumor effect: for the prevention and treatment of various leukopenia, particularly caused by chemotherapy, radiotherapy and benzene poisoning. Its phosphate stimulates - blood cell hyperplasia. It was found that Leukocyte recovered about 2-4 weeks after administration. It can extend the time of chemotherapy and prevent the occurrence of leukopenia if used before chemotherapy or simultaneously.

Anti tumor B: Pachyman
Structural formula:[13-D-Glcp- (1.-3) a 13-D.-Glcp- (1 - 3)] n

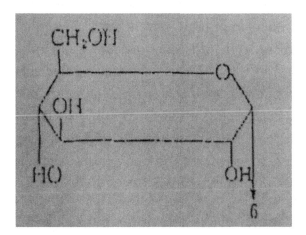

Antitumor effects: Studies have shown that: new Pachymaran: in 1970 Chihara etc slightly transform pachyman structure into pachymaran of removing the side chain β (1--6) with significant anti-tumor activity, but the poor water-soluble activity.

Carboxymethyl Pachymaran was synthesized by Hamuro etc. in 1971 with pachymaran carboxymethylation which has significant anti-tumor activity in animal experimeriments.

Hamuro, J and other experiments proved: new biological Pachymaran of pachyman such as CM-pachymaran and HM-pachyman 2-4, have significant anti-tumor actin activity of its agents and routes of administration have a great relationship and the appropriate route of administration of the optimal dose must be selected.

About pachyman antitumor mechanism of action and its derivatives, it has also reported: think no direct cytotoxicity; however through the host's intermediary it played anti-tumor roles which enhance the body's immune system.

Chaoqiaoli etc. observed inhibition of carboxymethyl Pachymaran mouse lung metastasis of inbred uterine cancer U_{615}. The results show that the non-transfer 64% tumor control group were 94%; metastasis inhibition rate of 75.68%, significantly higher than the control group, the experimental group tumor weight, inhibition rate was 23.58%, the above results suggest that: indeed carboxymethyl Pachymaran has some anticancer activity.

Data reported also: carboxymethyl tuckahoe polysaccharide is a good immune enham: and apply the treatment of various tumors.

Patent No. 4339435 reports: A Poria sclerotium obtained cultured mycelium, tilt-the mycelium of the water or that the water-soluble organic solvent such as ethanol extraction, to obtain an anti-cancer medicament "A-1", it is not only very good anti-cancer activity and no toxicity, 92% inhibition of the S_{180}, this anti-cancer substance accounted for 24.2% cultured mycelia. Xu Jin et al reported that a group of fat-soluble organic tetracyclic three, collectively known as Poria factors was isolated from Pachyman and significantly inhibited Ehrlich ascites carcinoma, S_{180} metastasis of Lewis lung carcinoma in mice. When administered with Cyclic amines and phosphorus, there is a certain synergy and it proved Poria increases immune function.

In 1986 Japanese scholars Jinshan isolated a water-soluble anti-tumor polysacchariL called Pachymaran H11 from cultured mycelia of Poria, accounting for about 0.69c dry mycelium. With 4mg / kg injection JCR / TCL mice subcutaneously x10 days S_{180} the inhibition rate was 94%, this report shows that there have been polysaccharide which has anti-cancer activity with no structural transformation in Poria.

There are also reports, after Poria cocos contained β- polyester (β-pachyman) was treated and approached to obtain Poria cocos glycan complex (abbreviated UP), it had a significant anti-tumor effect and the inhibition rate was 57%. It can extend tumor-mice survival time, improve the spleen index, and it has a direct effect on cancer cells.

Wu Bo and other scholars also conducted experiments to observe PPS's anti-tumor effect and mechanism on mouse S_{180} cells and human leukemia cells K5G2. It was that PPS has a strong suppression effect and discusses its anti-tumor mechanism of S_{180} cell membrane composition. The results showed that after PPS contacts with cells 24h, the membrane phospholipid content decreased and cell membrane sialic content increased, but the membrane cholesterol content, membrane fluidity membrane fatty acid composition is not affected. When PPS membrane put together with S_{180} under appropriate conditions, it was found that PPS interference of membrane of inositol phospholipid metabolism is critical step. Changes related to PPS antititumor mechanism and biochemical characteristics also have some reports. PPS significantly inhibited DNA synthesis in mouse L_{1210} cells with irreversible inhibition increased with the dose.

Poria has anticancer drug synergistic effect : on mitomycin and using inhibitory (mouse sarcoma S_{180}) was 38.9% (5-Fu alone 38.6%) ; in mouse leukemia L1210 cyclophosphamide alone amines life extension of 70%, combined with phosphorus domide was 168.1%.

PPS and thymus-related anti-tumor effect. Polysaccharides can nonspecifically stimulate the reticuloendothelial system function and enhance the host of cancer-specific antigen immunity to resist the effects of cancer.

Pachymaran with Poria known significant anti-tumor effect, can inhibit the growth solid tumors, extend survival time in mice S_{180} and Ehrlich ascites carcinoma. Pachymaran has distinct anticancer roles on cultured mouse sarcoma S180 cells and human chronic myelogenous leukemia K562 cell. Antitumor mechanism includes two aspects of increased immune system and direct cytokine roles. Antitumor mechanism y be suppressed by inhibiting tumor cell nuclear DNA synthesis and enhance production of tumor necrosis factor (TNF) from macrophage and the ability to enhance or cell killing effect.

Intraperitoneal injection of polysaccharides (PPS) 5-200mg / kg continuous 100, above 10mg, it inhibited S_{180} significantly. On S180 sarcoma in mice and Ehrlich ascites cinoma (EAC) orally taken 8d, it can enhance tumor necrosis factor (TNF) levels and significantly increase natural killer (NK) cell activity.

It significantly inhibited lung metastasis from U_{14} after mice were fed carboxymeth-. tuckahoe polysaccharide (250mg / kg/d) 25d. The mouse sarcoma S_{180} cells were seeded in ICR / JCL mice subcutaneously, 24 hours later 5mg / kg polysaccharides once daily once 10 days injected intraperitoneally. The results showed that inhibition rate was 95%.

Carboxymethyl Pachymaran strongly inhibited U_{14} in mice. Using 500mg / kg, 100mg / kg, 50mg / kg, the result of inhibition rate was 75.5%. 92.7% 78.7%, respectively, which 100 mg / kg dose was the best. Intraperitoneal injection carboxymethyl tuckah polysaccharide 100mg / kg/ d 10d extended lifetime was 23.49% compared with control in Ehrlich ascites carcinoma. It reduced the amount of ascites 7%, reduced total number of cancer cells 139.20%. PPS can inhibit DNA synthesis in Ehrlich ascites tumor cells. The inhibition role of PPS is related to the dose which using 100 / 50mg / kg, 5mg / kg 3 the results of tumor inhibition rates were 92.3%, 96.1%, 53.4%.

Z-C1-G GuF
Anti-tumor components A: Glycyrrhiza acid
Structure:

Existing parts: wooden grass roots, rhizomes.

Antitumor effects: The product can produce morphological changes on rat hepatoma and Ehrlich ascites carcinoma (EAC) cells and inhibit subcutaneous Yoshida sarcoma. Licorice as raw material soluble Monoaniniornum glycyrrhetate, namely licorice acid amine, can inhibit Ehrlich ascites carcinoma and muscle tumor. Meanwhile, licorice acid amine has some detoxification for certain toxic of anti-cancer drugs. Natural products such as having a certain anti-tumor effect: Caniptotliecine causes toxic reactions and limits the use of drugs, but a licorice acid amine can lower camptothecin toxicity by not reducing its efficacy and having a certain synergy. On animal experiments: the number of white blood cells caused by camptothecin, Glycyrrhizinate amine has protective effect.

This product is hot-water extract on human cervical cancer cells JTC-26 and inhibition rate is 70%- 90%.

Anti-tumor component B: Gycyrrhetinic aicd Struture:

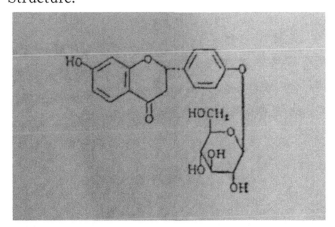

Existing parts: the herbal roots, rhizomes.

Antitumor effects: glycyrrhetinic acid inhibited transplanted Oberling-Guerin myeloma on rat. Its sodium salt has been inhibition on the growth of mouse Ehrhlich ascites carcinoma and sarcoma -45, even orally.

Anti-tumor components: Liguirtin

Structure:

Existing parts: the root herbal.

Antitumor effects: The product can inhibit morphological changes and also have anti-rumor effect on rat hepatoma and Ehrlich ascites carcinoma cells and rat mammary tumor. It has the preventive effect on rat stomach cancer, can reduce the incidence of rastric cancer. In addition, grass sweetener has inhibited aflatoxin B1-induced hepatic precancerous lesion.

Z-C-K LwF

Antitumor points: (Tetrainethylpyrazine, TTMP)

Anti-tumor effects: TTMP can inhibit TXA2 synthetase activity. Li Xue Tang et al reported: TTMP administered once has a certain anti-metastatic effect on hepatoma cell metastasis. Jin Rong and other reports: TTMP anti-tumor effect and its mechanism, the experimental results show that: TTMP at 20mg/d x 18d could significantly inhibit the artificial lung metastasis in B16-F10 melanoma and TTMP can enhance normal and tumor-bearing spleen NK cell activity in isotope incorporation assay in mice and antagonized cyclophosphamide inhibition of NK cell activity. TTMP anti-metastatic effect may be related to reduce plasma TXB content and to enhance NK cell activity.

Some academics have also been reported: isolated from this plant gland (Adenine), its pharmacological activity has been confirmed that stimulate white blood cell proliferation, prevent fine thrombocytopenia, particularly for leukopenia caused by radiotherapy or chemotherapy. TTMP has a certain anti-metastatic effect on liver cancer cells.

Z-C-L AMB
Anti-tumor component B: p-Sitosterol
Structure:

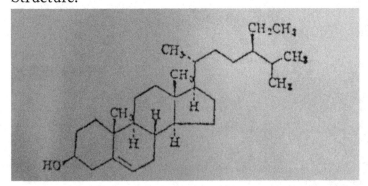

Existing parts: The root of the plant.

Anti-tumor effects: p-Sitosterol has an edge activity for lymphocytic leukemia P134; has effect on mouse adenocarcinoma 715, which inhibition rate of tumor weight (TWI) was> 58%; it has effects on Lewis lung carcinoma, its TWI was > 58%; for the rat carcinoma Wacker cancer 256 its TWI was > 58%.

Reports: AMB roots have in a certain amount of polysaccharide; AMB polysaccharide contains 1.34-2.04% and there are several polysaccharides. It has broad biological activity and has anti-tumor effect in vivo, but does not directly kill cancer cell in vitro which means that AMB polysaccharide works by enhancing immune function.

AMB can improve human and mouse plasma cAMP levels, can inhibit tumor growth, and make tumor cells even reversed; can promote animal leukocytosis; can recover leukopenia induced by chemotherapy or radiotherapy; can promote immune function and inhibit tumor cell killing effect. The inhibition rate of its water extract was 41.7% in vivo experiments on mice sarcoma -180. The alcohol extract AMB is currently used clinically as an anticancer drug righting.

ZhouShuYin reported: the results of AMB polysaccharide show in vivo experiments: APS 2.5mg/kg, 5mg/kg, 10mg/kg, 20mg/kg significantly inhibited on transplanted tumor S_{180} liver cancer; in vitro results showed that: APS and interleukin-2 can significantly improve the compatibility of applied rate LAK cell killing target cell P851 and Yae cells. Its anti-tumor mechanism is related to increasing immune function.

In vivo the inhibition rate of AMB hot extract was 41.7% on mice sarcoma S180; was 12.25% on human lung adenocarcinoma SPC-A- 1. The inhibition index Iodized oil was induced with MCA human-mouse lung which the injection group with MCA was 16.28%, the control group was 51.52% cancer, the difference is very significant. MCA can inhibit DNA synthesis in human ovarian cancer cells. When the concentration increases, the inhibition will strengthen and the duration of action of the drug will prolong and inhibition of DNA synthesis of cancer cells also will be enhanced. MCA polysaccharides have synergies on T lymphocyte activation at malignant ascites.

Z-G-M LIA

Fight tumor components: Ursolic acid
Structure:

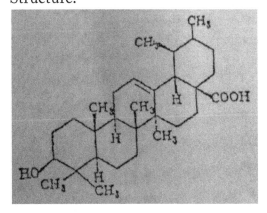

Exist parts: the leaves of the plant.

Anti-tumor effect: it has a very significant inhibition rate on cancer cells in vitro culture and can prolong the life on Hershey ascites carcinoma mice.

Pharmacological experiments show that: the goods flooding agent can inhibit certain animals transplanted tumor growth; it can increase immune function; it can recover leukopenia induced by chemotherapy and radiotherapy. There are also reported thr the active ingredient in this product is Oleanic acid.

Z-C-N CzR
Anti-tumor component A: Turmeric alcohol Curcumol
Structure:

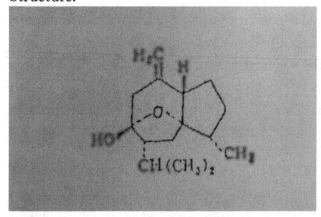

Exist parts: roots for the plants.

Anti-tumor effects: Curcumol has anti-tumor effect. At 75mg/kg the inhibition rate -Nis 53.47-61 .96% on mice sarcoma S37; at 75ug/kg the inhibition rate was 45.1-77.13% on mice cervical cancer U14; the inhibition rate was 65.8- 78.9% at the same doses on EAC. There is better effect on treating cervical cancer.

Antitumor Component B: Turmeric dione /Curdione
Structure:

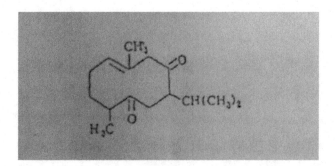

Exist parts: roots for the plants.

Antitumor effects: turmeric significantly inhibited mouse sarcoma 37, U_{14} and neck cancer and mouse Ehrlich ascites carcinoma and can make cancer cells degeneration end necrosis. After this product is processed in Ehrlich ascites carcinoma it can be successfully immunized mice to obtain initiative. The clinical results indicate that cervical cancer has a good effect.

There are also reports: In its same plant Curcuma wenyujin Y.H. Chen etc isolated β-elemene which has anti-cancer activity. The research proved that β-elemene could significantly prolong the survival time on Ehrlich ascites carcinoma and ascites reticulocyte cell sarcoma in mice and has strong killing effect on liver cancer cells in vitro. It also reduced nucleic acid content on EAC, especially in RNA content decreased more significantly. On leukocyte and bone marrow nucleated cells and Immune test: β-elemene has relatively small toxicity.

100% 0.3-0.5ml of Curdione has a good effect and the inhibition rate reached over 50% when it was injected to mice abdominal in S_{180}.

Z-C-Q LBP

Antitumor components:. Lycium burbarum Polysaccharides LBP Structure: The main components are arabinose, glucose, galactose, mannose, xylose, rhamnose and other components. Exist parts: to have come from the fruit.

Anti-tumor effect: Wangbekung etc proved: LBP enhanced immune function on normal mouse cells. At 10mg / kg it can improve the immune function and have inhibitory effect on S180 tumor-bearing mice, and synergistic anti-tumor effect with chemotherapy cyclophosphamide. There are also reports: LBP has a certain influence on the immune function. Lu Changxing and other reports: LBP showed significant radiosensitization with radiotherapy.

In addition, its roots and skins have Betaine, which also have anti-cancer function: with D-isoascorbic together it can inhibit mitosis in vitro on sarcoma 37, Ehrlich cancer and lymphoid leukemia L1210 which is stronger than alone medication. LB P contained (3- sitosterol, ascorbic acid, etc. which has anti-tumor effect.

There are also reports: LBP and interleukin-2 have the regulation effect on two anti-tumor LAK activity.

Z-C-R

Panax pseudo-Wall, var.notoginseng Hooet Tseng

Anti-tumor components: Notoginsenoside R1

Effective parts: that the roots of plants.

Antitumor effects: 180 µg/ml 5 days Panax saponin R can induce 68% HL-60 cell differentiation which proved Panax saponin R1 is a strong inducer of HL-6 0 cell lines and can induce HL-60 neutrophil cell differentiation. H-TdR incorporation assay results show: notoginsenoside R1 can induce differentiation of HL-60 cells while it affects DNA and RNA synthesis. There are also reports: during Cr release assay with soap studied Panax test it induced mouse spleen activity against tumor; have a strong anti-tumor effect with ConA / PHA together. Further experiments showed that soap Panax has no stimulation on proliferation of splenocytes, but changes the level of intracellular CAMP in spleen cells.

Z-C-Z1

Corioius versicolor Quel.

Anti-tumor components: Polysocohaitibe-piptide

Structure: a, R (1-4) dextran as main chain of Polysaccharide with 15% protein and kinds of amino acids

The presence of site: mycelium body

Antitumor effects: target cells: human gastric cancer cell lines (SGC79O1); hum:- lung adenocarcinoma fine lines (SPC); human monocytic leukemia cell line (SLY human skin cell lymphoma cell lines (MEI)

In vitro inhibitory test of PSK Application the results showed that: PSK has moderate inhibition of proliferation at a concentration dose 1000ug / ml on human lung adenocarcinoma cell line (SPC). The Japanese scholars shared PSK (Kiestin) has effects on sarcoma 180, liver AH-13, AH-7974, AH-66F, leukemia P388 in vivo by intravenous, intraperitoneal, subcutaneous, or oral administration and has almost no toxicity. Its mechanism is to improve the immune function through "host agency" role.

Li Jian and other scholars in the report: versicolor extract has no inhibition on ascites hepatoma on subcutaneously transplanted mouse while it has significant effects on the subcutaneous mouse ascites sarcoma S_{180}.

In clinical the extracellular polysaccharide PSK is used on primary liver cancer and alone n improve the clinical symptoms and prolong life, anticancer drugs; in combination with antitumor drugs it also reduces the toxic side effects of antitumor drugs. Japanese vood has developed into proteoglycan "PSK" anti-cancer drugs.

Lentinus edodes Sing

Anti-component A: Lentinan

Structure: The structure of p-D- (1 3) glucan backbone, C-6 has two fulcrum of every D- glucosyl, connecting p-D- (1 6) and p-D- (13) glucose branched-chain, also containing small amounts p-D- (16) branches.

Existing parts: its fruiting bodies.

Anti-tumor effects: Lentinan has some anti-tumor effect and improve the body's immune function. At a dose of 0.2, 1, 5, 25mg /kg, the daily cavity injection for consecutive 10 days, the inhibition rates were 78, 95.1, 97.5 and 73% on S180. It can Increase their compatibility of anti-tumor effect with chemotherapy drugs.

Lentinan can induce DNA synthesis and immune globulin and interferon-inducible, and non-specific cell-mediated cytotoxic effect in human peripheral mononuclear cells (PMNC, mainly lymphocytes); can enhance the cytotoxic response of NK cells of NK cell activity is very low and even absent in Leukemia patients; the general immune enhancer treatment increases the risk of cancer of the white blood cells. Lentinan can Increase the activity of NK cells. It induced β-IFN which has stronger anti-cancer effect than α and β -IFN, can enhance the phagocytic activity of white blood cells in patients with hormone production. At the same time, it can prevent patients with cancer from bacteria and viruses infection.

Shiio T et al reported: LNT and chemotherapeutic agents together can inhibit tumor metastasis in mice which the effect is the best when it is administrated after the surgery. Fachet T et al found Lentinan and their preparations A/ph(A/ph B10) F1hybrid mice A/ph, MC, S1 fibrosarcoma have significant anti-tumor alivity; however, Lentinan does not directly affect tumor growth in vitro. Shiio T et al also studied the inhibitory effect of Lentinan on cancer lung metastasis; intravenous Lentinan can inhibit Lewis system cancer (3LL), melanoma (B6) and fiber sarcoma (ML-CS-1) transfer.

Chapter 10 Clinical Data of XZ-C Immunoregulation in Treating Cancer

1. Statistics Table of Some Case Information(The epidemiologic study)

(We keep all of our patients' epidemiologic information and life habits and clinical information in detail in order to understand the cancers)

1) The Table of Some Cases of Treated liver cancer

Table 10-1 Statistics and Treatment of Hepatocellular Carcinoma Patients A

Number	Name	Medical record	Gender	Age	Native place	Occupation	Address	Diagnosis	in accordance with	Unit	Society habit			
											Smoking year	Amount of Smoking	Drinking years	Alcohol consumption
1	Shixx	x	M	57	Zhaoyan	Farmer	Zaoyang	Liver cancer	(CT, MRI) 98/6/22	Zaoyang City Hospital	30	1-2 packages a day	30	3-4 oz / per
2	Lan xx	x	M	35	Dawu	Teacher	Dawu	massive liver in liver right lobe	CT (98/08)	Dawu County Concord hospital			10	
3	Lunxx	x	M	38	Danyang	Land management cadre	Dangyang	After right liver cancer surgery	U/S, CT (98 /07)	Concord hospital	6-7	little		
4	Liu xx	x	M	30	Gongan	engineer	Gongen	massive liver cancer	U/S, CT (98/0707)	County Hospital Ezhou City Hospital	More than 10	One package/ day	10	2-3 oz / meal
5	Zhen Xx	x	M	50	Zhongyan	Farmers	Zhongxiang	primary liver cancer	CT (98/08)	Zhongxiang City People's Hospital				
6	Ke xx	x	M	54	Hongshi	Agricultural Bank staff	Yellowstone	liver cancer	CT (98/08)	Yellowstone Hospital Concord Medical hospital	More than 30	1-2 package/ day	More than 10	8oz / meal
7	Shong Xx	x	M	37	Yinchen	headmaster	Ying city	massive liver cancer	U/S, CT, MRI (98/07/01)	Ying City People's Hospital Concord Hospital				
8	Yanxx	x	M	51	Eizhong	Attending physician	Ezhou	After liver cancer surgery	U/S, CT(98/09)	Ezhou City Hospital Concord hospital				

#	Name		Sex	Age	Origin	Occupation	Location	Diagnosis	Exam	Hospital				
9	Jiangxx	x	M	57	Henan	Radio station welder	Xiaogan	massive liver cancer	U/S(98 /02 /10)	Sanjiang spaceflight Red Star Hospital Association	20	One package	More than 10	One pound/meal
10	Zhangxx	x	F	64	Shanhai	Accountant	Wuhan	hepatobiliary and pancreatic cancer with metastasis lung	U/S, CT(98 /0/25)	Railway Hospital				
11	Lixx	x	M	36	Huangpi	Farmer	Huangpi	left liver cancer with gallbladder invasion	U/S(98/07)	Union Hospital	10	2-3 package		
12	Wangxx	x	M	47	Wuhan	Cement factory worker	Wuhan	left liver cancer after surgery with lung	U/S(98/04)	Tongji Hospital	10	2 Package/day	10	often
13	Yangxx	x	M	46	Tongchen	Security Section	Wuhan	primary liver cells cancer	U/S, CT(98 /09/13)	Wuhan Second Hospital Concord hospital	20	12 cigrettes/day	10	
14	Yan xx	x	F	56	Tiangmen	Farmer	Tanmen	primary liver metastases	U/S, CT, MRI (98/05)	Concord Hospital				
28	Liu ixx	x	M	40	Zhaoyan	Cadre	ZaoyangZaoyang City Xiangyang Road Hongqi Village	Primary liver cancer	CT	Zaoyang City Hospital and concord hospital	20	40 cigarettes/per day	20	8 oz
29	Zheng xx	x	M	61	Henan	Selfemployed	Henan Huaiyang Beimen Township Jia camp aluminum factory	multiple liver cancer	CT	Henan Zhoukou Hospital	Decades	40 cigarettes/per day	several decades	8 oz
30	Wang xx	x	M	40	Shandong	Teacher	Wuhan Electric Power School	Liver cancer	U/S, CT	Concord hospital		5-6 cigarettes/day		
31	Xie xx	x	M	57	Gangxi	Professor	Wuhan xx	Metastasis liver cancer	U/S, CT	Concord hospital				
32	Zhen Xx	x	M	60	Zhanggan	Cadre	Huaxing	primary liver cancer	CT	Concord hospital	More than 20	20 cigarettes/day		
33	Cheng xx	x	M	49	Zhanggang	Cadre	xxx	The liver lumps in right lobe of Liver cancer and ascites	CT, U/S	Concord hospital			20-30 years	16oz
34	Liu Xx	x	F	65	Yinchen	headmaster	Ying city	Primary massive liver cancer	CT	Concord hospital	5-6years	10 cigarettes/day		
35	Zhangxx	x	M	66	Eizhong	Attending physician	Ezhou	Primary liver cancer	U/S, CT	Air force Hospital	40 year	20 cigarettes/day		

311

36	Hongxx	x	F	54	XX	Worker	xxxx	Liver cancer with bile duct bleeding	Pathology slides	Concord hospital				
37	Qing xx	x	M	58	Hongen	Cadre	Wuhan	Primary diffuse Liver cancer	U/S, CT	People Hospital	20	20 cigarettes/day		
38	Songxx	x	M	62	Enhui	Cadre	xxx	Multiple liver cancer	U/S, CT	Concord Hospital	10	2-3 package		
39	Huang xx	x	M	59	Hanchun	Peasant	xxx	Multiple diffuse liver cancer	U/S, X-ray and CT	Tongji Hospital	20-30	20 cigarettes/day		
40	Zheng xx	x	M	32	Hebei	Cadre	xxx	primary diffuse liver cells cancer	U/S, CT	Tongji Hospital	10	20 cigarettes/day	10	4oz
41	Wuxx	x	M	55	Shanghai	Cadre	XX	primary liver left lobe cancer	U/S, path slide	City three Hospital				

Table 10-1 Statistics and Treatment of Hepatocellular Carcinoma Patients B

Number	Water pickles	Salt pickles	Smoked meat	Dried salted fish	Dry pickle	sausage	Fried food	chili	garlic	onion	fresh vegatables	fruit	Fried food	Green tea	Strong tea	Other	The method of drinking water	meat	Ribs soup	Vegetarian food	General	Tension overcharged	Cheerful	Dull and irritable	Whether to love sports
1		√		√							√		√		√		well water	√ fatty meat							
2	√	√		√			√			√		√		√		Unsolicited water						√		√
3					√	√	√					√		√		Unsolicited water							√	No
4					√	√√	√					√		√		Unsolicited water						√		
5	√	√		√	√		√			√		√		√		Pool water						√	√	
6					√	√	√					√		√		Well water	√					√		
7												√		√		Unsolicited water	√			√		√	√	No
8												√		√		Well water							√	

Number	Water pickles	Salt pickles	Smoked meat	Dried salted fish	Dry pickle	sausage	Fried food	chili	garlic	onion	fresh vegatables	fruit	Fried food	Moldy food	green tea	Strong tea	other	Drinking Water	meat	Ribs soup	Vegetarian food	General	Tension overcharged	Cheerful	Dull and irritable	sports
9							√	√										Unsolicited water	√ fatty meat			√	√	√	√	No
10			√		√					√	√							Unsolicited water			√		√			
11								√										Unsolicited water	√	√		√	√		√	
12									√									Unsolicited water				√		√		No
13		√			√	√	√			√	Eatingmoldyrice							Unsolicited water	√	√	√	√	√	√	√	No
14	√						√											Well water	√√	√		√		√		No

Number	Wether to eat often														Wether to drink often			Drinking Water	Wether to eat often			jobs		characters		Whether to love sports
	Water pickles	Salt pickles	Smoked meat	Dried salted fish	Dry pickle	sausage	Fried food	chili	garlic	onion	fresh vegatables	fruit	Fried food	Moldy food	green tea	Strong tea	other		meat	Ribs soup	Vegetarian food	General	Tension overcharged	Cheerful	Dull and irritable	
28																					√		√			
29					√					√		√									√			√		
30					√																			√		No
31							√	√√	√	√	√	√			√			Unsolicited water						√		
32	√	√		√	√							√						Sugar water				√	√			
33							√	√		√			√					Well water	√					√		

34									√					water Unsolicited	√			√	√		√	No
35							√				√			water Well						√		
36									√	√			√	water Unsolicited	√ fatty meat	√	√	√	√			No
37							√							water Unsolicited		√		√		√		
38							√							water Unsolicited	√	√		√	√		√	
39						√								water Unsolicited				√		√		No
40		√			√	√	√		√	√	Eating moldy rice			water Unsolicited	√	√		√	√	√	√	No
41	√						√							water Well				√	√		√	No

Table 10-1 Statistics and Treatment of Hepatocellular Carcinoma Patients C

Number	Chronic disease History	Family three generation of cancer history	Application of pain medication situation			Mass reduction and disappear situation after medications	
			Disappear	Reduction	effective	Tumor location and size	Lump shrinkage after medication
1	In 1991 suffering from pleurisy and removing out the yellow liquid	No			√	In 98/06/22 Check 2 placeholder 1-3cm range in liver	

2	In junior high school suffering from jaundice hepatitis, Liver function is normal, in 1998 acute jaundice hepatitis	Father died because of esophageal cancer			98 /08/18 right palpable 12 x 10 cm2	Reducing to 11 × 8 cm2 in 98/08/30 on Physical exam
3	In 1983 had hepatitis B, in 1991,1996 and 1997 hepatitis B +	No				
4	Hepatitis B positive with nosebleeds history	No			On 1998/07/10 CT showed 2.5× 2.5 × 3cm3 in liver side leaves and 10 x 5 x 9 cm3 in right lobe of liver	
5	In 1989 found a large number of ascites and recurrent schistosomiasis in follow-up check health, had checked Hb-SAg (+), and sometimes negative	The third brother had liver cancer without removing; and extensive metastasis and Intubation did not work, 3 months after surgery, this brother died in 1983			In 1998/08 the right lobe of the liver was 8X 10 cm2	
6	check for schistosomiasis; in 1970 Tuberculosis cured	no				
7	In 1983 treatment with hepatitis B half Year and had been delayed intermittent service medicine	no			In 1998/07/01 liver right lobe 8.7 ×7.1cm2 size	
8	2 months ago checked hepatitis B	the father had cardia cancer, in 1997 death			98/09 liver mass 4. 3 ×4.4cm2 size	
9	In 1967 had hepatitis B in Sanyang hospitalization For three months and treatment did not turn negative; Tuberculosis has calcified; gastric ulcer	No			98/02/10 U/S showed 15 × 4 × 12cm2 lesion in hepatic right lobe	
10	Diabetic	No			98/09/29 Ultrasonographic liver right lobe 2.5x2.4 cm2; pancreatic head 3× 3.1 cm2	

11	Had a history of schistosomiasis for seven years with three positive in small lobe and not treated	No				98/08/03 CT showed in left liver 4.3× 9.9cm2	
12	In 1983 had acute jaundice liver Inflammation and had hospitalization for one month, sometimes liver area had pain, cholecystitis	Father died because of liver cancer					
13	In 1984 acute jaundice liver Inflammation, hospitalization for one month; after one month relapse	No					
14	In 1960s and 1970s has three hospitalization for histosomiasis late stage; endoscopy showed anemia gastric mucosa like	No					

Number	Chronic disease History	Family three generation of cancer history	Application of pain medication situation			Mass reduction and disappear situation after medications	
			Disappear	Reduction	effective	Tumor location and size	Lump shrinkage after medication
28	In 1991 suffering from pleurisy and removing out the yellow liquid	No		√		In 98/06/22 Check 2 placeholder 1-3cm range in liver	
29	In junior high school suffering from jaundice hepatitis, Liver function is normal, in 1998 acute jaundice hepatitis	Father died because of esophageal cancer				98 /08/18 right palpable 12 x 10 cm2	Reducing to 11 × 8 cm2 in 98/08/30 on Physical exam

30	In 1983 had hepatitis B, in 1991,1996 and 1997 hepatitis B +	No					
31	Hepatitis B positive with nosebleeds history	No				On 1998/07/10 CT showed 2.5× 2.5 × 3cm3 in liver side leaves and 10 x 5 x 9 cm3 in right lobe of liver	
32	In 1989 found a large number of ascites and recurrent schistosomiasis in follow-up check health, had checked Hb-SAg (+), and sometimes negative	The third brother had liver cancer without removing; and extensive metastasis and Intubation did not work, 3 months after surgery, this brother died in 1983				In 1998/08 the right lobe of the liver was 8X 10 cm2	
33	check for schistosomiasis; in 1970 Tuberculosis cured	no					
34	In 1983 treatment with hepatitis B half Year and had been delayed intermittent service medicine	no				In 1998/07/01 liver right lobe 8.7 ×7.1cm2 size	
35	2 months ago checked hepatitis B	the father had cardia cancer, in 1997 death				98/09 liver mass 4. 3 ×4.4cm2 size	
36	In 1967 had hepatitis B in Sanyang hospitalization For three months and treatment did not turn negative; Tuberculosis has calcified; gastric ulcer	No				98/02/10 U/S showed 15 × 4 × 12cm2 lesion in hepatic right lobe	

37	Diabetic	No			98/09/29 Ultrasonographic liver right lobe 2.5x2.4 cm2 ;pancreatic head 3× 3.1 cm2	
38	Had a history of schistosomiasis for seven years with three positive in small lobe and not treated	No			98/08/03 CT showed in left liver 4.3× 9.9cm2	
39	In 1983 had acute jaundice liver Inflammation and had hospitalization for one month, sometimes liver area had pain, cholecystitis	Father died because of liver cancer				
40	In 1984 acute jaundice liver Inflammation, hospitalization for one month; after one month relapse	No				
41	In 1960s and 1970s has three hospitalization for histosomiasis late stage; endoscopy showed anemia gastric mucosa like	No				

Table 10-1 Statistics and Treatment of Hepatocellular Carcinoma Patients D

Number	What kind of treatment done				Medication time, type and efficacy	Remarks
	Surgical approach	intervention	Chemotherapy	When the recurrence and metastasis and site size		
1	Not appropriate	For two liver intervention from 98/8/5 to 9/15			From 98/7/14 to 98/09/22 Night pain can not sleep, pain for the stinging 10AM-2PM; Taking XZ-C1, 4,5,2; XZ-C3 topical, after taking the medications, the appetite good; liver pain reduction, obvious medication significantly reduced pain after intervention; no any adverse reactions, hepatomegaly, lump reduced from 3 . 2 x 3. 9 cm2 to 2 . 2x 2 .4 cm2 size	
2		From 98/08 to 98/11 For two liver intervention f			Taking XZ-C1, 4,5; XZ-C3 topical medication ; having good appetite, eating a pound, walking activities such as ordinary people, the right upper quadrant mass much softer than before and reduced size, reduced from 12 × 10cm2 to 11 × 8cm2 size	Interventional of vascular occlusion abnormalities and vascular malformations; can not get up after the second intervention and can not eat right upper quadrant pain increased low back pain
3	On 98/08/05 had half of Liver resection				From 98 /08/19 to 98/11/15 taking XZ-C1, 4, 5, ; after the medication, the spirit is good medicine, appetite is good, the complexion is rosy as ordinary people	

4	Not appropriate	98 /07/21 home pump hemotherapy four times			98 /0 8/ 20-9/24 taking XZ-C1, 4, 5, XZ-C3 topical medication; after taking the medications, the appetite is good	Chemotherapy Mitoniyan5Fu heparin with right pulmonary tuberculosis induration
5					From 98 /09/07 -98/11/28 after taking XZ-C1, 4, 5, medication, the mental and appetite are improved than the previous, can get up and take a mile road, morning exercise, liver area is painful, sometimes tingling, mild ascites sign	Fourth younger brother of liver cancer for resection, two years after the death of ascites, mother cirrhosis ascites in patients with ascites blood hospital four times, treatment of schistosomiasis pirimicron three days therapy
6	98/08/20 laparotomy failed to resection	98 /08/30 for the pump in the hepatic artery secondary carboplatin doxorubicin		98/08/20 intraoperative intrahepatic metastasis	98/09/08 so far taking XZ-C1, 4, 5, after taking the medications, the spirit of improvement and the the appetite increased and the weight gain 8 pounds, walking activities as usual, self-care	
7	98 /07/02 surgical exploration failed to remove	98/07/27 and 98/08/27 for these two hepatic artery pump chemotherapy		98/10/08 chest right lower lung metastasis of two 1. 2 cm diameter lesions	98/0 9/20-98/10/18 taking XZ-C1, 4, 5, after taking the drug the generally good, good appetite; 98/07/27 the first pump chemotherapy with adriamycin cisplatin 5-FU digestive tract response, WBC ↓ 2300 ; 8/27 second chemotherapy response large WBC ↓ 1500 lesions have narrowed; 9/19 U/S 5.0 × 5.0cm 2	98 /07/01 sudden lower abdominal pain; 07/02 liver rupture bleeding emergency surgery; the exploration of liver cancer rupture tofu and failure to resection, ligation of liver A

8	98/09/15 for liver resection of the square leaf cholecystectomy				98/09/25- 11/30 taking XZ-C1, 4, 5, after taking the medications, the spirit and appetite is good, physical recovery gradually, AFP and CEA were normal while reviewing	
9	Not appropriate	98/02/18 to 98/11/ for six interventional response		98/09/15 CT considered possible intracystic metastases	98/09/27-98/11/18 after taking XZ-C4; consciously good, pain symptoms disappeared in the original liver area; before the patient had pain; cough does not hurt; if no moving, the patient is not painful;, cramp-like pain every day.	After the fourth intervention the patient can not speak, right shoulder can not move because of being painful
10	Not appropriate				From 98/09/30 on chest radiographs see lung metastasis	98/09/30- 98/10/11 after taking XZ-C1, 4, 5, and Jieshui Xiaotang, the spirit is better, the original muscle aches, and now pain, bloating and lower extremity swelling
11	Not appropriate	On 98/08/07 and 98/09/21 twice Intervention, liver pain after surgery			98/10/03-98/10/18 After taking the XZ-C1, 4, 5, the patient is generally good, good spiritual and appetite, walking activities such as complexion is rosy; in 98 after embolization and following up check up, there is the liver mass, 8 × 6.8cm2 slightly smaller	

12	On 98 /04/30 had the left liver resection	From 98/06/23 to 98/09/04 had three times Intravenous drug injection		Right liver metastases after secondary chemotherapy; on 98/ 10/19 in Chest X-ray lung metastasis	From 98/10/10-98/11/22 Taking XZ-C1, 4, 5, 2, application of XZ-C3 in decoction and decoction of decoction; after the drug the patient is generally good, good appetite, all of the symptoms such as right shoulder pain, bloating, vomiting and spit cough, dyspnea oliguria, a large number of ascites topical, were getting better.	
13	On 98/09/29 had the right liver leaf resection	On 98/11/09 had intervention, MMC + 5FU		On 98/11/13 liver ultrasound reviewed the left lobe and found that 1. 5 × 7.3cm2 occupying from the postoperative complex	On 98/10/11- 98/11/29 after taking the XZ-C1, 4, 5, the patient was in stable condition, generally good, good spiritual and appetite, walking activities as usual	
14	Not appropriate		98/10/06-98/10/31 had 5Fu+ CF +HCPT	98/05 liver cancer with peritoneum, pancreatic turnover shift	On 98/10/31- 98/12/07 After taking XZ-C1,4,5, XZ-C3 external application; the complexin is rosy and there was painful and had intermittent vomiting	

Number	What kind of treatment done					Medication time, type and efficacy	Remarks
	Surgical approach	intervention	Chemotherapy	When the recurrence and metastasis and site size			
28	Not appropriate	For two liver intervention from 98/8/5 to 9/15				From 98/7/14 to 98/09/22 Night pain can not sleep, pain for the stinging 10AM-2PM; Taking XZ-C1, 4,5,2; XZ-C3 topical, after taking the medications, the appetite good; liver pain reduction, obvious medication significantly reduced pain after intervention; no any adverse reactions, hepatomegaly, lump reduced from 3 . 2 x 3. 9 cm2 to 2 . 2x 2 .4 cm2 size	

29		From 98/08 to 98/11 For two liver intervention f			Taking XZ-C1, 4,5; XZ-C3 topical medication ; having good appetite, eating a pound, walking activities such as ordinary people, the right upper quadrant mass much softer than before and reduced size, reduced from 12 × 10cm2 to 11 × 8cm2 size	Interventional of vascular occlusion abnormalities and vascular malformations; can not get up after the second intervention and can not eat right upper quadrant pain increased low back pain
30	On 98/08/05 had half of Liver resection				From 98 /08/19 to 98/11/15 taking XZ-C1, 4, 5, ; after the medication, the spirit is good medicine, appetite is good, the complexion is rosy as ordinary people	
31	Not appropriate	98 /07/21 home pump hemotherapy four times			98 /0 8/ 20-9/24 taking XZ-C1, 4, 5, XZ-C3 topical medication; after taking the medications, the appetite is good	Chemotherapy Mitoniyan5Fu heparin with right pulmonary tuberculosis induration
32					From 98 /09/07 -98/11/28 after taking XZ-C1, 4, 5, medication, the mental and appetite are improved than the previous, can get up and take a mile road, morning exercise, liver area is painful, sometimes tingling, mild ascites sign	Fourth younger brother of liver cancer for resection, two years after the death of ascites, mother cirrhosis ascites in patients with ascites blood hospital four times, treatment of schistosomiasis pirimicron three days therapy
33	98/08/20 laparotomy failed to resection	98 /08/30 for the pump in the hepatic artery secondary carboplatin doxorubicin		98/08/20 intraoperative intrahepatic metastasis	98/09/08 so far taking XZ-C1, 4, 5, after taking the medications, the spirit of improvement and the the appetite increased and the weight gain 8 pounds, walking activities as usual, self-care	

34	98 /07/02 surgical exploration failed to remove	98/07/27 and 98/08/27 for these two hepatic artery pump chemotherapy		98/10/08 chest right lower lung metastasis of two 1. 2 cm diameter lesions	98/0 9/20-98/10/18 taking XZ-C1, 4, 5, after taking the drug the generally good, good appetite; 98/07/27 the first pump chemotherapy with adriamycin cisplatin 5-FU digestive tract response, WBC ↓ 2300 ; 8/27 second chemotherapy response large WBC ↓ 1500 lesions have narrowed; 9/19 U/S 5.0 × 5.0cm 2	98 /07/01 sudden lower abdominal pain; 07/02 liver rupture bleeding emergency surgery; the exploration of liver cancer rupture tofu and failure to resection, ligation of liver A
35	98/09/15 for liver resection of the square leaf cholecystectomy				98/09/25- 11/30 taking XZ-C1, 4, 5, after taking the medications, the spirit and appetite is good, physical recovery gradually, AFP and CEA were normal while reviewing	
36	Not appropriate	98/02/18 to 98/11/ for six interventional response		98/09/15 CT considered possible intracystic metastases	98/09/27-98/11/18 after taking XZ-C4; consciously good, pain symptoms disappeared in the original liver area; before the patient had pain; cough does not hurt; if no moving, the patient is not painful;, cramp-like pain every day.	After the fourth intervention the patient can not speak, right shoulder can not move because of being painful
37	Not appropriate				From 98/09/30 on chest radiographs see lung metastasis	98/09/30-98/10/11 after taking XZ-C1, 4, 5, and Jieshui Xiaotang, the spirit is better, the original muscle aches, and now pain, bloating and lower extremity swelling
38	Not appropriate	On 98/08/07 and 98/09/21 twice Intervention, liver pain after surgery			98/10/03-98/10/18 After taking the XZ-C1, 4, 5, the patient is generally good, good spiritual and appetite, walking activities such as complexion is rosy; in 98 after embolization and following up check up, there is the liver mass, 8 × 6.8cm2 slightly smaller	

39	On 98 /04/30 had the left liver resection	From 98/06/23 to 98/09/04 had three times Intravenous drug injection		Right liver metastases after secondary chemotherapy; on 98/ 10/19 in Chest X-ray lung metastasis	From 98/10/10- 98/11/22 Taking XZ-C1, 4, 5, 2, application of XZ-C3 in decoction and decoction of decoction; after the drug the patient is generally good, good appetite, all of the symptoms such as right shoulder pain, bloating, vomiting and spit cough, dyspnea oliguria, a large number of ascites topical, were getting better.	
40	On 98/09/29 had the right liver leaf resection	On 98/11/09 had intervention, MMC + 5FU		On 98/11/13 liver ultrasound reviewed the left lobe and found that 1. 5 × 7.3cm2 occupying from the postoperative complex	On 98/10/11- 98/11/29 after taking the XZ-C1, 4, 5, the patient was in stable condition, generally good, good spiritual and appetite, walking activities as usual	
41	Not appropriate		98/10/06- 98/10/31 had 5Fu+ CF +HCPT	98/05 liver cancer with peritoneum, pancreatic turnover shift	On 98/10/31- 98/12/07 After taking XZ-C1,4,5, XZ-C3 external application; the complexin is rosy and there was painful and had intermittent vomiting	

2) The Table of Some Cases of Treated pancreatic cancer

Table 10-2 Statistics and Treatment of Pancreatic cancer Patients A

Number	What kind of treatment done					Medication time, type and efficacy	Remarks
	Surgical approach	intervention	Chemotherapy	When the recurrence and metastasis and site size			
190	In 1994/11/22 had hand surgical exploration + drainage					In 1995/01/16-05/16 took XZ-C1, 4, XZ-C3; after taking topical medication the appetite and spirit are improved; after the local topical 3 the situation markedly improved	

191	In 1990/07/06 had radical surgery of intestinal cancer	In 1995/03/28 had posterior catheter chemotherapy for three courses		In 1990/07 had pancreatic metastasis (found in the operation) ; In 1995/03 magnetic resonance had bowel swelling tumors, small bowel transverse colon tumors	In 1995/09/06-present taking XZ-C1, 4, after taking medicine the mental and appetite are good; the physical recovery, walking and life as usual, life is not stable and still smoking	
192	In 1995/06 had abdominal exploration and the tumor can be removed due to cancer huge arterial adhesion			In 1995/06 found right neck lymph nodes metastasis	In 1995/10/26-1996/03/12 after taking XZ-C1, 4, XZ-C3 topical medication the appetite in improvement; in 1995/12 at the end of ascites drainage improved, with after topical lymphatic softening neck	In 1995/06 the color Doppler ultrasound before the aorta 6.1 x 5.4 cm2
193						In 1996/04/19-04/22 After taking XZ-C1, 4,5, the situation is still good and the jaundice is getting better than before
194	In 1996/03/15 had laparotomy exploration and anastomosis duodenal with total bile duct				In 1996/04/11-1997/11/23 after taking XZ-C1 medication the body weight have improved and the appetite is improved significantly, the mental and sleep is also good ; the jaundice decreased significantly, even to subside	

195	In 1995/11/27 had most of the stomach resections		After five courses of Chemotherapy to 1996/05	In 1996/06/04 CT review found that the pancreas was metastasis	In 1996/06/24-07/27 After taking XZ-C1, 4 the pain disappeared and the mass also disappeared, generally good. Before the patients had recurrent for paroxysmal pain, abdominal lump.	
196	In 1996/11/28 had abdominal exploration failed to remove				In 1996/12/11-1997/04/27 after taking XZ-C1, 4 medication, the patient's appetite was improving, the weight gain; there was no fever and no sweating while high fever when discharge; in the past eating a little food the patient had abdominal pain, drinking water is also pain, currently pain relief by medication obviously, jaundice has been subside	Another patient Tian Yang who is the friend husband was told that appealed full of red and can participate in manual labor and has normal work
197	In 1996/12/25 had abdominal exploration and found that the colon adhesion into blocks, failed resection		Postoperative two course chemotherapy	In 1996/12/25 intraoperative see the right lobe 3 ×3cm2 metastatic disease lesions were squamous cell carcinoma	In 1997/01/03-03/17 after taking XZ-C1, 4,5, the situation was improved significantly, the appetite were improved (due to Debiatics the food intake is limited); the hair turned black, physical also increased; On 02/10 had the second course of chemotherapy with strong. Before chemotherapy U/S showed liver metastases disappeared, pancreatic mass significantly reduced	

198	In 1997/01/20 had laparotomy exploration, due to liver metastases pancreatic tail drainage was done with Czech Republic diameter anastomosis	Postoperative intervention twice		In 1997/01/20 intraoperative showed liver metastasis	In 1997/01/27-10/19 after taking XZ-C1, 4,5 and water consumption, then had a course of chemotherapy, ten days after treatment did not eat, vomit and Spit for supportive therapy, abdominal pain, back pain and Continued paroxysmal worsening; in 1997/05 U/S showed the pancreatic tail 6.3x 5.1cm2 mass ;In 1997/07 had upper digestive tract Bleeding, the condition is very heavy, after treatment hemostasis in 1997/09 the condition improved significantly	Bleeding has been stopped, can play and out of the bed activities, appetite well, the medical staff recognized as is a miracle, waist to lower extremity with calf above swelling edema with dissipated ⌐ and, such as ordinary people
199	In 1997/02/18 had Laparoscopic exploration with the anastomosis between gallbladder and jejunum				In 1997/03/09-12/28 after taking the drug XZGC1, 4 the appetite was improved, physical recovery, jaundice subsided, the original swelling and fatigue had been subsided and can live on their own, for light degree of household ; In 1997/12 the patients vomiting spit mucus with Brown color and with duodenum compression, or adhesion caused Pancreatic head swelling uplift, there are umbilical pain	98/09/30-98/10/11 after taking XZ-C1, 4, 5, and Jieshui Xiaotang, the spirit is better, the original muscle aches, and now pain, bloating and lower extremity swelling
200	In 1997/02/27 had laparotomy Exploration of bile and intestinal anastomosis.			In 1997/07/14 U/S re-examination showed pancreatic head Lesions considered from the ampullary occupying disease	In 1997/03- 07/14 showed after taking XZ-C1, 4 the spirit and appetite were improved, weight gain, the body is better than before, Jaundice subsided, ruddy complexion, to restore part of the work, Pick 40-50 lb	

201	In 1997/07/12 had laparotomy Exploration and the tumor can not be removed				In 1997/07/30- 10/04 after taking XZ-C1, 4 the appetite has improved	
202	In 1997/08/19 had laparotomy Exploration and the tumor can not be removed	After operation, once Treatment with 5GFU, MMC	In 1997/08/19 intraoperative saw pancreatic cancer invasion of the posterior wall of the stomach with liver metastases, pelvic Peritoneal metastasis	In 1997/08/24- 11/22 after taking XZ-C1, 4, and Topical medication the spirit is good, appetite is still good, low back Increased pain, burning pain because of gastric ulcer can not take Medication, after taking topical medication the pain was getting better ; after chemotherapy the patient had poor appetite x	In 1997/12 had sudden Upper gastrointestinal out Blood, portal hypertension, Esophageal variceal rupture and Bleeding, no time to grab and Save, later the death	

Pancreatic cancer Table 2-B-1

Number	Whether to eat often												Whether to drink often				The method of drinking water	Whether to eat often			Jobs		Characters		Whether to love sports
	Water pickles	Salt pickles	Smoked meat	Dried salted fish	Dry pickle	sausage	Fried food	chili	garlic	onion	fresh vegatable	fruit	Fried food	Green tea	Strong tea	Other		meat	Ribs soup	Vegetarian food	General	Tension overcharged	Cheerful	Dull and irritable	
190											√											√			√
191								√						√								√	√		
192	√	√												√								√	√		
193		√	√	√			√	√	√	√	√						Well water	√ fatty meat	√	√		√	√		
194											√			√			Unsolicited Wter				√		√		
195			√	√	√			√	√		√			√			Unsolicited water	√					√		
196		√			√			√			√		rice	√			Well Water				√		√		
197	√	√	√	√	√			√	√		√						Milk / Well water			√	√		√		

198	√	√	√	√	√	√			√			√			Unsolicited water	√ fatty meat			√		√	
199	√	√		√			√		√	√					Unsolicited water				√		√	
200		√		√			√	√	√	√					Unsolicited water	√√ fatty	√	√			√	
201		√	√	√				√							Unsolicited water	√			√		√	
202								√	√						Unsolicited water			√	√		√	√

Pancreatic cancer Table 2-B-2

Number	Chronic disease History	Family three generation of cancer history	Application of pain medication situation			Mass reduction and disappear situation after medications	
			Disappear	Reduction	effective	Tumor location and size	Lump shrinkage after medication
190				√			
191							
192	10 year ago branch cough Have high blood pressure					In 1995/06 CT showed pancreatic body 6.88 x6.69 cm2 mass, pancreas; Tail 1.25 ×1.72 cm2 mass	Cervical lymph nodes turn soft but no significant change in size
193							
194		lover one year ago Gingival cancer				In 96/03/15 Intraoperative pancreatic head cancer 3 ×4cm2	

195							
196	check for schistosomiasis; in 1970 Tuberculosis cured	no					
197	In 1983 treatment with hepatitis B half Year and had been delayed intermittent service medicine	no				In 1998/07/01 liver right lobe 8.7 ×7.1cm2 size	
198	2 months ago checked hepatitis B	the father had cardia cancer, in 1997 death				98/09 liver mass 4. 3 ×4.4cm2 size	
199	have a history of gastritis	brother died of gastric cancer					
200							
201							
202	In 1930s had Schistosomiasis History, used Antimony agent of schistosomiasis 864, had blood Fluke liver cirrhosis and ulcer of ball collapse						

Pancreatic cancer Table 2-C

Number	What kind of treatment done				Medication time, type and efficacy	Remarks
	Surgical approach	intervention	Chemotherapy	When the recurrence and metastasis and site size		
190	In 1994/11/22 had hand surgical exploration + drainage				In 1995/01/16-05/16 took XZ-C1, 4, XZ-C3; after taking topical medication the appetite and spirit are improved; after the local topical 3 the situation markedly improved	
191	In 1990/07/06 had radical surgery of intestinal cancer	In 1995/03/28 had posterior catheter chemotherapy for three courses		In 1990/07 had pancreatic metastasis (found in the operation); In 1995/03 magnetic resonance had bowel swelling tumors, small bowel transverse colon tumors	In 1995/09/06-present taking XZ-C1, 4, after taking medicine the mental and appetite are good; the physical recovery, walking and life as usual, life is not stable and still smoking	
192	In 1995/06 had abdominal exploration and the tumor can be removed due to cancer huge arterial adhesion			In 1995/06 found right neck lymph nodes metastasis	In 1995/10/26-1996/03/12 after taking XZ-C1, 4, XZ-C3 topical medication the appetite in improvement; in 1995/12 at the end of ascites drainage improved, with after topical lymphatic softening neck	In 1995/06 the color Doppler ultrasound before the aorta 6.1 x 5.4 cm2

193						In 1996/04/19-04/22 After taking XZ-C1, 4,5, the situation is still good and the jaundice is getting better than before
194	In 1996/03/15 had laparotomy exploration and anastomosis duodenal with total bile duct				In 1996/04/11-1997/11/23 after taking XZ-C1 medication the body weight have improved and the appetite is improved significantly, the mental and sleep is also good ; the jaundice decreased significantly, even to subside	
195	In 1995/11/27 had most of the stomach resections		After five courses of Chemotherapy to 1996/05	In 1996/06/04 CT review found that the pancreas was metastasis	In 1996/06/24-07/27 After taking XZ-C1, 4 the pain disappeared and the mass also disappeared, generally good. Before the patients had recurrent for paroxysmal pain, abdominal lump.	

196	In 1996/11/28 had abdominal exploration failed to remove				In 1996/12/11-1997/04/27 after taking XZ-C1, 4 medication, the patient's appetite was improving, the weight gain; there was no fever and no sweating while high fever when discharge; in the past eating a little food the patient had abdominal pain, drinking water is also pain, currently pain relief by medication obviously, jaundice has been subside	Another patient Tian Yang who is the friend husband was told that appealed full of red and can participate in manual labor and has normal work
197	In 1996/12/25 had abdominal exploration and found that the colon adhesion into blocks, failed resection		Postoperative two course chemotherapy	In 1996/12/25 intraoperative see the right lobe 3 ×3cm2 metastatic disease lesions were squamous cell carcinoma	In 1997/01/03-03/17 after taking XZ-C1, 4,5, the situation was improved significantly, the appetite were improved (due to Debiatics the food intake is limited); the hair turned black, physical also increased; On 02/10 had the second course of chemotherapy with strong. Before chemotherapy U/S showed liver metastases disappeared, pancreatic mass significantly reduced	

198	In 1997/01/20 had laparotomy exploration, due to liver metastases pancreatic tail drainage was done with Czech Republic diameter anastomosis	Postoperative intervention twice		In 1997/01/20 intraoperative showed liver metastasis	In 1997/01/27-10/19 after taking XZ-C1, 4,5 and water consumption, then had a course of chemotherapy, ten days after treatment did not eat, vomit and Spit for supportive therapy, abdominal pain, back pain and Continued paroxysmal worsening; in 1997/05 U/S showed the pancreatic tail 6.3x 5.1cm2 mass ;In 1997/07 had upper digestive tract Bleeding, the condition is very heavy, after treatment hemostasis in 1997/09 the condition improved significantly	Bleeding has been stopped, can play and out of the bed activities, appetite well, the medical staff recognized as is a miracle, waist to lower extremity with calf above swelling edema with dissipated ⌐ and, such as ordinary people
199	In 1997/02/18 had Laparoscopic exploration with the anastomosis between gallbladder and jejunum				In 1997/03/09-12/28 after taking the drug XZGC1, 4 the appetite was improved, physical recovery, jaundice subsided, the original swelling and fatigue had been subsided and can live on their own, for light degree of household ; In 1997/12 the patients vomiting spit mucus with Brown color and with duodenum compression, or adhesion caused Pancreatic head swelling uplift, there are umbilical pain	98/09/30-98/10/11 after taking XZ-C1, 4, 5, and Jieshui Xiaotang, the spirit is better, the original muscle aches, and now pain, bloating and lower extremity swelling

200	In 1997/02/27 had laparotomy Exploration of bile and intestinal anastomosis.			In 1997/07/14 U/S re-examination showed pancreatic head Lesions considered from the ampullary occupying disease	In 1997/03- 07/14 showed after taking XZ-C1, 4 the spirit and appetite were improved, weight gain, the body is better than before, Jaundice subsided, ruddy complexion, to restore part of the work, Pick 40-50 lb	
201	In 1997/07/12 had laparotomy Exploration and the tumor can not be removed				In 1997/07/30- 10/04 after taking XZ-C1, 4 the appetite has improved	
202	In 1997/08/19 had laparotomy Exploration and the tumor can not be removed	After operation, once Treatment with 5GFU, MMC	In 1997/08/19 intraoperative saw pancreatic cancer invasion of the posterior wall of the stomach with liver metastases, pelvic Peritoneal metastasis	In 1997/08/24- 11/22 after taking XZ-C1, 4, and Topical medication the spirit is good, appetite is still good, low back Increased pain, burning pain because of gastric ulcer can not take Medication, after taking topical medication the pain was getting better ; after chemotherapy the patient had poor appetite	In 1997/12 had sudden Upper gastrointestinal out Blood, portal hypertension, Esophageal variceal rupture and Bleeding, no time to grab and Save, later the death	

3) The Table of Some Cases of Treatment of gastric cancer

Stomach cancer Table 3 -A

Number	Name	Medical record	Gender	Age	Native place	Occupation	Address	Diagnosis	in accordance with	Unit	Society habit			
											Smoking year	Amount of Smoking	Drinking years	Alcohol consumption
219	Zhou xx	x	F	64	Gongen	Women's Director	Gongen	Gastric Cancer	Gastroscopy	Gongen Hospital				
220	Dang xx	x	F	38	Jingshan	Cadre	Jingshan	gastric cancer and pelvic uterine fallopian tube cancer	Endoscopy B ultrasound (In 1994 and in 19 9 6)					
221	Liu xx	x	M	66	Wuhan	Food worker	Caiyue	stomach cancer, bladder cancer	Gastroscopy, barium meal	Concord hospital	40	1 package/ day	40	3oz
222	Shu xx	x	M	58	Henan Xinyang	Driver	Xinyang	The postoperative gastric cancer	gastroscopy, CT (In 1996/09)	Concord hospital, Xinyang City hospital				
223	Cai Xx	x	M	55	Suizhou	Public Security Bureau	Suizhou	gastric cardia cancer	Endoscopy and biopsy (in 1996/11/06)	Concord hospital	30	1 package/ day	30	1-2oz/ day
224	Xiao xx	x	F	18	Zhejiang	Student	Wuhan	antrum, gastric body cancer right ovarian metastasis	Endoscopic biopsy barium meal (96/10/25)	Concord Medical hospital				
225	Lu Xx	x	M	53	Hefeng County	deputy secretary	Enshi	gastric cancer lymph node metastasis		Concord hospital	20-30	One package/ day	20-30	Often
226	Yu xx	x	M	30	Dawu	Cadre	Dawu	postoperative	gastroscope (96/04/20)	Concord Hospital				
227	Wang Xx	x	F	37	Chongyang	deputy director of the Inland Revenue Department	Chongyang	antrum cancer, liver diffuse metastasis	Barium meal (97/01/0 1)	Concord Hospital			Often	16oz
228	Zhao xx	x	M	65	Shanxi	Teacher	Echeng	gastric cancer postoperative	barium meal	Finance and Trade Hospital				

338

229	Ding Xx	x	F	47	Hubei	administrative cadres	Echen	Postoperative gastroscopy,	biopsy, GI biopsy (97/01)	Concord Hospital				
230	Fong Xx	x	M	65	Huangpi 10 years 1 6 2	special note	Wuhan	gastric cancer with systemic metastasis of large amounts of cancer ascites	endoscopy	Tongji Hospital			10	6oz/day
231	Li xx	x	M	67	Hannan Xingcounty	Cadre	Xingxian	stomach gastric cardia, esophageal cancer liver metastases, a small amount of ascites, pleural effusion	endoscopy (97/ 03 /20) of	Xinyang City Hospital Concord Hospital	40	a package		

Stomach cancer Table 3-B-1

Number	Whether to eat often													Whether to drink often			The method of drinking water	Whether to eat often			Jobs		Characters		Whether to love sports
	Water pickles	Salt pickles	Smoked meat	Dried salted fish	Dry pickle	sausage	Fried food	chili	garlic	onion	fresh vegatables	fruit	Fried food	Green tea	Strong tea	Other		meat	Ribs soup	Vegetarian food	General	Tension overcharged	Cheerful	Dull and irritable	
219											√											√			√
220							√								√							√		√	
221	√	√													√							√		√	
222		√	√	√			√	√	√	√	√						Well water	√ fatty meat	√	√	√	√		√	
223											√			√			Unsolicited Wter					√		√	

339

224		√	√		√		√	√		√			√		Unsolicited water	√				√		
225		√		√			√			√	rice	√			Well Water			√		√		
226	√	√	√	√		√		√	√		√				Well water / Milk		√		√	√		
227	√	√	√	√		√		√			√			√	Unsolicited water / √ fatty meat				√		√	
228	√	√			√			√		√	√			√	Unsolicited water				√		√	
229	√	√	√	√		√		√	√		√				Unsolicited water / √√ fatty	√	√	√			√	
230	√	√		Moldy tofu	√							√			Unsolicited water / Jamic flower	√				√		No
231	√	√	√	√		√	√	√	√	√	√	√	√	√	√	Unsolicited water				√	√	

Stomach cancer Table 3-B-2

Number	Whether to eat often													Whether to drink often				The method of drinking water	Whether to eat often			Jobs		Characters		Whether to love sports
	Water pickles	Salt pickles	Smoked meat	Dried salted fish	Dry pickle	sausage	Fried food	chili	garlic	onion	fresh vegatables	fruit	Fried food	Green tea	Strong tea	Other		meat	Ribs soup	Vegetarian food	General	Tension overcharged	Cheerful	Dull and irritable	
219											√											√			√

220					√						√						√		√	
221	√	√									√						√		√	
222		√	√	√		√	√	√	√	√				Well water	√ fatty meat	√	√		√		√
223							√		√			Unsolicited Wter					√		√	
224			√	√		√		√	√		√			Unsolicited water	√				√	
225		√		√			√		√	rice √			Well Water				√		√	
226	√	√	√	√	√		√	√		√			Milk	Well water		√		√	√	
227	√	√	√	√	√		√		√		√			Unsolicited water	√ fatty meat			√		√	
228	√	√			√		√		√	√				Unsolicited water				√		√	
229	√	√	√	√	√		√	√		√				Unsolicited water	√√ fatty	√	√			√	
230	√	√		Moldy tofu √							√	Jamic flower	Unsolicited water	√				√		No
231	√	√	√	√	√	√	√		√	√	√	√	√	√	√	Unsolicited water			√	√	

Stomach cancer Table 3-C

Number	What kind of treatment done					Medication time, type and efficacy	Remarks
	Surgical approach	Postoperative pathological examination	intervention	Chemotherapy	When the recurrence and metastasis and site size		
219	In 1996/09 had gastric cancer surgery	There are 10 lymph nodes metastasis to peripancreatic lymph nodes				In 1996/10/03-97/03/01 taking XZGC1; in 04 after medication the general good, normal meals and sleep, can get up for the light housework	
220	In 1994 Surgical resection of gastric cancer(most) (and in 1996 pairs ofOvarian Cancer Resection.	In 1996 see the uterus wide adhesion (intraoperative) and Can not be removed		In 1994 had the postoperative chemotherapy of the sixth course of chemotherapy with the strong reaction		In 1996/10/19-1997/05/13 After Taking XZ-C1, 4 medication the general good, good appetite; after eating 3-9 Weitai the Bell pain, abdominal pain went away	
221	In 1991 had bladder cancer resection					In 1996/11/14-12/20 taking XZ-C1,4 with XXX, the spirit and the appetite are good, can eat the general food	

222	In 1996/09/17 for stomach Total removalIn		1996/9/9 Lymphatic metastatic with External invasion of lymph nodes and completely removed		In 1996/11/14 chemotherapy	In 1997/03 in the supraclavicular fossa and cervical root two peanuts large lymph nodes can touch, no significant tenderness	In 1996/11/14-1997/03/08 after Take XZ-C1,4, XZ-C3 topical medication the general is good, can eat and had the spirit, Sleep well
223	In 1996/11/27 had Gastric cancer Radical surgery and left chest Under the arch anastomosis	Gastric mucus adenocarcinoma, stomach Wall full-layer and esophageal one Segment with small curvature of the lymph metastasis			In 1997/01/21 CT saw a small amount of abdominal ascites, retroperitoneal lymph nodes, in Ascites the cancer cells can be checked and lymphatic node is 2.5 × 2.5cm2	In 1996/12/23-97/02/28 after taking XZ-C1, 4 and xxx, the situation improved, the appetite is good, there was reduction of ascites	
224			In 1996/11/18 had magnetic therapy guiding treatment with four times interventions	In 1998/11/13 oral Adriamycin	In 1996/12 U/S showed a small amount of ascites and Pleural effusion, ovarian lesions were found with 1. 5 × 1.7cm2 (right side)	In 1996/12/29-1997/01/05 after taking XZ-C1, 4, XZ-C3 topical and Xiaoshuitang decontamination for ascites, the symptoms were significantly reduced and increased urine output	

225	In 1996/12/23 had stomach Radical surgery	Had Gastric poorly differentiated denocarcinoma, Invasion of stomach full-thickness, Gastric pylorus and common hepatic artery and Portal vein posterior lymph metastasis				In 1997/01/12-03/16 after taking XZ-C1,4 medication, the spirit and appetite got better
226	In 1996/05/01 for gastric cancer Resection			In 1996/06, 07 and 10 three chemotherapy, WBC down to 3200 should not be made		In 1997/01/17-1998/04/18 after taking XZ-C1, 4, the spirit and appetite was good, the weight increased
227	In 1997/01/14 for gastric cancer Radical surgery	Clean the lymphatic liver within the multiple metastases	In 1997/06/08 for Chemotherapy with response seriously, and had palpitation Significantly		In 199702/16 Chemotherapy 5-FU carboplatin, reaction strongly with unfinished that is suspended, in 1997/10 for a treatment Of chemotherapy, reaction with Unfinished suspension	In 1997/01/22-1998/10/30 after taking C1, 4, 5, the general condition is good and the spiritual and appetite were good, walking activities as usual; in 1997/02 One week after chemotherapy, hair all lost, WBC down to 1600; after taking our medication the WBC up to 3600, In 1997/06/06 CT showed liver metastases were multiple.

228	In 1996/11/27 for the partial excision of the stomach and the small intestine and Sweep lymph nodes There were lymph nodes in	Gastric antrum, pylorus, cardia and small intestine, Stomach abdominal cancer, invasion of muscle Full-thickness, small gonad Lymphatic metastasis		Postoperative mitomycin + 5GFU chemotherapy After a total of four courses		In 1997/01/26-09/30 after taking XZ-C1, 4, the spirit and the appetite were good, poor eating, Can get out of bed activities lower extremity edema	
229	In 1997/01/23 for the stomach Cancer laparotomy	Poorly differentiated adenocarcinoma, large and Small mesentery and gastric fundus cardia cancer		Generally poor and could have Chemotherapy		In 1997/01/14-04/06 after taking XZ-C1,4, the spirit and the appetite were improved, before had eating Obstruction, difficulty swallowing, after the medication take the patient the semi-flow noodles, abdominal distension, low back pain Limb swelling subsided and black stool got ;the next Abdominal touch than a large mass of fist	

230					In 1997/01 under the left subclavian palpable lymph nodes, right in the lower abdomen Palpable and large mass, U/S had ascites	In 1997/02/04-04/13 after taking XZ-C1, 4 and Water soup the spirit and appetite got better; the original had A large number of ascites and after taking 10 Xiaoshu all of these symptoms subsided. In additional in abdominal mass had significantly prominent with the ball was large, fixed soft, the original completely can not Eating, tea could not enter, after taking medications the patient could eat.	The original bedridden, is now available For getting up to go, the original doctor said no hope, preparation of funeral, now Stable condition improved
231					In 1997 /03/20 CT showed there were liver two metastatic foci with a small amount of ascites and pleural effusion	In 1997/03/25-04/04 after taking XZ-C1, 4, the spirit and appetite were improved	

4) Some cases of the treatment of lung cancer

Lung cancer Table 4-A

Number	Name	Medical record	Gender	Age	Native place	Occupation	Address	Diagnosis	in accordance with	Unit	Society habit			
											Smoking year	Amount of Smoking	Drinking years	Alcohol consumption
305	Dain xx	x	M	68	Hubai		Liupinguang	Upper right lung Cancer	Chest x-ray, CT (99/01)	Concord hospital	30	1 package/ day	No	
306	Cheng xx	x	M	70	Wuhan	Worker	Hangyang	Right lung cancer with obstruction pneumonia and bone metastasis	Chest x-ray, CT	Tongji hospital	40	1 package/ day	40	
307	Pen xx	x	F	53	Xiangfan	Housewife	Xiangfan	Right lung cancer with huge fluid in chest	CT, U/S (99/01)	Xiangfan railroad hospital	No		no	
308	Shu xx	x	M	18	Henan	Student	Xingxian	The lung metastasis from liver cancer	CT (99/02)	Concord hospital	NO		NO	
309	Dengxx	X	M	37	Zhijiang	Technician	Zhijiang	Right lung cancer with diagraph and lung and pleural metastasis	Chest x-ray, CT (99/02)	Zhijiang hospital	20	1 package/ day	occasionally	
310	Fang Xx	x	F	41	Tianmen	Worker	Tianmen	Left upper lung cancer postoperation	CT (98/ 10/09)	Province people's hospital	No		No	
311	Zhou xx	x	M	70	Gualin	Driver	Wuhan	Left lower lung cancer	CT (99/01)	Tongjin	50	1 package/ day	50	1 bottle/ day
312	Wang Xx	x	M	73	Wuhan	secretary	Hankou	Lung cancer with decending aorta aneurysm	Chest x-ray(99/04)	The fourth wuhan hospital	20	One package/ day	40	3oz /day
313	Zhao xx	x	M	44	Hannan	Police office	Xiaogan	Lung cancer with high pressure in portal vein and splenomegly and high function of spleen	U/S, color Doppler ultrasound, CT, AFP	Concord Hospital				
314	Liu Xx	x	M	30	Hubei	Worker	Jinmen	Righ upper lung cancer	Chest x-ray, Pathology slides(98/08)	Concord Hospital	Occassionally		no	

Lung cancer Table 4-B-1

Number	Whether to eat often												Whether to drink often				The method of drinking water	Whether to eat often			Jobs		Characters		Whether to love sports
	Water pickles	Salt pickles	Smoked meat	Dried salted fish	Dry pickle	sausage	Fried food	chili	garlic	onion	fresh vegatables	fruit	Fried food	Green tea	Strong tea	Other		meat	Ribs soup	Vegetarian food	General	Tension overcharged	Cheerful	Dull and irritable	
305											√	√	√			√	Unsolicited Wter					√	√		
306					√					√	√	√			√		Well water	√				√	√		
307	√	√													√							√	√		
308		√	√	√		√	√	√	√	√	√						Well water	√ fatty meat	√	√		√	√		
309											√				√		Unsolicited Wter				√		√		
310			√	√		√	√	√			√				√		Unsolicited water	√					√		
311		√	√				√				√		rice		√		Well Water				√		√		
312	√	√	√	√	√			√	√		√						Milk / Well water		√			√	√		

313	√	√	√	√	√		√			√			Unsolicited water	√ fatty meat			√		√	
314	√	√		√			√		√	√			Unsolicited water				√		√	

Lung cancer Table 4-B-2

Number	Chronic disease History	Family three generation of cancer history	Application of pain medication situation			Mass reduction and disappear situation after medications	
			Disappear	Reduction	effective	Tumor location and size	Lump shrinkage after medication
305	Chronic bronchus Inflammation with emphysema, Stomach bleeding, enteritis	Father suffering from esophagus Cancer died		√			
306	59 years suffering from blood Worm disease, after treatment of alcohol liver hard						
307		Dad died of stomach cancer					
308							
309							
310		Uncle died of nose and throat cancer					
311	Haptitis and arthritis						
312							
313	In 1995 years of schistosomiasis Cirrhosis, in 1989 hepatitis B (small three positive)	Father died of lung cancer					
314							

Lung cancer Table 4-C

Number	What kind of treatment done					Medication time, type and efficacy	Remarks
	Surgical approach	Postoperative pathological examination	intervention	Chemotherapy	When the recurrence and metastasis and site size		
305	Not appropriate		Not appropriate	Not appropriate	1999/01/07 CT howed: right upper lung cancer with mediastinal lymph nodes	In 1999/01/21-99/08/09 After taking XZGC1 +4 +7 medications, the patient was in stable condition, the spirit and the appetite were good, every day 3-4 meal, each meal 1-2 two; do not breathe, withdrawal to panting, in cold days or hot days the symptoms increase and hemoptysis, Mostly white sputum, no fever	Exam: lung type III tuberculosis, chronic bronchitis and emphysema, chronic schistosomiasis, cirrhosis, bilateral pleural adhesions
306	Not appropriate		Not appropriate	In 1999/01/14 Chemotherapy : DDP + VPG16 (3 days) HCPT (1 day) DDP + VPG16 (3 days) HCPT (1 day)	In 1999/01 X-ray review: left lung and lower lobe lung cancer, T8-9 vertebral metastatic carcinoma, ECT: L5 bone metastasis	In 1999/01/31-2000/07/31 After taking XZ-C1 +4 +7 MDI medications, the general condition was good, good appetite, illness was stable effect and could work, X-ray results: lung swelling and Tumor had disappeared, in 2000/07/31 at 11:30 pm had bleeding stroke and died	After Patient had chemotherapy for one course, the review of X-ray showed most of the right lower lung inflammation reduced, right diaphragm had hypertrophic adhesion angle

307	Not appropriate		Not appropriate	Not appropriate	In 1999/01 Thoracic puncture showed bloody pleural effusion and there were cancer cells	In 1999/02/03-1999/03/03 taking XZ-C1 +4 + 7	Drawing pleural effusion three times for the bloody and there were cancer cells, the current physical weakness with shortness of breath
308	Not appropriate		Not appropriate	Not appropriate	In 1999/02/11 CT showed liver multiple lesions, the largest 11.6 × 7.cm2, in chest there were scattered patchy shadows with Hilar widening, lymphatic metastasis	In 1999/02/11 -1999/04/11 after taking XZGC1 +4 +7 LMS.Indo. and XZ-C3 topical medication, the spirit and the appetite and sleep were good, 2oz/meal, walking activities as usual, laughing as usual, there were secondary liver pain, no other discomfort, the appearance was the same as healthy people	In 1999/03/07 families from Henan New County made a special trip to pick up the medications
309	Not appropriate		Not appropriate	Not appropriate		In 1999/02/27-1999/03/27 after taking XZ-C1 +4 +7 +2 LMS the spirit and appetite were good;	Patient professional was the painter, car spray Paint for 10 years, nitro paint was harmful; after spraying paint, the gas mist made the patient cough
310	In 1998/11/23 had left low Lung and right lung lobe removed		In 1998/12/30 for X remove	In 1998/12/21-1998/12/30 had Radiation therapy for 10 days, In 1999/01/19-1999/01/26 intra vein Therapy (VPG16, DDP600mp)		In 1999/03/07-1999/04/07 after taking XZGC1 +4 +7 LMS/Indo the spirit and appetite were good	Disease detection: upper left lung squamous cell carcinoma stage II, tongue lobe Lymph nodes (1) and hilar lymph nodes (2) were cancer metastasis

311	In 1967 had Stomach perforation and Subtotal gastrectomy		Not appropriate	Not appropriate		In 1999/04/20-1999/05/22 after taking XZ-C1 +4 +7, XZ-C3 topical, the general situation is still good; in the past had more cough and sputum, however at present Breathing smoothly, up and down the fourth floor and could take care of themselves	The patient has four girls, the old couple often argued, heart muffled every day and liked to eat fermented bean curd and Pickles
312	Not appropriate		Not appropriate	Not appropriate	report: descending aortic aneurysm 3.0 × 1.5cm size with hilar spherical lesion diameter was 5.8cm	In 1999/04/2- In 1999/04/26 after taking XZGC1 +4 +7 medications, the spirit and appetite were good	
313	patients with schistosomiasis Liver cirrhosis + hepatitis B liver cirrhosis+ alcohol liver cirrhosis(Not surgery)		Due to hypersplenism Progress, Not appropriate	Not appropriate		In 1999/04/21-1999/11/29 after taking XZ-C1 +4 + 8+LMS blood soup, Xiaotang Tang medications, the general situation was good, the appetite and sleep were good, three meals a day, a meal 2oz, weight Increase 2.5 kg; on 10/01 had "cold", a few days later there was abdominal distension, and had abdominal water and urine situation were getting worse	AFP: 355. 7 ng / ml
314	In 1998/08/25 had top right Lobectomy		Postoperative chemotherapy III Cycles(had strong gastrointestinal reaction		There was palpable right cervical lymph	In 1999/06/10-1999/07/10 after taking XZ-C1 + 4, XZ-C3 External application of medication the patient had a good appetite	Exam: the right upper lung large cell poor differentiation, Adenocarcinoma, 1/5 lymph node had cancer

5) Some of Cases of Esophageal cancer and cardia cancer

Esophageal cancer and cardia cancer Table 5-A

Number	Name	Medical record	Gender	Age	Native place	Occupation	Address	Diagnosis	in accordance with	Unit	Society habit			
											Smoking year	Amount of Smoking	Drinking years	Alcohol consumption
394	Cai xx	x	M	55	Shuizhou	Public Security Bureau	Shuizhou	Gastric Cardia Cancer	Endoscopic biopsy (96/11/06)	Concord hospital	30	1 package/day	30	1-2oz
395	Liang xx	x	M	54	Hunan	power supply bureau	Xiangyang	The lower esophageal cancer	Endoscopic biopsy of esophagus in(96/10)	Concord hospital	30	1 package/day	30	6-10oz
396	Li xx	x	F	56	Nanzhang	Teacher	Nanzhang	esophageal cancer after surgery with Liver metastasis	Swallow barium	Nanzhang County Hospital				
397	Wang xx	x	F	45	Xiangyang	Peasant	Xingxian	The middle Esophageal surgery with Post-pulmonary metastasis	CT(99/02) Endoscopic biopsy (97/01/10)	Finance and Trade Hospital	NO		5-6	2-3oz
398	Huang xx	X	M	70	Huangpi	Boiler worker	Wuhan	cardia postoperative	CT, endoscopy (97/01)		30	1 -2 package/day	20	16oz
399	Li Xx	x	M	61	Xingzhou	Metallurgical Industry Company workers	Xingzhou	Postoperative recovery of cardia cancer	Swallow barium angiography	Fanicail hospital				

Esophageal cancer and cardia cancer Table 5-B-1

Number	Water pickles	Salt pickles	Smoked meat	Dried salted fish	Dry pickle	sausage	Fried food	chili	garlic	onion	fresh vegatable	fruit	Fried food	Green tea	Strong tea	Other	The method of drinking water	meat	Ribs soup	Vegetarian food	General	Tension overcharged	Cheerful	Dull and irritable	Whether to love sports
394												√	√				Unsolicited Wter	√				√	√		
395		√				peanut				√	√	√	√				Well water	√				√		√	
396	√	√											√									√		√	
397			√				√	√	√	√	√						Well water √ fatty meat	√	√			√	√	√	
398											√		√				Unsolicited Wter				√			√	
399			√	√	√		√	√			√		√				Unsolicited water	√					√		

Esophageal cancer and cardia cancer Table 5-B-2

Number	Chronic disease History	Family three generation of cancer history	Application of pain medication situation			Mass reduction and disappear situation after medications	
			Disappear	Reduction	effective	Tumor location and size	Lump shrinkage after medication
394		Father suffering from esophagus Cancer died		√			
395	Renal Diatics	In 1950s Granpa died for esophageal cancer					
396	uterine muscle Tumor surgery	Father because of brain swelling Tumor pain suicide Mother died of uterus cancer					Shrink softening
397	In 1986 had haptitis B with jaundice and three positive						
398	chronic gastritis for years without the system treatment						
399							

Esophageal cancer and cardia cancer Table 5-C

Number	What kind of treatment done					Medication time, type and efficacy	Remarks
	Surgical approach	Postoperative pathological examination	intervention	Chemotherapy	When the recurrence and metastasis and site size		
394	In 1996/11/27 had gastric cardia cancer cure and left thoracic arch anastomosis				In 1997/11/27 intraoperative found that gastric cardia mucinous adenocarcinoma, invasion of the stomach wall full-thickness and lower esophagus, with the lymph node metastasis of small curvature(10/10); in 1997/01/21 CT showed a small amount of ascites, check the retroperitoneal lymph nodes metastasis 2.5 × 2.5cm	In 1996/12/23- in 1997/02/28 after taking the medication the mental, the appetite and the physical strength had improved; taking XZ-C1,4 Brucea javanica	
395					In 1998/11/07 MRI showed upper left lung 2.2x2.5x 3.2 cm3 metastases	In 1996/12/25 after taking XZ-C1,4, the spirit and appetite, were good, the complexion rosy, could work, and consciously digest well, but could be not supine after eating because of nausea phenomenon	

396	In late 1993 had esophageal cancer by thoracotomy			Had one year of radiotherapy and chemotherapy	In 1995/05 found liver metastasis, barium see 5-6cm2 esophageal recurrence	In 1997/01- 04/06 after taking XZ-C1,4,2 ;XZ-C3 topical, had good appetite with the original obstruction, is gradually better; the original had cough seriously withspit, now the cough spit got better, but not much food, malnutrition; the neck Lymph node got shrinkage, softening after application	
397	In 1997/01/25 had esophageal cancer radical surgery, in 1997/06 had left supraclavicular lymphadenectomy				In 1997/06left subclavian lymph node metastasis; in 1998/03 had the left edge of lymph node metastasis; in 1999/01/28 chest x-ray showed lung several metastases	In 1997/02/19 after taking XZ-C1,4, 2 XZ-C3 topical medication, the general was good; from 97/03 to 98/10 the patient stopped medications, then had lymphatic metastasis and took the medications again; in 1997/0 6 had left scapular diffuse Limited swelling, 10 × 2cm2 tenderness, local pain, food can be satisfied, the spirit was poor, can walk	

| 398 | In 1997/01/13 had cardia cancer radical surgery | | | | In 1997/01/13 intraoperative saw lymph node metastasis (4/7) in right supraclavicular lymph nodes with the metastasis | in 1997/02/27-03/30 after taking XZ-C1,4, 2, XZ-C3 external application for two months, the general is good; in 1997/03 examination found the right neck string of fixed lymph, fusion into a plate, hard, right armpit 3 fingers;The size of the right shoulder lymph nodes can not lift ⌐ 97 ⌐ Yuan ⌐ 9CT suspect retroperitoneal lymph nodes and mesenteric lymph node metastasis | |
| 399 | In 1997/04/04 had gastric cardia surgery of left thoracic and thoracic esophageal gastric anastomosis | | In 1998/03/29-04/12 had fatigue, nausea and vomiting, dizziness after chemotherapy | | In 1998/04/15 barium showed local stenosis;In 1998/06/15 and in 1998/09/21 swallow barium saw esophagus and gastric anastomosis, below the small curvature of the stomach with irregular filling defect recurrence | In 1997/04/29 after taking XZ-C1, 4 the appetite was still good, there is the phenomenon of reflux, eating without obstruction but pain, shoulder pain, and weather-related, for rheumatoid arthritis, left neck tenderness; when eating the hot food, feeling sternal pain | |

6) Some cases of the treatment of Breast cancer

Breast cancer Table 6-A

Number	Name	Medical record	Gender	Age	Native place	Occupation	Address	Diagnosis	in accordance with	Unit	Society habit				
											Smoking year Smoking	Amount of Smoking	Drinking years	Alcohol consumption	
447	Jing xx	x	F	75		Teacher	Huangpi	Right side Breast		Concord hospital					1-2oz
448	Peng xx	x	F	47	Wuhan	Worker	Wuhan	Right side breast	Biopsy (95/02/16)	Red community hospital					6-10oz
449	Gui xx	x	F	40	Nanzhang	Teacher	Nanzhang	esophageal cancer after surgery with Liver metastasis	Biopsy and pathology (95/02/28)	Red community hospital					
450	Li xx	x	F	47	Xiangyang	Peasant	Xingxian	The middle Esophageal surgery with Post-pulmonary metastasis	CT, Biopsy (94/11/)	Red community hospital					
451	Cheng xx	X	F	44	Huangpi	Boiler worker	Wuhan	cardia postoperative	Biopsy	Concord hospital					
452	Fang Xx	x	F	45	Hubei	Peasant	Xiaochang	The lymphatic metastasis of the left axillary and the supraclavicular fossa of postoperative breast cancer	Pathology (94/12)	Concord hospital					

Breast cancer Table 6-B-1

Number	Water pickles	Salt pickles	Smoked meat	Dried salted fish	Dry pickle	sausage	Fried food	chili	garlic	onion	fresh vegatables	fruit	Fried food	Green tea	Strong tea	Other	The method of drinking water	meat	Ribs soup	Vegetarian food	General	Tension overcharged	Cheerful	Dull and irritable	Whether to love sports
447																									
448										√	√	√			√		Well water	√				√	√		
449	√	√													√							√	√		
450							√	√	√	√	√	√					Well water	√ fatty meat			√		√	√	
451		√				√					√			√			Unsolicited Wter					√		√	
452										√															

Breast cancer Table 6-B-2

Number	Chronic disease History	Family three generation of cancer history	Application of pain medication situation			Mass reduction and disappear situation after medications	
			Disappear	Reduction	effective	Tumor location and size	Lump shrinkage after medication
447				√			

Number	(continued)						
448	In 1986 had stomach disease						
449							
450	In 1984 had appendectomy						
451							
452							

Breast Cancer Table 6-C

Number	What kind of treatment done						Medication time, type and efficacy	Remarks
	Surgical approach	Postoperative pathological examination	intervention	Chemotherapy	When the recurrence and metastasis and site size			
447	In 1994 /10 had the right Cancer resection						94/11/14-02/17 after taking XZ-C1,4, he general situation is good	
448	In 1995/03 had Right breast cancer with Radical surgery						In 1995/03/27-04 After taking XZ-C1, 4 for two month, in October the patient came to tell us that the patient was in good condition and because of economic difficulties the patient stopped medication	
449	In 1995/03/29 Left breast cancer Radical surgery						In 1995/0 3/29 – 04/25 after taking XZ-C1, 4 the appetite and sleep were good; In 1995 had little white milk in the right breast	
450	In 1994/11 had the right breast Radical surgery						In 1995/04/14-04/30 after taking XZ-C1, 4, for a month the spirit was good	

451	In 1995/02/20 had the right breast Radical surgery				In 1995/05/11-98/02/26 after taking XZ-C1, 4, the appetite was good; in 1995/11 had no abnormal in chest X-ray, ruddy weight increase of 10 pounds	
452	In 1978 the right breast cancer surgery and in 1990 the left breast Cancer surgery (November)			In 1990/11 had left breast metastasis and in 1993 left armpit Lymph node metastasis; in 1995 underarm (left) 8 × 6 × 6cm3 size, left supraclavicular lymph node metastasis	In 1995/05/08- 08/25 after taking XZ-C1, 4, bruce milk external application, the general was good, the appetite was good; the patient looked good, the wound was significantly reduced, less	

7) The Table of Some Cases of the Treatment of Rectal and Colon cancer

Rectal and colon cancer Table 7-A

Number	Name	Medical record	Gender	Age	Native place	Occupation	Address	Diagnosis	in accordance with	Unit	Society habit			
											Smoking year	Amount of Smoking	Drinking years	Alcohol consumption
482	Li xx	x	M	67	Wuhan	Worker	Wuhan	Recurrence of rectal cancer and had surgery twice	Rectoscopy (95/10)	Concord hospital	30	A package/ day	30	occasionally
483	Yao xx	x	M	62	Hubei	CADRE	Wuhan	Rectal cancer	Pathology (96/12)	Concord hospital	20	A or two package/ day		occasionally
484	Gui xx	x	M	68	Heilongjiang	Cadre	Wuhan	Rectal cancer	Pathology (96/11/13)	Concord hospital				
485	Li xx	x	F	42	Xiangyang	Cadre	Xingxian	sigmoid colon cancer	U/S	Concord hospital				
486	Cheng xx	X	F	39	Huangpi	Peasant	Wuhan	Colon cancer	U/S (97/03/15)	Concord hospital				

| 487 | Fang Xx | x | M | 51 | Wuhan | Procuratorate cadre | Wuhan | Colon cancer with liver metastasis | (96/03) | Concord hospital | | | |

Colon and rectal cancer Table 7-B-1

Number	Whether to eat often													Whether to drink often			The method of drinking water	Whether to eat often			Jobs		Characters		Whether to love sports
	Water pickles	Salt pickles	Smoked meat	Dried salted fish	Dry pickle	sausage	Fried food	chili	garlic	onion	fresh vegatables	fruit	Fried food	Green tea	Strong tea	Other		meat	Ribs soup	Vegetarian food	General	Tension overcharged	Cheerful	Dull and irritable	
482			√				√										Unsolicited Wter	√				√			no
483	√	√	√	√	√	√		√	√	√	√	√			√		River water	√				√		√	
484	√	√													√							√		√	
485							√	√	√	√	√						Well water	√ fatty meat	√			√		√	
486		√					√				√			√			Unsolicited Wter					√		√	
487													√												

Colon and rectal cancer Table 7-B-2

Number	Chronic disease History	Family three generation of cancer history	Application of pain medication situation			Mass reduction and disappear situation after medications	
			Disappear	Reduction	effective	Tumor location and size	Lump shrinkage after medication
482	Calcification of tuberculosis with gastritis history of gastritis			√			
483	years of coronary heart disease old myocardial infarction						
484	On 199205\18 stroke, left hypothalamic hemorrhage, right hemiplegia						
485	a history of chronic gastritis						
486	History of chronic headache constipation						
487	In 1982 hepatitis, chronic gastritis history, colitis ; in 1994 barium enema, sigmoid colon mucosal disorder	Father esophageal and cardia Ca; in 1974 passed away					the lump got smaller than before

Colon and rectal cancer Table 7-C

Number	What kind of treatment done					Medication time, type and efficacy	Remarks
	Surgical approach	Postoperative pathological examination	intervention	Chemotherapy	When the recurrence and metastasis and site size		
482	In 1995/10/17 had rectal resection and anastomosis; in 1996/12/20 had sigmoid fistula		In 1996/09 intubation pump, injection only once	Postoperative chemotherapy 4 times, each time 10 days	On 1996\12\20 during fistula surgery the rectum Ca was found with invasive of the sacrum	On 1997\01\14-02\14 XZ-C1,4, XZ-C3 for external application, after taking the drug the patient had significantly changed, could not get out of bed, there were still red and white frozen; after removing these bloody things, the patient was improved on bloating difficulties and hematuria	Drinking pond water has high incidence of cancer and, the Yangtze River water has the pool sediment
483	On 1997\01\20 for rectal ca radical surgery					On 1997\02-1997\03\16 after taking XZ-C1,4 medication the patient had a good appetite, physical strength had been restored so that the patient could go up and down the stairs, now their own downstairs, on the garden	
484	On 1996\12\09 had rectal caDixon operation					On 1997\02\23-04\22 after taking XZ-C1,4 medications the patient had a good appetite, physical recovery, such as preoperative, blood pressure is not high, good memory, right hemiplegia	

485	On 1997\02\23 had sigmoid colon ca radical surgery	A course of chemotherapy after surgery				On 1997\03\22-04\27 After Taking XZ-C1,4 the spirit of appetite was good, face as usual	
486	On 1997\04 had laparotomy, left colon resection				On 1998\10\28 had laparotomy and abdominal wall and small intestine tumors, invasion and full-thickness abdominal wall and omentum nodular metastasis	On 1997\04\26-06\13 and on 1998\11 \0 5 after taking XZ-C1,4 medications the patient was generally good; on 1998\08 found left abdominal mass ; On 1998\10\28 had laparotomy and found invasion of abdominal wall tumor and full-thickness abdominal wall and omentum Nodule metastasis so that the patient had intestinal tumor resection and anastomosis	
						In 1997/06/03-06/29 After taking the XZ-C1, 4,5, XZ-C3 topical, the patient had good spirit and appetite, looking good; after topical the lump was reduced compared with before; after the drug WBC was up from 6. 4 × 109 /l to WBC7. 0 × 109 /l; on 97 \06\15 physical examination mass was 12 × 9cm2, on 97\06\ 29 tumor mass was significantly reduced to 7 × 17cm2	

8) The Table of Some Cases of the Treatment of Cholangiocarcinoma

Cholangiocarcinoma Table 8-A

Number	Name	Medical record	Gender	Age	Native place	Occupation	Address	Diagnosis	in accordance with	Unit	Society habit			Alcohol consumption	
											Smoking year	Amount of Smoking	Drinking years		
650	Zhang xx	x	F	31	Wuhan	Street Office Director	Wuhan	common bile duct papilloma malignant transformation of liver metastases	Color Doppler ultrasound, CT (94 /0 4)	Concord hospital	1-2	10 cigerattee/ day			
651	He xx	x	M	51	Xishui	CADRE	Wuhan	Liver hilar cholangiocarcinoma	Pathology (95/04)	Concord hospital	20	10 cigerattee/ day		15	2-3 oz
652	Jiang xx	x	M	76	Wuhan		Wuhan	hilar region bile duct cancer surrounding the ampulla	Exploration surgery (95/02)	Concord hospital					
653	Zheng xx	x	F	61	Huanghu	Peasant	Huanghu	gallbladder cancer	U/S (1995/ 10/08)	Tongji Hospital					
654	Zhang xx	X	F	58	Wuhan	Agricultural Bank cadre	Wuhan	hilar cholangiocarcinoma	U/S, CT (95/11)	Concord hospital					
655	Yang Xx	x	M	28	Guizhou	Painter worker	Wuhan	hilar cholangiocarcinoma	(color Doppler ultrasound, CT(95/12))	Concord hospital	7-8	A package/ day			

Cholangiocarcinoma Table 8-B-1

Number	Whether to eat often												Whether to drink often			The method of drinking water	Whether to eat often			Jobs		Characters		Whether to love sports
	Water pickles	Salt pickles	Smoked meat	Dried salted fish	**Dry pickle**	sausage	Fried food	chili	garlic	onion	fresh vegatables	fruit	Fried food	Green tea	Strong tea	Other		meat	Ribs soup	Vegetarian food	General	Tension overcharged	Cheerful	Dull and irritable	

No.																						
650						√		√						Unsolicited Wter	√				√			
651	√	√	√	√	√	√	√	√	√	√	√		√	River water	√ fatty meat			√		√	no
652										√											
653																					
654		√	√	√		√		√		√				Unsolicited Wter			√			√	
655					√									River water	√ fatty meat						

Cholangiocarcinoma Table 8-B-2

Number	Chronic disease History	Family three generation of cancer history	Application of pain medication situation			Mass reduction and disappear situation after medications	
			Disappear	Reduction	effective	Tumor location and size	Lump shrinkage after medication
650	In 1989 Found T.B and recovery after 2 months treatment			√			
651	Often cough						
652							
653	There was Schistosoma with Abdominal pain Recurrence more than 20 years	Spouse had brain tumor and died in 1979				In 1995/10/08 U/S showed there was 6. 5x4.5 cm2 mass	
654							

655	history of gastritis, had gastroscopy which showed gallbladder and biliary Stone and Biliary colic in 1993						

Cholangiocarcinoma Table 8-C

Number	What kind of treatment done						Medication time, type and efficacy	Remarks
	Surgical approach	Postoperative pathological examination	intervention	Chemotherapy	When the recurrence and metastasis and site size			
650	In 1994/08/24 had tumors Resection with anastomosis of bile duct and jejunum				In 1994/04 found bile duct tumor with liver metastasis		In 1995/03/15-03/25 after taking XG-C1, 4; in 01 XZ-C3 outside application, local topical analgesic effect is still good, but less urine, ascites	
651							In 1995/04/23-07/29 after taking XZ-C1, 4 the Appetite was good, abdominal fullness after meals; otherwise, no discomfort; in 1994 gain weight 148 pounds, and now was 114 pounds	
652	In 1995/03/17 had surgery of Exploration due to duodenum and hilar adhesions				In 1995/03/17 found Tumor occupying in hilar and biliary duct, cystic duct, gallbladder ampulla		In 1995/03/22-12/17 after taking XZ-C1, 4 the spirit was good, yellow Jaundice subsided, physical recovery, but poor appetite due to bile completely external drainage	In 1995/02/0 2 had jaundice, yellow urine, one week ago had fever and found obstructive and jaundice Hilar cholangiocarcinoma

653	No application				In 1995/10/08 U/ S showed right hepatic lobular gallbladder Squamous cell lesions of gallbladder invasion	In 1995/10/16-11/15 after taking XZ-C1, 4, the appetite and the spirit had improved, weight gain of 3 pounds	
654	In 1995/12/29 Abdominal exploration of bile enteric anastomosis with Internal drainage					In 1996/01/31-03/29 after taking XZ-C1, 4, the appetite was improved; 39 °C fever for three days due to cold; after the temperature went down, the patient had still jaundice.	
655	In 1995/12 had exploration Surgery; due to adhesion the pieces were unable to cut					In 1996/02/11-02/25 after taking XZ-C1, 4, 5, the general situation was well; the wound flew yellow water which every day 3-4 gauzes were used; the whole body was yellow without change, the body depth of yellow, urine dark yellow as tea	

2. Typical Cases

1) The typical cases of inoperable, nor radiotherapy and chemotherapy, simply taking Z-C immunomodulatory anticancer medicine treatment

Case 1 Mr. xxx, male, 68year-old, Changzhou, officer

Diagnosis: the central lung cancer on the right upper of the lung with the metastasis

Disease courses and treatment: in Octocber 1998 he coughed two weeks with the pain in the right shoulder and was treated with inflammation. In Jan 1999 his cough is getting worse and this appetite is decreased and fatigure and getting weak. On CT there is mass on the right upper lung showing the central lung. He had endoscope and biopsy which showed that lung adenocarcinoma in the xxxxxx. He and his family member don't want to have operation. In Feb 1999 after chemotherapy for one course, his reaction to the chemotherapy was strong and stopped to use it. This patient had metastasis in the left lung which showed there are two lesions and he coughed with mucous and blood sputdu and difficult walking. On April 23 2000 he started to take the XZ-C1+XZ-C4+XZ-C7, LMS+MDZ for three months and his general condition is good and he is lively and his appetite is great. In December 2000 his medical condition is stable, and he is lively. His appetite is good and his breath is smooth and his face is red. He walked as the normal person and sometimes he coughs. He persistently takes this medication for more than four years and when he comes back to follow up during the five years, his general condition is great and he walked as the normal healthy person.

Comments: this patient has the central lung cancer in the right upper lung. In April 2000 he started to use XZ-C1+XZ-C4+XZ-C7. XZ-C1 is used to kill the cancer cells only without kill the normal cells; XC-C4 protect the thymus and increase the thymus weight and to protect the bone marrow, XZ-C7 inhibit the lung cancer cells and protect the lung and solve the suptid. After short-term chemotherapy he started to take the XZ-C to strengthen his long-term therapy. XZ-C improve the whole body immune system and he is lively and his appetite is good and his spleen is great and help the patients against the diseases and help the patient's organ functions and the nutrition condition and metabliztion recover so that the patients' healthy condition is recovery.

This patient didn't have the operation. In Feb 1999 he had chemeotherapy, however there is left lung metastasis after chemotherapy. Afterh that, he only took the XZ-C to control the metastasis. He persistently took the medicine for more than four years and his medical condition is great without any complaints. He followed up with us for more than seven years. In May 2005 when he came back to follow up, his general medical condition is great and his appepital is good without other symptoms. His walking and activities and he talks cheerfully and humorously.

Case 2 Mrs. xxxxx femal, 66 year-old, Wuhan han yan

Diagnosis: the squamous carcinoma of the low esophagus

Disease courses and treatment: in December 2000 the patients started to vomit and to have progressively swallow difficultly and only swallow the half of xxxx food. EGD showed that there was narrow in the low esophagus, congestion, ulcer and xxx. Pathology showed squamous carcinoma in the lower esophagus. According to his medical condition he should be treated for a surgery, however because he could afford to the medical cost, he started to take XZ-C. After one month, he is energetic and his appetite is getting better and can eat the soft food, noodle and rice soup. After she continued to take these medicine for six months, he is vagour and his appetite is good and can eat the soft food and noodle and rice soup. Until June 2003 she took the medicine more than two and half years and his health condition is good and can eat the regular rice and felt fine as the normal healthy persons. However she stopped to taking the medicine for more than four and half months. Until Octocber 16 2003 he suddenly had the difficulties to swallow the food and vomit the brown food. She could not eat for more than three days. After adding her some fluids and continued to take XZ-C until Octocber 31 2003 she can eat the food again. After that, she never stopped taking the medicine again. Now she is 70 year-old and healthy the same as the normal persons. She is energetic and her appetite is good and can eat regular food. She lived in the seventh floor and everyday she will come down the first floor and sometimes she help others to fill the bicycle wheels.

Comments: This patient had the low grade squamous carcinoma in the low esophagaus which was diagnosed by EGC and pathology. At that time he could only eat the liquid food and half of XXXX food. She makes her living by filling the bicycle wheels and didn't have money for her surgery so that she started to take XZ-C medicine. After taking the medicine half of year her symptoms turned good. Aftertaking the medicine two andhalf years she recovered as the normal person and didn't have any complain. Because of her incoming condition, she didn't get any other tests and treatment. When she came back to followup, she had taken the medicine more than five years and her condition is good.

To take XZ-C for longterm can improve the patients immune function and the pateitns energy level will increase and the appetites will increase and the sleep will be good. XZ-C4 can protect the bone marrow and thymus to improve the nutrition and the metabolism will turn good and will get rid of the free bases to control and to repair the diseases.

Case 3 Mrs xxx, female, 65year-old, Huangpi in Hubei

Diagnosis: the middle esophogus carcinoma

Disease courses and treatment condition: In April 2001 the patient had difficulty swallowing and chest and back pain and gradually increased. Until June only can eat the liquid food and vomit the mucous staffs. On June 6 2001 the barium swallow tests in the xxx showed under the aorta branch xxxx 2cm there is a 10cm lenghth narrow and 6cm xxxxxlump in the left wall and the muscous stop. Because of the cost, she didn't have the operation, radioactive and chemotherapy. On June 25 she started to take XZ-C. After three months, her general condition is better and her appetite is getting better and the difficultying swallowing is getting better and can eat the rice soup, noodle. She continued taking the medicine until March 2002 then can take the rice and regular food. In July 2003 she just took XZ-C4+XZ-C2. In April 2005 when she followed up with us, she is energetic and her appetites was great at that time she had been taking XZ-C for more than five year. He condition is stable and can eat the regular food and can do light house work.

Comments: This patient had esophageal cancer which she only took XZ-C to control her condition without the operation, radiactiv therapy and chemotherapy. For more than four years, there was no metastasis and her condition had been controlled and can eat the regular food and rice. She is as healthy as other old persons and can do some choresevery day.

She kept taking her medicine regularly.

Case 4 Ms. xxx, female, 65 year-old, Jianxian in Hubei, officer.

Diagnosis: primary huge liver carcinoma

Disease course and treatment: Because of discomfort in upper abdomen, the patient had CT in XieHe hospital which found that a 6.7 cm x 7.1 cm x 9 cm nodule in right liver, then diagnosed as primary liver carcinoma. She refused to take operation and chemotherapy. In July 11, 1995 she started to take the XZ-C1+XZ-C5. After 2 months, her emotion and appetite get better and her weight increased. In September 20, 1995 on follow-up ultrasound, the nodule was reduced. In November 1995 she had a chemoembolization and didn't have any other therapy. She continues to take the XZ-C for more than 6 years and continues to follow-up more than 10 years. This patient's condition is good. In May 2005 this patient is as healthy as a normal person.

Comments: On July 4, 1995 this patient was diagnosed with primary liver carcinoma by CT and then took XZ-C after 1 week. After 2 month, the CT scan showed that the nodule become smaller. On November 21 the chemotherapy procedure was conducted, and then she continued to take XZ-C regularly and persistently for 10 years. Now this patient is as healthy as a normal individual.

Implication: The chemotherapy+XZ-C have good results on liver carcinoma treatment. The chemotherapy can stop the blood supply to the cancer nodule and chemotherapy can kill some of the cancer cells. There are living cancer cells inside and under the tumor nodule membrane after chemotherapy; the tumor cells didn't die completely and then grew fast after circulation built up. XZ-C can protect thymus and improve the immune ability, protect the bone morrow function and improve the body immune function. In addition, 85% hepatic cancer occurred in the cirrhosis patients so chemotherapy will damage the liver function. XZ-C will protect the liver. The combination of chemotherapy+XZ-C will inhibit the tumor and protect the host to improve the long-term treatment. This is called "take out the bad and keep the good" in Chinese.

Case 5. Mr. xxx, male, 53 year-old, Wuhan.

Diagnosis: primary huge liver cancer, liver cirrhosis after hepatitis, the later stage of Japanese blood fluke, Portal hypertension.

Disease course and treatment: Patient's appetite decreased and he felt uncomfortable in his abdomen. In September 2000 CT showed a 13.6cm x 11.8cm lesion in the right liver lobe. In September 7, 2000 MRI showed a huge 13.1cm x 11.4cm x 12.5cm lesion in right lobe, diagnosed as huge liver cancer in right lobe. The patient had hepatic arterial chemoembolization (HACE) and embolization (HAE) and the chemoembolization medicine were xxxx 25mg+xxx1000g: xxxx10ml+xxxx10mg. Currently his general condition is good. The change of his liver lesions are the following which are stable and getting small: CT showed a 11.1cm x 11.8cm lesion in the right liver lobe on October 12, 2000, a 10.8cm x 9.8cm lesion in the right liver lobe on December 14, 2000, a 10.5cm x 9.5cm lesion on Feb 2001 and a 9.8cm x 8.9cm lesion on September 3, 2001 in the right liver lobe. This patient started to take XZ-C1+XZ-C4+XZ-C5 on January 9, 2002 and his general condition is good, just as his emotion, appetite and sleep are very good. He comes back for check-up every month and takes his medicine regularly. On October 21, 2002 during his follow-up, his general condition is good, emotion is stable, and appetite is good and bowel movement is good and his routine is regular and he exercises regularly. He reports not having had a cold during the last four years. He lived as a normal healthy person.

Comments: This case is primary huge liver carcinoma which had five times embolization and the lesion was getting smaller and had very good response. Last embolization is on November 12, 2001 and the lesion is 9.8cm x 8.9cm. He started to take XZ-C1+XZ-C4+XZ-C5 on Jan 9, 2002. The XZ-C1 can kill the cancer cells and not kill the normal cells; XZ-C4 protects thymus and inhibits thymus shrinkage; XZ-C5 protects liver function. This patient continues to take this medicine for more than 3 years, however when he came back for follow-up in the fourth year, his health condition is general, disease is stable and there is no metastasis and no further development. His emotion is stable, his appetite is good, and he walks as a normal healthy person. The experience from this case is for primary huge liver cancer, first embolization treatment are given to make this lesion smaller and stable, later use XZ-C to support the long-term therapy and to protect the liver function and to improve the immune system and to control the metastasis.

Case 6. Mr. xxx, male, 51 year-old, Yin Zheng, officer.

Diagnosis: primary liver cancer

Disease course and treatment: There is a 4.6cm x 3.6cm nodule in left liver and a 1.6cm x 1.6cm nodule in right liver after the patient had CT on October 30, 1997. Diagnosis was liver carcinoma. There is a 5.9cm x 4.0cm x 5.4cm nodule in the left liver lobe and a 2.1cm x 1.8cm lesion in the right liver lobe when the patient had Ultrasound in the XieHe hospital. Liver angiography showed that the patient had liver cancer. HBsAg(+), AFP(-). Because this patient's liver function was poor, he couldn't stand the operation and put on the tube for chemotherapy. This patient is alcohol drinker for 40 years (250ml/per meal average). In 1996 he had Hepatitis B. In 1966 he had blood fluke. On November 25 the patient starts to take XZ-C1+XZ-C4+XZ-C5. In 1998 and 1999 the patient continued to take the medicine. The patient's condition is good, and his face is red and smiles. On November 2, 1999 he came to follow-up and the ultrasound showed the lesion was reduced. He can do light work and feels very well. For more than 2 years, he continues to take XZ-C1+XZ-C4+XZ-C5. After these medicines the patient's energy level is improving and appetite is improving. In June 2002 he went to Beijing for treatment (before he went to Beijing, he was good and walking as the normal person). During the operation there is a 5cm x 6cm nodule in the liver which is the same as 5 years ago and there are cancer cells in the common duct and now metastasis, and no fluid in the abdominal cavity. There is no metastasis in the liver, however because the nodule is close to the hepatic artery entrance, it is very difficult to remove the cancer nodule and then place the drainage tube. After surgery, this patient didn't have urine and had acute renal failure. He passed away on day 6.

Comments: On October 30, 1997 CT showed a 4.6cm x 3.6cm nodule in left liver and in November 1997 there is a 1.6cm x 1.6cm nodule in right liver. Because the liver function was poor, the patient didn't have operation and tube placement and other treatment. On November 25 he started to take XZ-C1+XZ-C4+XZ-C5 and continued for 5 years. His health condition was fine.

Implication: XZ-C can improve the host immune system ability (including the cell and antibody immune function) to protect the central and peripheral immune organs, to protect the liver and kidney, and to produce anticancer factors an dprevent cancer cells metastasis and spread. XZ-C is a medication with no side effects which helps the patient in "fight with bad and help the right". In addition the patient's disease condition was under very good control without metastasis so that therapeutic effect was very good. This patient took XZ-C for 5 years, during which time his condition was stable and the liver cancer lesion was not increasing and there were no metastasis. His general condition was good and not uncomfortable and the patient walked as a normal person. He went to Beijing and was diagnosed as liver cells carcinoma which was in the entrance of the liver and couldn't be removed because of the cancer cells in the common duct. The patient underwent surgery for the placement of the T-tube for chemotherapy. After the operation, this patient didn't have urine and died of acute renal failure. If he had not had the operation which destroyed the liver and kidney function, he might have survived to the present day.

2) Surgical exploration cannot remove tumor, nor do radiotherapy and chemotherapy

Case 1 Mr.xxx, male, 64 year-old Hubei Xin Zhou, officer

Diagnosis: the tumor of the mesentaic membranexxxx.

Disease courses and treatment condition:On January 6 1999 the patient suddenly had the uncomfortable in chest and pain and vomit. The emergency diagnosis was "actual GI infection", the surgeons thought of that he had the pancreatitis. On March 3 EGD showed the obstractle of the duodenum. On March 6 1999 during the survey of the abdomen, the tumor which was behind the abdominal membrance including big vessals which during the operation a 6cmx9cm lump in the roots of the small intestine membreance xxxx of hard, stable, fixed and unsmooth on the surface, connected to aorta and the xxxx arterial and pressed the duodenum which it was difficult to remove so that the connection of the duodenus and colon was done because the tumor can not be removed and the patients was told to be treated by the combination of the western and Chinese therapy. On April 1999 she started to take XZ-C1Z+C4. From May 15 1999 to February 2002 she continued to take the medicine and refill her medicine. She is stable and her medical condition is good.

Comments: On March 6 1999 the tumor from the abdomen membrane was foundby the survey of the operation. Because it is connected to the small intestine membrance including the big artery, this tumor can not be removed. But the surface of the tumor was firm and stable, which implied malignant. After taking Z-C years, the patients is stable and no development and no metastasis and healthy.

Case 2. Mr. xx, male, 50 year-old, Hubei Lou Tang, peasant.

Diagnosis: Postoperative Pancreas cancer

Disease course and treatment: Because of discomfort in upper abdomen for more than three months, he had jaundice and had opening abdomen surgery showing: No stones in the bile system and enlargement of the pancreas. The tumor couldn't be removed and Pathology showed pancreatic cancer. CT showed enlargement of pancreas head and dilation of the bile duct in liver. After the operation the jaundice extended persistently. On December 11, 1996 he started to take the XZ-C and after one month his medical condition got better and his appetite increased, however he still had little jaundice and weakness and sweating. After taking XZ-C and soup two months the jaundice and pain reduced and got better. After four months, the jaundice was gone completely and his appetite and energy level were good. His pain in abdomen was mild. In July 1998 he returned to work and did mild labor work and his face looks red. He continues to take his medicine for many years. On April 6, 2004 his family introduced a new patient to us and told us that this patient is fine and his activities are as a normal person's and he does his chores very well.

Comments: This patient has pancreas head cancer and jaundice. On November 28 1996 during the operation, this tumor cannot be removed and the Pathology is pancreas cancer with the dilation of the bile duct system in the livers. On December 11, 1996 this patient took ZX-C and soup. After seven months his jaundice is reduced and he continues to take medicine to improve his immune system. Until July 1998 his condition is completely normal. He continues to take his medicine for more than four years and later changed to taking the medicine periodically to support his healthy condition. This patient has followed up for more than nine years and his condition is very good

3) The Typical cases for recurrence after radical surgery with Z-C immunomodulatory anticancer medicine treatment

Case 1 Mr. xxx, male, 48 year-old, Taimen, officer.

Diagnosis: Primary liver carcinoma

Disease course and treatment: On August 1, 1994 because the patient felt fatigued, he had ultrasound in the local hospital and found a 4.1cm x 4.5cm nodule in the left lobe of the liver. On August 26, 1994 the left lobe of the liver was removed in the Xian Ha hospital. Pathological slides showed: liver cell carcinoma without any treatment. After operation, the patient was treated with anticancer immunological traditional medicine **XZ-C1+XZ-C4+XZ-C5** in our outpatient center. After taking these medicines, the patient's appetite increased, energy level increased and he was happy. He takes medicines regularly and comes to our office every month for follow up and refilling of the medicines. He feels very well and goes back to his work. On December 14, 1996 there was another 1.3cm x 1.8cm nodule which was found by B ultrasound in the edge of the left liver. On December 30, 1996 he had that nodule removed. After the operation, he continued to take the medicine. After that, the patient took his medicine persistently and regularly. In May 2010 when he came to follow-up, his general condition was good and his face was glowing with health, his body was as strong as a healthy person's and the patient returned to work for more than 11 years. His appetite is great and his emotion is very good. He eats 600g food per day and his ultrasound is normal.

Comments: On August 26, 1994 this patient had a 4.1cm x 4.5cm nodule removal of left liver. After the operation, the patient received XZ-C for treatment. On December 30, 1996 another 1.3cm x 1.8cm nodule was found and removed. After that, this patient continued to take XZ-C. When he came back for 16-year follow-up, his health condition is good and he can do labor work for many years. This patient is still alive and very well at the time of writing this book.

Case 2 Mr. xxx, male, 65 year-old, Wuhan, retired officer.

Diagnosis: Adenocarcinoma in the pyloric area of the stomach and recurrence after surgery in the remaining stomach

Disease course and treatment: This patient had pain in the upper abdomen for more than one year and in June 1993 he was diagnosed as stomach cancer and had removal of the great curvature in the stomach. After the operation, he had FM chemotherapy once which caused anemia and weakness and wbc is 1900. 8 months after operation, the patient had abdomen pain with vomiting and had left upper abdominal pain for half year. On March 25, 1994 the Barium showed: there was no filled on the upper area of the stomach and part damage of the membranes and the narrow change in the cutting parts. A barium swallow showed recurrence of the stomach cancer. On May 3, 1996 ultrasound showed that there is no lesion inside the liver. Because this patient couldn't eat rice and just eats noodles and liquid food so that he had fatigue and no energy, he didn't want to have operation. In June 1996 he started to take XZ-C. After that he is fine and his appetite is increased and he takes this medicine regularly for more than four years. On May 6, 2000 when he came back to follow-up, his general condition is great and his face looks red and healthy. Walking and activities are normal as the others and he eats rice soup and banana often as his meal.

Comments: In June 1993 the patient had stomach removal. In March 1994 the cancer recurred and the junction part turned narrow. After taking XZ-C+XZ-C4 only, for more than six years his health condition is great.

Implication: For the recurrence of the stomach cancers, the junction of the surgery was not closed completely and the patient could still eat food. After taking the medicines to improve thymus function to control the tumor growth and prevent the tumor growth and metastasis XXXX. The patient's medical condition is stable and he is still alive.

Case 3: Mr. xxx, male, 62year-old, Wuhan, engineer

Diagnosis: Renal pelvis carcinoma in the right kidney and the recurrence after the bladder carcinoma operation.

Diseases courses and treatment: the patient had cytoscopy which showed the bladder carcinoma in November 4 1995 afterthe bloody urine for two years. On November 21 1995 CT showed that rght renal pelvis tumor. On December 6 1995 the right kidney and urother were removed and his bladder was removed by the xxx and after the operation the local xxxx chemotherapy was used for seven times. On March 8 1996 the cystoscopy showed there was the hard lump in the left wall of the bladder in order to prevent the reccurrence of the tumor, he started to take XZ-C1+XZ-C4+XZ-C6. After taking this medicine he is well and his appetite is getting better. On June 24 1996 the cytoscopy showed that the bladder walls are smooth and the surface is smooth and the new things were gone. He continued to take XZ-C medicine to prevent the recerence and metastasis. Until June 11 1997 the cystoscopy showed the bladder is normal. On December 28 1998 the cystoscopy is normal. On June 26 1999 when he came back to follow up, his condition is stable and he continues to take the XZ-C1+XZ-C4+XZ-C6 for more than ten years to prevent the recurrence and metastasis. On May 6 2005 when he follow-up, he is stable and his condition is good and is the same as the normal individuals.

Comments: this case is the recurrence of the bladder cancinoma after the operation. After taking this medicine more than ten years to prevent the recurrence and metastasis, his medical condition is good and after many cystoscopy, the bladder is normal.

Suggestion: XZ-C can improve the patients immune function and prevent the tumor recurrence and metastasis and control the primary lesions. He is healthy and is in the good condition.

Case 4. Mr. xxxx, male, 68year-old, Wuhan, Professor

Diagnosis: the recurrence of the bladder cancer operation.

Disease courses and treatment conditions: After the removal of the bladder cancer was done in April 1994 in the hospital, Pathology showed: transitional cell carcinoma. After the operation the bladder was poured with chemotherapy. Because of the decrease of the white blood cells the chemotherapy stopped. In 1996 he came back to check up and found the cancer recurrence so that the second operation was done by the removal of eight tumors. After the surgery the patient's bladder was poured with XXX+XXXX twice every month for three months. After three months, repeat these medicine for another three months. Twice per month until 1997. In May 1998 the cystoscopy in the XXX hospital showed the xxx in the bladder. In December the ultrasound showed the bladder infection. In April 1999 because of the bloody urine, the cystoscopy showed that there were a four cm2 of the tumor and CT biopsy showed that bladder cancer. In May 1999 the arterial chemotherapy was poured. In June the second time of the poured the XXXX+XXXX+XXX was done. After that the white blood cells decreased into 2x109/l. In September the third time of the poured medicine with xxx+xxxx+xxx, the white blood cells decreased into 1.2x109/L, then inject the XXX to increase the white blood cells. His medical history: stroke in 1992, Hypertension(160/90mmHg), Diabete. In 1984 he had hepatitis and in 1998 had cirrhosis. Family history : two brothers had hepatitis B and then liver cancer, another brother had rectal cancer.

In July 1999 because of the white blood cells decrease after the chemotherapy, he started to take xxxx to protect the bone marrow and take XZ-C1+XZ-C4+XZ-C6. After taking them more than six months, the whole blood count come back again. His energy level is increased and his appetite is getting better and continue taking the medicine. In July 2000 the cystoscopy showed that the bladder was filled well and a 1.3cmx0.6cm xxxxx in the xxxx ranges, considering as the recurrence of the tumors and continued to take the medicine until June 2001, because of the prostate enlargement which caused the frequency and urgency of the urine. CT showed that this lesion was getting bigger than before(in February in 1999), then had arterialy poured once. He continued to take XZ-C1+XZ-C4+XZ-C6 untill July 2002 CT showed that the lesion in CT shrinkled. After taking the medicine, his general medical condition is better and his appetites is good without the bloody urine. He kept coming back to followup and take his medicine for more than six years. His lesion in his bladder is stable without metastasis and enlargement.

Comments: This case is transitional cell carcinoma. After the removal of the cancer, the long- time chemotherapy didn't stop the recurrence. Because of many years of the poured bladder and many times of the cystoscopy with the enlargement of the prostate and the narrowness of the urother, the cystescopy is difficult to be done. After taking XZ-C such as XZ-C1+XZ-C4+XZ-C6, the neoplasm in the bladder didn't develop and didn't metestes. Since he had this disease, it has been 11 years. His general medical condition is well and his appetite is getting better. When he walked more, sometimes the bloody urine occurred.

Case 5 Mrs. xxx, female, 67year-old, Shiyiazhoung, worker

Diagnosis: The recurrence after the surgery of the abdominal cavity serous tumors

Disease courses and treatment conditions:because of the belly was getting bigger and ascites, in May 1999 he was hosptilized in Tongjing and ascite(++) and his belly was like to frog and the tumor can be touched. On April 9 the surgery found that there were very many different sizes of the tumor, which were gel-like lump full of the abdominal cavity. One by one were removed, the total weight are 2.5g. During the operations, the chemotherapy tube was put with XXX 500mg. After the operation of four days xxx500MG once/per day and continued to use five days and xxx 100mg once/per day and continuing three days. On June 16 1999 he started to take XZ-C1+XZ-C4 andd after two months she is vigour and her appetite is good and her weight increases. PE: there were no lymph nodes in the superclavial, the abdomen is soft and flat, the ascite(-) and continue to take the XZ-C and refilled her medicine every month until November 26 2000, PE: there was a lump of the fit=size, hard, many nodual on the surface and deep and the clear edges which showed the tumor recurrence. The patient refused to the operation again and to chemotherapy, however he continued to take the XZ-C medicine: XZ-C1+XZ-C4+LMS+MDZ and the anticancer gel on the skin patched. Until Febrauay 24 2002 PE: there was on abnormal and her abdomen was soft and there was a lump which was hard, deep and clear edge and the size is smaller than before and her medical condition is stable. Until December 15 2004 her medical condition is good and her appetite is good and her abdomen is little enlarge and her ascite(++) and there is a fit-size lump with unsmooth surface and many nodule and deep and fix without the metastasis further. After her operation until now she has been following up with us more than six years and her medical condition is stable and the tumor is not metasatasis further.

Comments: This case is the serous tumor in the abdominal cavity. After the removal, the tumor recurrence. After the chemotherapy one week, the reaction is great so that in June 1999 she started to take XZ-C1+XZ-C3+XZ-C4 and she continued to take this medicine for more than six years and her medical condition is stable without the far metastasis and the tumors didn't grow big. She lives well with the tumors.

4) The typical cases of extensive bone metastasis with Z-C immunomodulatory anticancer medicine treatment

Case 1 Mrs xxx, female, 68year-old, Shengyang

Diagnosis: multiple bone metastasis after the removal of the breast cancer.

Disease courses and treatment: in 1984 the patient had the removal of the right breast cancer I stage, the pathology showed that simple breast cancer without lymph node metastasis. After the xxx +xxxx chemotherapy for two years, she started to use some immune enhancing drug. In January 2001 she felt the right shoulder pain and ECT showed that multiple bone metastasis and the supericlavical lymph nodes enlargement. Since March 27 she had 25 times radicacto therapy on the sites of the right superoclaviceal lymph nodes and the whole blood counts decreases and the white cell counts decrease into 2.9x109/L. After the radiactherapy, her condition stable.

On June 15 2001 he started to take XZ-C such XZ-C1+XZ-C2+XZ-C4+LMS+MDZ+VS for two months and her symptom significantly increased. After six months ECT was normal and she is stable. On September 2 2002 on the phone she told us that she is stable and takes her medicine regularly for more than four years. In April 2005 She called us that she is energetic and her appetites is great and walking as the normal healthy persons. On her physical examination, Ultrasound of her liver and gallbladder, Chest X-ray, ECT etc she is normal.

Comments:this patient had right breast cancer after the operation for more than 17 years with bone metastasis and right shoulder pain. After the radiactiv therapy her medical condition is getting better. After taking XZ-C for a long period to protect thymus and bone marrow function, her metastasis was controlled well.

Case 2 Mr. xxx, male, 66 year-old, Wuxiu, officer

Diagnosis: right kidney clear cell tumors with the bone marrow metastasis and superclavaical lymph node metastasis.

Disease courses and treatment condition: Because of the pain in the right should, the diagnosis was "the inflamtion of the sourround shoulder", which there was a lump as big as XXX behind the right clavical and stern bone, the biopsy showed adenocarcinoma. After CT of abdomen and chest Ultrasound, there was no lesion found. On March 2002 he started to take the XZ-C such as taking XZ-C1+XZ-C4 and plastic XZ-C3. After the plastic gels, the lump was getting soft and shrinkle into small. On March 24 2002 Ultrasound showed a lump of 3.1cmx4.3cm in the right kidney. CT showed : L2, L4 had bone damage and still took the XZ-C and GEM+XXX chemotherapy once. On May 16 2002 the right renal was removed which there was a lump of the size of table tennis. Pathology showed clear cells. Because he was on the immune function medicine, his medical condition was stable and his appetite is good. Although he had the metastasis of his whole body, he still walked as the normal persons. In 2002,2003 and 2004 he came back every month to refill his medicine and his medical condition is stable. Until July 2004 he suddenly lost the ability of speech and headache. CT showed that the bleeding of the brain. After three weeks of the hospitalization, his medical condition was stable and CT showed that the brain bleeding was absorbed and he continues to take XZ-C1+XZ-C2+XZ-C6+LMS+XXX+XXX+xxxx etc. His medical condition is good and he is vigour and his appetite is good.

Comments: this case is the right metastasis lump of the clavic bone with L2 and L4 bone metastasis, the biopsy showed the metastasis adenocarcinoma. After the whole examination the right kidney tumor was found. On May 16 2002 he was diagnosed as right kidney clear cell cancer and the kidney was removed. On March 16 2002 he started to use the XZ-C by taking and plastic. After three years his medical condition is stable and his appetite is good and he is vigour.

5) The cases of simply using Z-C anti-cancer traditional Chinese medicine after radical surgery without chemotherapy and radiotherapy

Case 1 Ms xxx, female, 49 year-old, Changsha in Hunan, teacher

Diangosis: breast infiltrating ductal cancer.

Disease courses and treatment condition: in February 2005 a left breast lump was found which is 2cmx1.5cm, biopsy showed that high degree mutation. On March 8 2005 she had CAF. On May 30 2005 the breast cancer was removed partially, pathology showed the breast cancer so that the breast cancer radiact removal was performed Pathologyshowed that left breast cancer infiltrated ductal cancer. LN0/20 with the C-erB2(++), P53(+), PR(-), ER(-), nm23(+). After the surgery the chemotherapy was used for six cycles. On Octocber 22 2005 she started to take XZ-C to strengthen the curative effects and to prevent the recurrence and metastasis.

Comments:in this case before the operation the lymph nodes under armpit were palpatited. Chemotherapy for six cycle was used before the operation and after the operations to strengthen the long time curative effect. She persistently takes these medicine more than six years and her healthy condition is stable.

Case 2 Mr. xxx, female, 71 year-old, Wuhan, teacher

Diagnosis: ascending colon carcinoma

Disease courses and treatment: Because of abdomen pain and bloody stool, the patient was diagnosed as colon cancer by colonoscopy with biopsy. On December 19 1994 he had half of the right colon removal. Pathology showed the medium grade of colon adenocarcinoma involved in serosa. After the operation, he didn't accept other therapy. On July 4 1995 he started to take XZ-C1+XZ-C4 as assistant therapy to prevent the recurrence and metastasis. He only takes XZ-C more than ten years and his healthy condition is very good. In April 2005 when he was 81 years old and came back to follow up with us, he was healthy and played the card every day in the afternoon.

Comments: this case is that after the removal of the ascending colon, the patient just takes XZ-C medicine as the assistant therapy to protect recurrence more than 10 years and his condition is stable.

Case3 Mr. xxx, male, 49year-old, Wuhan, officer

Diagnosis: lung cancer in the right low labor

Disease courses and treatment: In 1996 the patient started to have cough and chest tightness and low fever and difficult breath and was treated as the Cold. In April 1997 he suddenly started to cough blood and X-ray and CT showed the right lung cancer in low lobe. And at the same month he had right low lobe lung removal and Pathology showed that lung low grade adenocarcinoma. After the operation, his condition is stable and didn't have chemotherapy and radioactive therapy. On May 15 1997 he started to take XZ-C:1,4,7, vitamin C, B6 E, A. After he took these medicine his energy level is increase and appetite was great and his face is red and there were no recuurence and metastasis and no complaints. In June 2004, the patient came back to follow up with us he continues to take these medicine more than three years. Everything is stable. So far his condition is stable as the normal healthy person after he took his medication more than eight years.

Comments: this patient has right low lobe low grade adenocarcinoma. After the operation, he didn't have radioactive and chemotherapy treatment and he only takes the XZ-C medication XZ-C1+C4+C7. After taking these medicine more than eight years, his energy level is high and appetite is good and his healthy condition is great.

Case 4 Mr. xxx, male, 52 year-old, Wuhan, driver

Diagnosis: right lung low grade adenocarcinoma with lymph node metastasis

Disease courses and treatment: because of bloody cough he had the CTscan which showed that right low lung tumor and the bronchoscopy didn't show abnormal. On December 12 2001 he had the removal of the right middle and lower lobe and one lymph node between lobe and two lymph node in the entrance were found. Pathology showed that low grade adenocarcinoma with lymph node mestastasis. After the operation he has once chemotherapy. In 2002 he started to take XZ-C to prevent the tumor recurrence and metastasis. He continues to take the XZ-C1+C4+C7+LMS+MDZ for more than three year and his condition is stable and he is energetic and his appetite is great.

Comments: this patient has the right low lobe adenocarcinoma with lymph node metastasis. After the chemotherapy once, then using the XZ-C1+C4+C7 as the supplement treatment. XZ-C1 kills the cancer cells without killing the normal cells. XZ-C4 protects the thymus and bone marrow; XZ-C7 to protect the lung function. He continues to take his medication for more than three years and there was not metatastasis. When he came back to follow up for his fourth year treatment, his condition is stable and his appetite is great and walked as the normal healthy person.

Case 5 Mr. xxx, female, 60 yr, Huangpu

Diagnosis: sigmoid colon cancer and the removal of half of the left colon.

Disease courses and treatment: In August 1998 the patient had bloody stool and was treated as hemorrhoid. In Octocber 1999 when he had the colonoscopy in Xiehu hospital which there is narrow in the 32cm from the anus. On December 3 1999 he had the removal of half of the left-colon. Pathology showed:sigmoid xxxx adenocarcinoma involved in the whole layers of the colon and the metastasis of the nearby lymph nodules(6/8). On Jan 12 2000 he started to take XZ-C: XZ-C1+XZ-C4+LMS+MDA+VT to protect recurrence and metastasis. After he continues to take the XZ-C more than three years and eight months, his son came to refill the medicine on August 4 2003 and told us that his medical condition was good and did the chores every day and planted a lot of different kinds of flowers and vegatables watering them with ten buckles of water. The patient has been in the good condition and happy and has good energy. After his operation, he continues to take the XZ-C medicines only everyday without other chemotherapy. When he followed up with us, he already took the medicine more than five and half years.

Comments: the case is that sigmoid colon carcinoma with metastasis of the nearby lymph nodes. After the removal of the operation the patient didn't have chemotherapy because of the decrease of the white blood cells so that he took the XZ-C as the assistant therapy to protect the bone morrow and thymus to improve the body immune system to protect the reccurrence and the metastasis. After five and half years, his condition was good.

Case 6 Ms. xxx, female, 63year-old, Jiling, officer

Diagnosis: the rectal adenocarcinoma

Disease courses and treatment: in Octocbor 1999 the patient has the bloody stool and the the rectaoscopy showed there is a flower-like tumor in the 10cm distance from the ana and Pathology showed the rectal cancer. On November 22 1999 the rectal radioactive surgery was done in the affliatite hospital with Dixon ways. After the operation the patient's condition is stable. On December 2 the chemotherapy was done(urine xxxx 1.0g/day, for five days, xxx 100mg/day for three days). On December 9 the white blood cell counts decrease into 0.09x109/L, on December 10 the white blood cells decrease into 0.06x109/L, injection of the medicine of increasing the white blood cells for five days, the white blood cells into1.1x109/l and had the pneumonia and fever with 40C. On January 2 xxxx after treatment with xxxx+xxxx, the patient still has fever and had the throat infection with three bacteria and can not eat and drink anything. After using XXX for five days, the temperature dropped into 38C. Because this patient had hypertension, diabetes and lung diseases, her medical condition is weak and severe and had twice warrancy from the hospitals. After two months of the treatment, she is stable. On March 20 2000 she started to take XZ-C for half of the years and her medical condition is stable and can do a little chores and can support her daily life by her own. On September 2000 she recurred very well and can shop in the nearby market and do little chores. She has been taken the medicine for more than five years consistently. In May 2005 her daughter come to refill the medicine and told us that she is totally fine and still do some house chores as healthy as other normal healthy individuals.

Comments: this case is the radial rectal cancer removal and the chemotherapy. After these her immune function and bone morrow function were inhibited so that she had throat and both the lung infections, which later are two fungus infections. After the treatment her condition started to get better and started to take the XZ-C which XZ-C1 only inhibited the tumor cells without affecting the normal cells and improve the immune fucntions, XZ-C4 to protect thymus and bone marrow to improve the immune function. The chemotherapy can inhibit the bone marrow so as to lead the bone marrow inhibition to some degrees which can affect the patients for more than 2 to 3 years so that XZ-C which have protect thymus and bone marrow function need to be taken for several years to benefit the bone marrow and immune functions

Case 7 Ms xxx, female, 39 year-old, Shichuang Luchang, officer

Diagnosis: Thyroid cancer

Disease course and treatment: On April 27 1999 after the removal of the right neck lump, diagnosed as lymphocyte thyroid cancer. On May 6 1999 he had the radical total removal of the thyroid, then he had hourse voice and didn't have chemotherapy. On July 24 he started to take XZ-C:XZ-C1+XZ-C4, LMS, VS and follow-up with us every month and continue to use more than half years. Until Jan 2000 his voice gets better and after continue to take XZ-C another three months his voice come back to the normal. His general conditions get better and his emotion is stable and appetite is good and his energy level came back and he can go back his work. He persistently takes XZ-C1+XZ-C4 to improve his immune function and followed with us more six years and in May 2005 when he came back to us, his general condition is very good.

Comments: this patient has capillary thyroid cancer. After operation his voice was housral and didn't have radiology and chemoactive therapy. He only took the XZ-C to improve his immune function and to prevent recurrence and metastasis.

Case 8 Mrs. xxx, female, 67year-old, Shiyiazhoung, worker

Diagnosis: The recurrence after the surgery of the abdominal cavity serous tumors

Disease courses and treatment conditions:because of the belly was getting bigger and ascites, in May 1999 he was hosptilized in Tongjing and ascite(++) and his belly was like to frog and the tumor can be touched. On April 9 the surgery found that there were very many different sizes of the tumor, which were gel-like lump full of the abdominal cavity. One by one were removed, the total weight are 2.5g. During the operations, the chemotherapy tube was put with XXX 500mg. After the operation of four days xxx500MG once/per day and continued to use five days and xxx 100mg once/per day and continuing three days. On June 16 1999 he started to take XZ-C1+XZ-C4 andd after two months she is vigour and her appetite is good and her weight increases. PE: there were no lymph nodes in the superclavial, the abdomen is soft and flat, the ascite(-) and continue to take the XZ-C and refilled her medicine every month until November 26 2000, PE: there was a lump of the fit=size, hard, many nodual on the surface and deep and the clear edges which showed the tumor recurrence. The patient refused to the operation again and to chemotherapy, however he continued to take the XZ-C medicine: XZ-C1+XZ-C4+LMS+MDZ and the anticancer gel on the skin patched. Until Febrauay 24 2002 PE: there was on abnormal and her abdomen was soft and there was a lump which was hard, deep and clear edge and the size is smaller than before and her medical condition is stable. Until December 15 2004 her medical condition is good and her appetite is good and her abdomen is little enlarge and her ascite(++) and there is a fit-size lump with unsmooth surface and many nodule and deep and fix without the metastasis further. After her operation until now she has been following up with us more than six years and her medical condition is stable and the tumor is not metasatasis further.

Comments: This case is the serous tumor in the abdominal cavity. After the removal, the tumor recurrence. After the chemotherapy one week, the reaction is great so that in June 1999 she started to take XZ-C1+XZ-C3+XZ-C4 and she continued to take this medicine for more than six years and her medical condition is stable without the far metastasis and the tumors didn't grow big. She lives well with the tumors.

Case 9. Mr. xxx, male, 76year-old, Henan, officer

Diagnosis: left renal clear cell cancer.

Disease courses and treatment condition:in 1996 there is a kidney cyst, in 2000 on PE there is a 7.5cmx6.5cm cysts in the left renal. CT and MRI showed that left kidney tumor. On August 31 2000 the removal of the left kidney was done in Tongjing hospital. Pathology showed that middle degree of kidney clear cells carcinoma. After the surgery he started to take the xxxx without chemotherapy and radiactvie therapy. On September 28 2000 she started to take XZ-C1+XZ-C4+XZ-C6 to protect thymus ad bone marrow. After taking the medicine one month, he is vigour and his appetite is still low and contine taking the medicine for three months, his general condition is good and his energy level is high and his sleeping is good. After taking the medicine for one year, Ultrasound of the abdomen, Chest X-ray, and others regular tests are normal and he continues to take XZ-C1+XZ-C4+XZ-C6 to prevent the metastasis and recurrence. After five years of taking these medicine, his healthy condition is stable. On April 10 2005 when he follow-up with us, he is healthy and his face is glowing of the health and his voice is xxxx, and he is energetic and had the hear decrease due to his age. His medical condition is100 by CCCCCC.

Comments: this case is left kidney clear cells. He was 76 year-old when he had his surgery. Because of his age, he didn't have the chemotherapy and radioactive therapy and only take the XZ-C immune therapy as the supplement therapy to protect his thymus and bone marrow to improve the immune functions and protect the recurrence and metastasits. He has been taking the medicine for more than five years and when he came back to followup he was 80 years old. His general medical condition is good and his appetite is good and his face is glowing of the health and his energy level is high and his voice is xxx as the normal healthy person.

Case 10 Mr. xxx, female, 44 year-old, Wuhan

Diagnosis: Breast adenocarcinoma

Disease courses and treatment: right breast lump was found for three months which the needle biopsy showed breast cancer. On February 20 1995 she had the removal of the breast cancer and once radioactive therapy after the operation. Because of the weakness, she couldn't tolerate it. On May 11 1995 she started to take XZ-C1+XZ-C4 and continued to take them for more than three years. After she took the medicine, her energy level was improving and her appetite was increasing and her weight is increasing. Following up with us every month and her medical condition is stable.

Comments: this patient had the removal of the breast on Feb 20 1995 and once radioactive therapy after the operation. Because of the weakness the radiative therapy was stopped. In May 1995 she started to take the XZ-C1+XZ-C4. After three years her condition is stable. When she came back for her five year follow-up, she is healthy.

Case 11 Ms. xxx, female,33 year-old, Changda in Hunan, worker

Diagnosis: Left simple breast cancer.

Disease courses and treatment: On November 29 1996 she had the removal of the breast cancer in Changda which showed the right armpit lymph node metastasis(3/5). After one month, CMF was done which she used once/week, for more than four weeks.

On December 25 1996 she started to use XZ-C to protect her bone marrow. After taking the medicine, her whole blood went back to the normal level. From April 2 1997 to May 14 1997 she had radioactive 15 times in right breast inner line, 15 times under the armpit right and 25 times in the right breast outside lines. XZ-C were taken as the supplement therapy without the side effects. The patients is stable and reaction small and even no side effects when she took XZ-C with radiactherapy and chemotherapy. In June 2004 she only took XZ-C. Every three months she came to Wuhan to refill her medicines. Her condition is stable. In Dec 2004 when she came back to follow up with us, she is energetic and appetite is good and her face is glowing of the health. Acting is as the normal healthy persons. She came to refill her medicine from XXXX to WuHAN.

Comments: the curative experience of the treatment:1). During the radiacti and chemotherapy the XZ-C4 can reduce the reaction, during the interval time between the radiac and chemotherapy and after them XZ-C can strengthen longterm curative effects to protect the recurrency.2)after the surgery about six months the radia+chemotherapy +XZ-C can kill the remaining tumor cells or the small tumor lesions, meanwhile to protect the host immune organs. After taking the medicine for six months, the patient's general condition is good so that XZ-C can get rid of the wrong and strengthen the long-time curative effects. After 9 years of the operation, XZ-C can strengthen the long-term therapy.

Case 12 Ms xxx, female, 49 year-old, Changsha in Hunan, teacher

Diangosis: breast infiltrating ductal cancer.

Disease courses and treatment condition: in February 2005 a left breast lump was found which is 2cmx1.5cm, biopsy showed that high degree mutation. On March 8 2005 she had CAF. On May 30 2005 the breast cancer was removed partially, pathology showed the breast cancer so that the breast cancer radiact removal was performed Pathologyshowed that left breast cancer infiltrated ductal cancer. LN0/20 with the C-erB2(++), P53(+), PR(-), ER(-), nm23(+). After the surgery the chemotherapy was used for six cycles. On Octocber 22 2005 she started to take XZ-C to strengthen the curative effects and to prevent the recurrence and metastasis.

Comments:in this case before the operation the lymph nodes under armpit were palpatited. Chemotherapy for six cycle was used before the operation and after the operations to strengthen the long time curative effect. She persistently takes these medicine more than six years and her healthy condition is stable.

Case 13. Mr. xxx, male, 66year-old, Wuhan, accounting

Diangosis:rectal carcinoma

Disease courses and treatment conditions:occasionally diarria and constipation with bloody stool for two years. The rectal examination showed that there was a 3cmx3cm lump at the 6 clock point in the xxxx position. On January 20 1998 the colonoscopy showed the polypoid mutation of the rectal colon. On January 24 1998 Dixon which the 40cm of the colon were cut off was done in the xiehae hospital, Pathology showed that rectal cancer with middle division and invade into the muscular layer without lymph nodes metastasis and the margin clear. After thesurgery, on March 3 1998 he started to use the XZ-C and took this medicine persistenly for more than eight years and he come back to work for more than five years He is stable and still continued to use these medicine.

Comments: this case is rectal adenocarcinoma. In January 1998 Dixon was done and Pathology showed that rectal adenocarcinoma, middle-degree. After the operation he only took the XZ-C1+XZ-C4 for more tha eight years. His medical condition is stable.

Suggestions: After the rectal Dixon without the chemotherapy, he only took the immune regulation medicine XZ-C to protect his thymus and bone marrow to improve his immune functions to improve the life quality and prevent the recurrence and metasatasis. He was stable.

Case14 Msxxx, female, 32year-old, Zhaoyang, accounting

Diagnosis: rectal villious adenocarcinoma

Disease courses and treatment condition: the patient had bleedy stool. In September 1997 the Colonoscopy and biopsy showed the rectal cancer. On September 17 1997 she had the rectal radial operation which showed that the lump was 1.0cmx1.0cm on the bases and was 4cm distance from the ana. Pathology reported the rectal villious adenocarcinoma and invaded into the all of the wall of the intestines with the menstema lymph node metastasis. After the operation she had chemotherapy once. Because of the decrease of the white blood cells she stop chemotherapy and started to use XZ-C1+XZ-C4. Her medical condition is well and stable. She continued to take the medicine for more than eight years only without chemotherapy and other therapy. She did her chores as the normal persons.

Comments:this case is the rectal radial removal on September 17 1997, during the operation, the metastasis were found in the mestaen membrane lymph nodes and invades the whole wall of the intestines. After the operation she had the chemotherapy once which had been stopped because the side effects were severe. Since December 3 1997 she started to take XZ-C only for more than eight years to prevent the reccurrence and metastasis after the surgery. Her medical condition is well.

Case 15 Mr. xxx, Male, 69year-old, Heilunjing, officer

Diangosis: the bladder transitional cell cancer

Diseases courses and treatment condition: The bloody urine on Februay 27 in 1998. On March 2 the cystoscopy and ultrasound showed that there was the round lump in the front wall, which is 1.6cmx1.4cm and growed toward to the cavity of the bladder and is the neoplasum of the front wall of the bladder. On March 10 in 1998 the surgery removed the tumor tissues in the bladder and Pathology showed that the bladder transitional cell tumors. He was told that this tumor is the recurrence of the tumors. After the surgery, he had once chemotherapy(on May 26 1998). His reaction to chemotherapy is severe such as the vomiting, nausea, and the whole body is uncomfortable. The left testicule enlarges so that he stop chemotherapy. On June 18 1998 he started to take the XZ-C. He follow up with us very month and his condition is good and his urine is normal and he doesn't have any other symptoms. He follow up with us for more than six years and he is healthy.

Comments: in this case on March 10 1998 the surgery removed three tumors in the bladder and Pathology showed that bladder transitional cell carcinoma. After the operation once chemotherapy was done which the patient had severe reaction to this chemotherapy. On June 18 1998 he started to take the medicine XZ-C1+XZ-C4+XZ-C6. He continued to take this medicine for more than seven years and his healthy condition is good without other therapy and without the recurrence and metasatasis.

Case 16 Ms. Zhang, female,39 year-old, Wuhan, account

Diagnosis: the stomach cancer from the stomach ulcer, low differential adenocarcinoma

Disease courses and treatment: in March 1994 because of the uncomfortable in the upper abdomen for one month and getting worse for one week so that the endoscopy showed the stomach ulceration. On April 20 1994 the major stomach was removed and had chemotherapy for six courses of the treatment after the operation with xxxxx+xxxxx to protect the livers. Pathology showed the low differential stomach canciroma and had lymph nodes metastasis. On November 22 1995 he started to take

XZ-C1+XZ-C4+XZ-C8 only to protect the bone marrow and follow up with us for more than ten years. He doesn't have metastasis and recurrence and his condition is great.

Comments: this patient had low degree adenocarcinoma in the stomach and lymph node metastasis. On April 20 1994 he had the removal of his major stomach, then he had six courses of the chemotherapy. On November 22 1995 he took the medicine only and followed up with us for more than ten years. His medical condition is great.

Suggustions: After the operation the combination of the chemotherapy and XZ-C medicine can improve the long-term treatment. XZ-C can prevent the cancer recurrence and metastasis.

Case 17 Mrs xxx, female, 65year-old, Huangpi in Hubei

Diagnosis: the middle esophogus carcinoma

Disease courses and treatment condition: In April 2001 the patient had difficulty swallowing and chest and back pain and gradually increased. Until June only can eat the liquid food and vomit the mucous staffs. On June 6 2001 the barium swallow tests in the xxx showed under the aorta branch xxxx 2cm there is a 10cm lenghth narrow and 6cm xxxxxlump in the left wall and the muscous stop. Because of the cost, she didn't have the operation, radioactive and chemotherapy. On June 25 she started to take XZ-C. After three months, her general condition is better and her appetite is getting better and the difficultying swallowing is getting better and can eat the rice soup, noodle. She continued taking the medicine until March 2002 then can take the rice and regular food. In July 2003 she just took XZ-C4+XZ-C2. In April 2005 when she followed up with us, she is energetic and her appetites was great at that time she had been taking XZ-C for more than five year. He condition is stable and can eat the regular food and can do light house work.

Comments: This patient had esophageal cancer which she only took XZ-C to control her condition without the operation, radiactiv therapy and chemotherapy. For more than four years, there was no metastasis and her condition had been controlled and can eat the regular food and rice. She is as healthy as other old persons and can do some choresevery day.

She kept taking her medicine regularly.

Case 18 Mr. xxx male, 66year-old, Huanpi, officer Diagnosis: the middle and low esophagous carcinoma

Disease courses and treatment:in March, he had the difficulty to swallow and the barium swallow test showed that the middle and low esophagum cancer. In May 1996 he had the removal of his cancer without other therapy. On June 19 1996 he started to use the XZ-C as the supplemental therapy to prevent the reccurrence and metastasis. He only takes XZ-C to protect his thymus and bone marrow for more than three years, then he changed into periodly taking the medicine. He is energetic and his appetite is good and walking and other activities are the same as the normal persons. In April 2005 when he came back to follow up with us, his condition is stable.

Comments: after the operation of his esophague, this patient only took XZ-C to assisting his therapymore than nine years, his condition is stable.

6) Chemotherapy plus Z-C Chinese medicine treatment of typical cases of acute lymphoblastic leukemia

Case: Mr.xxx, female, 34 year-old, Wuhan, officer.

Diagnosis: Acute leukemia

Disease course and treatment: On Novermber 29 the patient was diagnosed as acute leukemia in Beijing hospital and was treated by chemotherapy for seven months. In August 2000 he was treated by bone morrow transplantation, however the results were not good after that because WBC, RBC and platelets are low. Such as wbc0.5x109/l, platelets were 5x100/l, HB46g/l. He depended on the blood transfusion, which were performed once per 8-9 days for 250ml. During his inpatient in Beijing, He had 10 times blood transfusion and 14 times platelets (once per 10 days). In Feb 2001 he came to Wuhan and on Feb 2, 2001 he started to use XZ-C1+XZ-C2+XZ-C8 to protect his thymus and his bone morrow. In April 2001 his WBC and RBC and Pletelets increase and stop to get transfusion. He takes XZ-C1+XZ-C2+XZ-C4 for more than one year and seven months and feel fine and he looked good and healthy and appetites increases and walking and runnig as the normal individual. In September 4 2003 he traveled to America and took his medicine XZ-C1+XZ-C2+XZ-C4 with him and he takes his medicine persistently.

In 2004 he immigrate into Canada and took his medicine XZ-C1+XZ-C2+XZ-C8 regularly and increase blood soups which will be filled once per 3 months. In April 2005 He called me and told us that he was healthy and his medical condition was controlled very well and appetite and sleep very well and started to work on business and energy level is perfectly well.

Comments: This patient has ALL and after seven months chemotherapy in August 2000, he had bono marrow transplantation. However the treatment results were not good because his blood counts were still low which he depended on the blood transfusion. On Feb 2 2001 he started to take XZ-C1+XZ-C2+XZ-C4. And increase blood soups etc. and after four months his blood counting went back the normal. After one year and seven months his blood counting keeps normal and he is healthy and has taken these medicine for more than 4 years and work in the business field and energy level is normal.

Suggustion: All can be treated satisfiedly by chemotherapy and XZ-C to protect the bone marrow and improve the immune system function. Now he has been followed up more than seven years and his healthy condition is very well.

To overcome cancer and to launch a general offensive

Prevention and Control and Treatment Together

Chapter 11 The initiative of conquering cancer and launching a general offensive

The overall strategic reform of cancer treatment

1. The requisite to launch a general offensive

1). Overview

Cancer is a common enemy of all mankind, should mobilize the world's scientists, leaders, the masses to be involved in, should call on the mobilization of the whole world to overcome cancer, the current is the time, it is imperative.

The goal of conquering cancer is to reduce the morbidity, to reduce the mortality rate, to improve the cure rate, to prolong the survival time, to improve the quality of life and to reduce the complications.

The current cancer hospital or oncology treatment of cancer is mainly concentrated on the late stage, the treatment effect is poor.

The way out of cancer treatment is "three early": early detection, early diagnosis and early treatment. The patients in the early stage have good results. It will improve the therapeutic effect so as to inevitably reduce the cancer mortality and improve the cure rate.

If we can treat the cancer in the precancerous lesions or the early stage, the cancer treatment is very good, and then the progression of the invasion or metastasis in the late stage of the patient will reduce, this will reduce the incidence of cancer.

If you ignore the precancerous lesions, the early patients, it is impossible to reduce the incidence of cancer. The key to cancer treatment is in the "three early", and how to deal with precancerous lesions is a critical stage of cancer prevention and treatment.

I have been engaged in clinical tumor surgery for 57 years. The more treatment, the more the patients; the incidence of cancer is also rising, so I deeply understand that cancer should not only pay attention to treatment, but also to prevention in order to stop at the source.

Cancer is not only a serious threat to human health, but also an important factor in the rapid rise in medical expenses. China's annual direct cost of cancer treatment is nearly 100 billion yuan, so that patients and the whole community bear a huge financial burden.

Although countries have invested heavily in the treatment of cancer patients, but in the past 20 years, 5-year survival rate of some common cancer was no significant improvement, such as the United States 1974-1990, 5-year survival rate of esophageal cancer rose from only 7% to 9%, gastric cancer from 16% to 19%, liver cancer increased from 3% to 6%, lung cancer from 12% to 15%, while pancreatic cancer is still basically no change it is still 3%.

What should be done? The way out of anti-cancer is prevention.

For malignancy tumor the prevention is better than treatment. Through the adjustment of public health resources and strategies, strategic shift, focus from treatment to prevention, develop both of prevention and treatment tighter, develop the active, effective and early warning and early intervention and intervention studies to reduce cancer incidence and to improve the cure rate, which has become a global consensus on cancer researchers.

How do we overcome cancer? How to overcome cancer?

XZ-C launches the general idea of attacking cancer and the total attack design, as well as the total attack of the planning, route, blueprint of conquering cancer.

What is the total attack? That is anti-cancer, cancer control, cancer treatment, keeping pace, both of prevention and treatment.

We should reform the whole strategy of cancer treatment, reform the prevention and treatment of cancer from lightening the anti-cancer prevention and focusing on anti-cancer treatment to focus on both of prevention and treatment. We should update our thinking, update our understanding, advance in reform, innovate in reform and develop in reform.

2). To conquer cancer has been urgent

Why should I put forward a general attack? Why is it imperative? Status: Look at the current situation:

(1) The incidence of cancer is that the more treatment, and the more the patients. The current incidence of cancer in China is that the new cases of cancer every year have the 312 million cases, for the average daily the new cancer cases are 8550 cases, in China there are 6 persons which are diagnosed with cancer per minute.

(2) The status of cancer mortality is high, has been the cause of death in urban and rural areas first, the number of cancer deaths per year is up to 2.7 million people, an average of 7,500 people die of cancer every day, in every 7 deaths one dies of cancer.

(3) The status of treatment: Although the application of the traditional three major treatments for nearly a hundred years, tens of thousands of cancer patients bear the radiotherapy and chemotherapy, but the results?

So far, cancer is still the first cause of death, although patients have a regular, systematic radiotherapy and / or chemotherapy, it still failed to prevent cancer metastasis, recurrence and has little effect.

(4) The current status of cancer hospital or oncology hospital model

①go all out to focus on treatment; for the middle, or late, it has poor efficacy which depleted human and financial resources, and failed to reduce mortality and to improve the cure rate and reduce morbidity.

② only cure, or focusing on treatment without prevention, the more treatment, the more the patients.

③ ignored the "three early", ignoring the precancerous lesions.

④ ignore the prevention.

⑤ masses: talk about cancer discoloration

Patients and their families: powerless

Doctors and nurses : cannot be resistant to cancer and medical treatment stays in the three treatments and the effect is wandering.

People's attitudes: a lots of chemicals, physicals and biology environment carcinogenic things appear. A variety of carcinogenic substances into the human body or a variety of carcinogens affect the human body, it seems people are enveloped in the environment of carcinogens in the ocean; when some people talk about cancer their color changes. Cancer is not terrible, however the terrible thing is that we do not have this simple knowledge with this basic knowledge, the vast majority of cancer can be avoided and can be prevented.

⑥ Many large hospitals, university hospitals have not established laboratories, can not carry out basic research on cancer or clinical basic research, because if there is no breakthrough in basic research, clinical efficacy is difficult to improve. "Oncology" is still the most unadvanced subject in the current medical subjects because the pathogenesis, pathophysiology, pathophysiology are not yet clear understanding. Its pathogenesis and the mechanism of cancer metastasis are still a lack of adequate understanding; the complex biological behavior of cancer cells is still not clear. Lack of adequate knowledge, so the current treatment program is still quite blind, it is necessary to establish a laboratory for basic research and clinical basic research.

3). The concept and the general goal of conquering cancer

General attack is to aim at anti-cancer, cancer control, cancer treatment, and three-phase of the whole process of the cancer development carried out in full swing, that is: anti-cancer – before the formation of cancer

Control Cancer - a malignant tendency to precancerous lesions

Treatment of Cancer--- has formed a cancer foci or metastasis

The goal of General attack : to reduce cancer incidence, to reduce cancer mortality, to improve the cure rate, to prolong survival, to improve quality of life and to reduce complications.

2. The feasibility of launching a general offensive

We propose to launch a general offensive, that is, anti-cancer, cancer control, cancer treatment and three-phase work carried out in full swing, simultaneously.

As we all know: how to reduce cancer mortality? How to improve the cure rate? How to prolong survival?

--- The way out of cancer treatment should be in the "three early" (the early detection, the early diagnosis, the early treatment). The result of the early cancer treatment is good and it can be healed more, especially if the precancerous lesions are treated well, it can be cured.

Whether are there the scientific basis or not now proposes to attack cancer? Whether are there the medical foundation? Although the nearly a century, the traditional therapy failed to conquer cancer, the traditional therapy of radiotherapy and chemotherapy can not rely on to overcome the cancer, can not overcome the cancer. Because it can only ease, it can not be cured, but also a lot of achievements and experience are made. We should be based on this medicine in-depth study to expand the results.

1) First, it has made a wealth of experience in the treatment of cancer

1. Human being has made great strides in surrendering cancer

Since December 1971, President of the United States, Nixon, signed the «National Cancer Act», which is considered to be a formal declaration of war by mankind.

In the past 42 years it has elapsed after a review of what has been achieved and shows that human cancer has made great strides in its journey to cancer: statistics show that the incidence of cancer in the United States has decreased significantly since 1996, cancer mortality since 1990 has dropped by 17%, cancer 5-year survival rate increased by 18%, and achieved significant new results, indicating that cancer is likely to be gradually surrender.

2 Now parts of the cancer have found a way to prevent it

(1) The study found that chronic inflammation is the leading cause of cervical cancer, liver cancer, gastric cancer, the main reason for cervical cancer are more based on chronic cervicitis; liver cancer is more based on chronic hepatitis, cirrhosis; gastric cancer is more based on chronic gastritis and gastric ulcer.

Part of the inflammation or eradication of pathogenic factors (such as stomach, intestinal cancer treatment of Helicobacter pylori) may prevent the occurrence of cancer.

(2) As we all know, lifestyle is one of the key factors of cancer incidence, especially tobacco. Promotion of smoking campaign and healthy eating habits can prevent the occurrence of lung cancer and other cancers. The promotion of anti-cancer lifestyles are: smoking, alcohol, weight loss.

3. Screening can prevent or treat parts of the cancer

(1) the occurrence of colorectal cancer is based on polyps, polyps can prevent the occurrence of cancer, and colonoscopy, you can reduce the incidence of colorectal cancer and mortality. Any intestinal symptoms or blood in the stool should be For colonoscopy.

(2) cervical smear can be effective in detecting precancerous lesions of the cervix, by treating precancerous lesions can prevent cancer.

(3) breast molybdenum target X-ray screening of early breast cancer.

Above three kinds of cancer, such as early detection, the vast majority can be cured.

4. The combination of Chinese and western medicine and the immune regulation and treatment are expected to obtain a major breakthrough

As mentioned earlier, immunosuppression is the key to cancer progression regardless of the complexity of the mechanisms behind cancer, and the removal of immunosuppressive factors and the restoration of cell recognition by cancer cells can be effective against cancer. Through the regulation of the body's immune system, it is possible to achieve the purpose of cancer control through the activation of the body's anti-tumor immune system to treat tumors, is currently the field of excitement of the majority of researchers and may become a major breakthrough in the treatment of cancer.

To explore the cause of cancer, pathogenesis, pathophysiology, we conducted a series of animal experiments.

As a result of the experimental study, we found that the thymus of the cancer-bearing mice showed progressive atrophy, impaired central immune organ function, decreased immune function and low immune surveillance. Therefore, the therapeutic principle must be to prevent thymic atrophy, promote thymic hyperplasia, Improve bone marrow hematopoietic function monitoring; the immune regulation treatment of cancer provides a theoretical basis and experimental basis.

Based on the above causes of cancer and the pathogenesis of the experimental results, the new ideas and new methods of XZ-C immune regulation and treatment are proposed. After 16 years of cancer specialist out-patient clinics in more than 12000 cases of advanced cancer patients in clinical validation observation, it confirmed that the principle of treatment of increasing thymus function is reasonable, the effect is satisfactory. Application of immune regulation of traditional Chinese medicine achieved good results, improved life Quality and significantly prolonged survival.

5. The molecular targeted drug treatment is eye-catching

Philadelphia chromosome opened targeted cancer door. In 1960 the United States Philadelphia researchers found that chronic myeloid leukemia (CML) patients with a chromosomal abnormalities, a few years later, the researchers found that Is the result of long arm translocation on chromosomes 9 and 22. Since this chromosomal abnormality was first detected in Philadelphia, it was named Philadelphia (ph) chromosome, which also became a target for CML targeted therapy that was available 40 years later. In 2001 it the the first time to verify the drugs that have been shown to be resistant to Philadelphia chromosome molecular defects - imatinib - are currently available in the following categories.

1. The monoclonal antibody ① cetuximab; ② panitumumab; trastuzumab; bevacizumab; rituximab.

2. The small molecule tyrosine kinase inhibitors ① imatinib; ② gefitinib; ③ erlotinib.

3. multi-target small molecule targeted drugs ① Sauenafenib; ② Lapatinib; ③ Vandetanib; ④ sunitinib.

4. anti-angiogenic drugs ① vascular endostatin; ② thalidomide; ③ PTK787.

5. other small molecule targeting drugs ① bortezolamizole; ② CCIG779.

Subsequently, the target drug like trastuzumab targeted to human epidermal growth factor receptor 2 (HER2), was used to treat HER2-positive breast cancer; to target VEGF and to target EGFR Cetuximab in the treatment of colorectal cancer. Genitibine and erlotinib targeting EGFR were used in the treatment of non-small cell lung cancer.

Molecular targeting drugs are cell stabilizers, most patients can not achieve CR, PR, but stable condition and improved quality of life. Except to gefitinib, erlotinib, imatinib, most of them are the need to combine with chemotherapy drugs.

Molecular targeted drugs represent a new class of anti-cancer drugs. Gleevec is a typical example, can control cancer by inhibiting the abnormal molecules to control cancer, without damage to other normal nuclear tissue. A growing number of molecularly targeted drugs are used in cancer therapies, such as Rituximab for B cell lymphoma, Trastuzumab for breast cancer, and Gifitinib and Erlotinib for lung cancer etc. Targeted therapy brings anti-tumor hope.

6. Advanced cancer has been seen as a chronic disease

Like hypercholesterolemia and coronary heart disease, advanced cancer has a variety of drug options, there are many kinds of molecular targeted drugs as a candidate, as well as biological therapy, immunotherapy, immunomodulatory treatment, combined Chinese medication with western medical treatment; through the above jointing treatment, some patients with advanced cancer can survive for many years with tumor.

7. Vaccine development

The vaccine of treating cancer becomes possible and the human papilloma virus (HPV) can cause cervical cancer and HPV vaccine discovery

In 1983, Professor Hausen discovered a new HPV DNA in a biopsy of cervical cancer, and discovered a new HPV16 virus. In 1984, it cloned HPV16 and HPV18 from cervical cancer patients, and later proved that all of the whole world there are about 70% of cervical cancer patients who are carrying these two viruses.

In 1991 a large-scale epidemiology confirmed that HPV is the causative agent of cervical cancer, and the study of HPV vaccine progressed into clinical research.

In June 2006, the preventive vaccine for cervical cancer was approved by the US Food and Drug Administration (FDA).

HPV vaccine are divided into two types of preventive vaccines and therapeutic vaccines, the current research is successful preventive vaccine.

Cervical cancer caused by HPV infection can be vaccinated to prevent, which makes people finally realize the dream of possession of cancer vaccines.

8. To change the strategy and both prevention and treatment together will change the status

Cancer has gone beyond cardiovascular and cerebrovascular diseases, which is the primary reason of urban and rural people died, mainly due to focusing on treatment and ignore prevention, or even just cure without prevention; census not a wide range of promotion; The proportion of cancer early diagnosis is very low, not pay attention to (three early), did not attach importance to the treatment of precancerous lesions, as well as anti-smoking campaign is not effective and environmental pollution is increasingly serious. It can be expected that the situation of cancer prevention and control in the future quite long time is still grim. In view of this situation, therefore, should be made to attack cancer attack, namely, anti-cancer, cancer control, cancer treatment, three carriages go hand in hand; both prevention and treatment together will gradually change the status.

9. Both prevention and control as a body and reducing cancer has example

The prevention and control of hepatitis B, that is, prevention and control of primary liver cancer; primary liver cancer in China is mostly on the basis of cirrhosis lesions.\

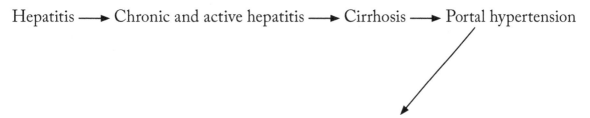

Hepatitis ⟶ Chronic and active hepatitis ⟶ Cirrhosis ⟶ Portal hypertension

Splenomegly / Ascites/ Jaundice /Hepatic encephopathy

Prevention and control of primary liver cancer is appropriate to have prevention and control of hepatitis B.

Hepatitis B is not only seriously affect the health of patients, but also to the family, society, causing a heavy financial burden, is an important public health problem endangering the health of the people. China is a high incidence of hepatitis B, in 1992 the national hepatitis B epidemiology Survey showed the crowd chronic hepatitis B virus (HBV) carrying rate is 9.75%, which means that every 10 people have a person for hepatitis B.

Prevent the occurrence of primary liver cancer is appropriate to prevent cirrhosis of the liver caused by hepatitis B and in high-risk groups of hepatitis B and cirrhosis the patients are should be actively treated to prevent its malignant transformation.

Hepatitis B vaccine is an important measure to control hepatitis B in newborns. Through the implementation of hepatitis B vaccination of newborns, it can effectively protect children against HBV infection and prevent and control hepatitis B significantly.

Prevention and control of hepatitis B also are that prevention and control of liver cancer caused by liver cirrhosis and hepatitis B.

2) The current timing is very favorable

(A) building an innovative country, prosperity and technological innovation

At present, China is building an innovation-oriented country and is promoting scientific and technological innovation. The National Conference on Innovation in Science and Technology has deepened the reform of science and technology system and decided to enter the innovation-oriented country in 2020. Its goal is to achieve a breakthrough in scientific research in key fields; to leapand bound the high technology field; on a number of new achievements in the field to enter the world; universal scientific quality generally improved, into the ranks of innovative countries.

How to build an innovation-oriented country? Innovation-oriented countries should not only prosperity and innovation, but also prosperity of the original innovation, not only should catch up with the international advanced level, but also the international leading level.

Cancer is the enemy of all mankind, the complexity of cancer beyond the human imagination, which is the hottest biomedical field, gathers the world's largest, elite research team and research elite.

Cancer is not only a disease, but a similar characteristic of a large class of diseases, although the cancer treatment has been more than a century, has now entered the 21st century, the second 10 years, but "oncology" is still the current medical subjects which is the most backward of the disciplines, why? Because the Oncology for scientific research, or a scientific virgin land, need to have a large number of basic scientific research, and clinical basic research.

To overcome the cancer as the main direction of research, experimental and clinical anti-cancer research should be the key areas of scientific research, to achieve original breakthrough.

According to the National Cancer Registry's «2012 China Cancer Registration Annual Report», about 312 million new cases of cancer each year, an average of 8550 people per day, the country on the 6 per minute diagnosed with cancer.

The number of cancer deaths in the country is 2.7 million per year, with an average of 7,500 deaths per day. Such alarming data should be included in scientific research in the key areas of science and technology innovation.

I think we should propose to overcome the general concept of cancer and the basic design, "to declare war on cancer" is the time, should launch a general attack.

Our physician's shoulders have two tasks, one is to treat patients, one is the development of medicine, we should overcome the cancer in this strategic high-tech fields to achieve leapfrog development, taking the characteristics of anti-cancer and anti-transfer technology innovation, Innovation, and strive to enter the world.

(B) Attention to environmental protection, prevention and control of pollution

At present, the country is implementing the spirit of the 18th CPC National Congress and building a well-off society in an all-round way to ensure the grand goal of building a well-off society in 2020. Its main contents are "resource-saving and environment-friendly society" and the goal is pollutant discharge. The total amount decreased significantly, the stability of the ecosystem was enhanced, and the people's environment is improved obviously.

Building a well-off society; people have improved health knowledge; being aware of that more than 80% of the cancer are caused by environmental factors or closely related to; building a moderately prosperous society has a great relevance with cancer prevention and cancer control; the intervention measures for environmental pollution and other risk factors will effectively reduce the cancer-related incidence.

"Two-oriented society," its purpose and effect can achieve the role of cancer prevention class I. We must seize this golden opportunity. I engaged in tumor surgery experimental basic research and clinical practice for half a century; to achieve the purpose of cancer prevention and control, we must rely on government-led efforts of experts and scholars to mobilize the masses to do. It is only by raising awareness of cancer prevention so as to to achieve the results of anti-cancer, cancer control and reducing the incidence rate of effect.

To strengthen the natural ecological system and environmental protection, adhere to the prevention, comprehensive management, to address the damage to people's health and to highlight the environmental issues can be as the focus.

In the construction of a moderately prosperous society, rural urbanization work, to develop the outline of preventing cancer and anti-cancer, to put forward and formulate anti-cancer, anti-cancer measures; to develop new towns, new rural cancer prevention and control planning and measures.

Our dreams are to overcome cancer, to build a well-off society, everyone's health, away from cancer.

3. The XZ-C program of overcoming cancer and launching a total attack

First, the necessary of building the organization

"To declare war on cancer," to launch a general offensive, should be cancer prevention, cancer control and cancer treatment going hand in hand and at the same time prevention and control and treatment ; it must be supported by the state and all levels of government and establish the appropriate organizations.

It is necessary to have the establishment of the "Working Committee to overcome cancer in China", the creation of "Cancer Prevention Science City", the establishment of "Wuhan, Hubei capture cancer workstation" "set up several research group", the first pilot.

From the clinical point of view, the following subjects are related to cancer research: immune and cancer-related groups; virus and cancer-related group; endocrine and cancer- related groups; fungi and cancer-related groups; chronic inflammation-related group; molecular biology and cancer-related group; gene and cancer-related group; environment and cancer-related group.

Second, to build a model hospital for the prevention and treatment of cancer throughout

The current oncology hospital or oncology are focusing o treatment and ignore prevention or only cure, while the fight against cancer must be both of prevention and treatment.

I entered the Central South Tongji Medical College in 1951, has been 62 years experience and witnesses the work of cancer prevention and treatment of the whole process of a century. We recall the 20th century, China and the world's hospitals, although also to prevent cancer, anti-cancer work, but in fact have focused on the formation of primary cancer treatment ; and parts of anti-metastatic treatments are staying in the invasion stages and the late treatment stages which the results are poor.

So far to the second decade of the 21st century, the world's hospitals, our province's Tumor Hospital, Affiliated Hospital of Oncology, the top three hospitals are oncology treatment hospital, cancer hospital are clinical treatment, the hospital model are for the treatment of hospitals; oncology, academic journals are clinical diagnosis and treatment of clinical basis, although there are several for the cancer prevention and treatment, but very little anti-cancer work article about the cancer prevention. In short, the 20th century tumor hospital and the University Hospital Of the Department of Oncology are focusing on treatment and ignore prevention, or only on treatment without prevention.

Looking back and reflection of cancer prevention and anti-cancer work, for a century in the cancer prevention what have we done research or work? What has been achieved?

The current status: for a century it is focusing on treatment and ignoring prevention, or only treatment without prevention. Prevention of cancer, anti-cancer is the work of mankind, but over the years we only did many anti-cancer treatment researches and lots of work, but the work of anti-cancer prevention is done very little, almost did not do.

Medical school textbook teaching content does not attach importance to cancer prevention knowledge.

Hospital model does not attach importance to anti-cancer science set.

Medical school or hospital research projects do not attach importance to anti-cancer research projects. The cancer medical journal does not attach importance to anti-cancer work papers. In short, anti-cancer did not attach importance to prevention.

As before said, the prevention of cancer and anti-cancer work were not paid attention to, or had not been implemented.

Third, The key of overcoming cancer and launching the general offensive attack is personnel training (Chapter 13)

They must not only have the specialized knowledge and technology, but also should have multi-disciplinary comprehensive knowledge, cultivate both ability and political integrity of the scientific research personnel, to build real talent to learn the scientific research team, is to develop a contingent of high-level professionals and anti-control, Capture the key to cancer.

Now, oncology talent, basically focus on surgery and radiotherapy and chemotherapy. In the future, medical education must be to overcome the cancer attack general training to train multidisciplinary talents, and apply their knowledge. To build an innovation-oriented country, in order to overcome cancer, save the patient life Outcome.

Training of personnel must attach importance to the construction of the laboratory; with a good laboratory it can be derived from the main innovation or original innovation of scientific research. With the laboratory and with talent it can have the result of scientific research.

Fourth, To converse the scientific and technological innovation into clinical medicine

With the results of scientific and technological innovation, it must be converted to clinical medicine in a timely manner to improve the medical level so that patients have benefit.

The basic ideas and design of XZ-C (XuZe China, Xu Feng - China) launches the general attack as the following:

Basic Design

The dawn of scientific research spirit

Work hard ------18 years of cold window and hard work

↓

Recall and reflection ------Following-up and reflection of the lessons of failure: summary of the successful experience

↓

Open up and innovation-------- Selecting 48 drugs with good cancer inhibition from 200 chinese herbs and Z-C immune regulation application for 11 years and stand up to the new concept and models and theory knowledge

↓

Facing the future medicine------ Releazing the shortage and problem of 20 centuries and making 21 centuries direction

↓

Look forward ---------Suggestion: build up the new molecular oncology university and hospital and institutes and drug factory

Fifth The planning and steps of launching a general offensive to overcome cancer (such as schematic)

How to overcome cancer?

↓

Where is the way?

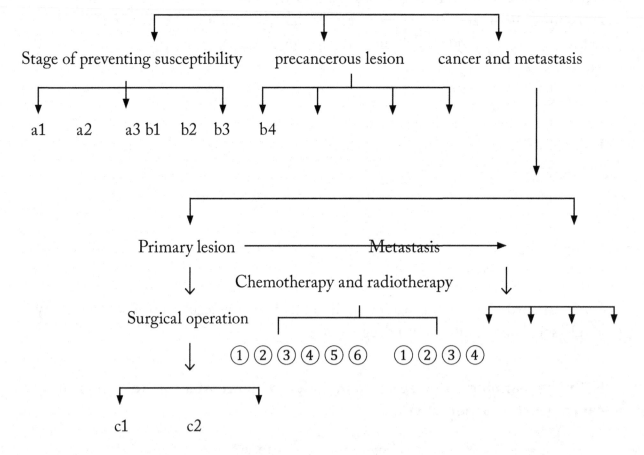

↓

Our thought, strategy and experience should be divided into three parts

↓

Before the formation of cancer——prevention part——anti- mutation

↓

Precancerous lesion with possible tendency of
malignant change——intervention part

↓

The therapeutic part of primary cancer with the
formation of focus and anti-metastasis

Stage of preventing susceptibility   precancerous lesion   cancer and metastasis

a1   a2   a3 b1   b2   b3   b4

Primary lesion ——————— Metastasis ——————→

Chemotherapy and radiotherapy

Surgical operation

① ② ③ ④ ⑤ ⑥   ① ② ③ ④

c1   c2

c1 c2

a1. "Two-oriented society" contains essences and measures

a2. "Lift scientific research" makes plans and measures of cancer control a3. Propaganda, education and study of popular science

b1. General investigation of physical examination

b2. Selective examination of high risk group

b3. Outpatient service of "early detection, early diagnosis and early treatment"

b4. Induced differentiation

c1. Improve free-tumor technique

c2. Prevent intraoperative implantation of cast-off cells

① with indication

② individuation

③ scientization

④ drug sensitive test

⑤ try to reduce untoward reaction

⑥ "intelligent resistance to cancer" of target administration

① targeted therapy

② anti-metastasis and anti-relapse therapies

③ BRM biological therapy

④ immunoregulation therapy

Sixth, focusing on action to conquer cancer

What should we do next? Now we propose of conquering cancer and launching the general attach. We hope to get support from leadership in cancer prevention and control purposes. Pay attention to work and open our steps. We deeply know that in order to the purposes of prevention and treatment of cancer it must get all of government leadership, government-led, experts, scholars efforts, mass participation, mobilization of the whole people, thousands of households involved in to achieve the goal.

No matter how far and how long the road of overcoming cancer is, we must avoid the empty talk; do heavily hard work and should start to walk; thousands of miles begins with a single step, just go forward, and eventually will walk out.

Chapter 12 to strengthen anti-cancer prevention and control research and to change the status of focusing on cancer treatment and ignoring cancer prevention

1. Recognizing the current problems and Clearing direction

First, To understand what the current treatment problems are

1 Postoperative recurrence and metastasis are clinically practical problems

The traditional three treatments of cancer have been applied for nearly a hundred years; however, cancer mortality is still the first, how should we do?

(1) The recurrence of the problem is still very serious. Patients and their families are afraid of postoperative recurrence; after surgery some patients are suspense and panic all day; how does the surgeon prevent recurrence, to prevent postoperative metastasis is worthy of our study?

(2) The metastasis is the core issue of cancer, is the key to survival, everyone is afraid of cancer metastasis. How effective anti-cancer metastasis, control of cancer cell metastasis should be done on our basic and clinical research.

2 The current problems in the treatment

(1) Chemotherapy should have further study and improvement. Whether the postoperative adjuvant chemotherapy is to prevent from metastasis or recurrence or not and how to help prevent postoperative recurrence and metastasis are worthy of our thinking and our having deeper research and improvement.

(2) Radiotherapy remains to be further research and improvement; radiotherapy is for local treatment and the metastasis is a systemic problem. How to play its role in anti-metastatic treatment and how to further study and improve are worthy of our thinking.

(3) The "radical surgery" design needes to be further research and improvement to reduce postoperative recurrence and metastasis. Since it is "radical surgery", why cannot it achieve the purpose of radical surgery? Since doing a lymph node dissection, why are there metastasis? How to pay attention to the intraoperative tumor-free technique, how to reduce and prevent the shedding off of intraoperative cancer cells, how to reduce the intraoperative transfer of cancer cells, how to reduce spread from the tumor vein, which are the questions that clinicians practice should pay attention to. The operation should be light, stable, accurate, and carry out basic experimental research, and experimental study of animal models of tumor surgery. The first and foremost thing of the operation is to prevent metastasis.

Second, the anti-cancer research is necessary for the current status of Oncology and we must recognize what are the problems of the current status of Oncology

(1) "Oncology" is the most backward subjects of medical subjects, because the cause of oncology, pathogenesis, pathophysiology are not clear; for oncology scientific research, it still is a virgin land and need to be a lot of basic scientific researches.

(2) Despite the large amount of funds invested in the treatment of cancer patients, despite the traditional three major treatment for almost a hundred years, but the cancer mortality rate is still the first cause of death for China's urban and rural residents, the main reasons are the following:

① the cause of cancer is not entirely clear; people on the pathogenesis of cancer cell metastasis mechanism is still a lack of adequate understanding.

② the complexity of the biological behavior of cancer is still a lack of adequate knowledge.

③ treatment program is still quite blind.

④ diagnostic methods behind, once discovered, that is, it is already in the middle, late stages and poor treatment.

⑤ many large hospitals have not established laboratories, cannot carry out basic research on cancer, cancer metastasis, and relapse; it must be carried out the basic study on cancer-bearing animal model and we should use nude mice to establish a variety of cancer metastasis animal model to study the rules and mechanisms of cancer metastasis.

Second, take the Chinese characteristics of anti-cancer research and innovation

Anti-cancer academic research focuses on the study of unknown knowledge, research workers should look forward, facing the future of science, science is an endless frontier, scientific research must be the development of vision beyond the old knowledge, constantly updated, and constantly go beyond under the guidance of the scientific concept of development, taking the Chinese characteristics of anti-cancer metastasis scientific research and innovation of the road.

As the clinical medical workers, especially professors, chief physicians, we have a double task on the shoulders, one treatment of patients; the second is the development of medicine. Published papers are to develop medicine, medical science hall by brick.

1. Medical research should be oriented to the future with the development of vision with the spirit of innovation, vision forward with future-oriented medicine and the cancer metastasis prevention and treatment. 20 century oncology is the cellular level, the 21st century oncology should be molecular level. The research and development of oncology must surpass the knowledge of the predecessors, the generation surpasses the generation, surpasses the blue and surpasses the blue.

2. The research should be based on the patient

   Based on research in patients with new results, new methods to improve the quality of care, reduce patient suffering and prolong the survival of patients. Medical quality refers to the medical effect; the medical effect of cancer patients is to live for a long time, good quality of life, patients with small pain.

3. To strengthen basic research, to find an effective way to solve the recurrence of cancer metastasis

To do biological basic research of molecular biology and genetic engineering, to carry out basic clinical research and clinical follow-up retrospective analysis of the study; to carry out evidence-based medicine to do evaluation of experimental studies and clinical validation data to assess the long-term efficacy evaluation; to study and to explore cancer metastasis, relapse mechanism and to find effective measures to control. The animal experimental surgery is extremely important in the development of medicine; is the key to open the medical closed area, can promote medical career. Many new drugs, new technologies are based on the success of animal experiments, then were applied to clinical.

The second The fight against cancer focuses on prevention and treatment and the effects lie on the "three early"

First, the focus of anti-cancer strategy forward

The focus of cancer prevention and control strategy forward, its meaning has two aspects, one is by changing lifestyle and improving environmental pollution prevention means, the other is for the treatment of precancerous lesions, to stop its development to the invasion or the late.

Cancer's production and growth will go through stage of susceptibility, precancerous lesion and invasive stage. All the present tumor hospitals or tumor departments mainly focus on the cancer treatment in middle or advanced stage. The Therapeutic effects are poor. If patients in middle or advanced stage can accept surgical operation, then they will be treated surgically. But if not, they will only receive palliative treatment. Therefore, cancer treatment lies in "early detection, early diagnosis and early treatment". Generally, patients in the early stage will get a better therapeutic effect. The increase of therapeutic effect will certainly reduce the fatality rate of cancer. Consequently, we must put much emphasis on the study of early-stage diagnostic and therapeutic methods, and on the treatment of precancerous lesion for lessening medium-term or terminal patients in the invasive stage.

Occupying lesion can be seen through CT or MRI, middle or advanced stage

stage of susceptibility	precancerous lesion	early stage	no metastasis	have metastasized	
				local position	amphi position
①	②	③	④	⑤	⑥

① Cancer prevention

② Outpatient service of "three kinds of earliness"

③ Surgical operation

④ Place surgical operation first, radiotherapy, chemotherapy and biological TCM second

⑤ Possible to undergo surgical operation

⑥ To give treatment as carcinomatous metastasis

If patients have been treated well in the stage of precancerous lesion or early stage, then the number of patients in middle or advanced stage of invasion and metastasis will fall off. Thus, the cancer incidence rate will also decline. Therefore, we hold that the present tumor hospitals in various places mainly focus on the cancer treatment in middle or advanced stage. Even though the therapeutic result is effective, it can only bring the reduction of cancer mortality rate. But if ignoring the stage of susceptibility, precancerous lesion or early stage, it will be impossible to reduce the cancer incidence rate. Therefore, we must put much emphasis on the whole process of cancer production and growth. After all this is the real global change of strategic importance.

The writer has engaged in surgical oncology for over fifty years. More and more patients suffer from cancer, and the cancer incidence rate also rises. The writer deeply feels that people should emphasize not only therapy but also prevention. Only in this way could the cancer be killed in the source. Cancer treatment lies in "three kinds of earliness" (early detection, early diagnosis and early treatment); anti-cancer method lies in prevention.

As stated above, the strategic center of gravity of tumor treatment and prevention moves forward. There are two aspects in its meaning. One is to prevent cancer by changing life style and improving environmental pollution; the other is to cure precancerous lesion for inhibiting cancer's development to the invasion stage, middle stage or advanced stage.

In 1990, our institute's specialist out-patient department of tumor surgery once opened the outpatient service of "three kinds of earliness" to carry out various endoscopies and biopsies, through which have found many atypical hyperplasia of stomach, intestinal metaplasia, atrophic gastritis and hyperplasia of mammary glands, etc. These "precancerous lesions" are difficult to treat. Then how to handle these precancerous lesions or precancerous conditions so as to prevent their cancerations urgently needs clinical researches to look for better treatment methods.

Second. Put emphasis on fundamental and clinical researches of precancerous lesions with diagnosis and treatment techniques.

"Three kinds of earliness" is the key to cancer treatment. While how to handle precancerous lesion is the key stage for cancer prevention and treatment.

The present cancer diagnosis mainly depends on image examinations of type-B ultrasonic, CT and MRI. But as soon as the cancer comes to light, it has reached the middle or advanced stage. Many patients have lost the chance of radical excision. Although the complex treatment has been done, the therapeutic effects are still poor. If the cancer is in the early stage or belongs to the carcinoma in situ, then the curative effect of operation will be better and the cancer can be cured. Therefore, the cancer treatment should strive for "three kinds of earliness", which refers to early detection, early diagnosis and early treatment.

Because cancer's pathogenic factors are not very clear, the primary prevention is still quite difficult.

Studies in recent years indicate that malignant tumor rarely has a direct carcinomatous change in normal tissues. Before the occurrence of tumor in clinical diagnosis, cancer often goes through quite a long evolution stage, which is the stage of precancerous lesion. Early identification and control of these precancerous lesions will bring positive significances for the secondary prevention of cancer.

What is precancerous lesion? The precancerous lesion is a histopathology concept, which refers to a kind of tissues with the dysplasia of cells. Precancerous lesion has the potential to become cancerous. If there is no cure in a long period, precancerous lesion will evolve into cancer. In other words, precancerous lesion just has the possibility of changing into cancer. But not all the precancerous lesions will eventually become cancer. Through proper treatments, precancerous lesions may return to their normal states or have a spontaneous regression.

Canceration is a developing process with several stages. There is a stage of precancerous lesion between normal cells and cancer. It is a slow process from precancerous lesion evolving into cancer, which needs many years or even more than ten years. The length of canceration course is closely related to the strength of carcinogenic factors, individual susceptibility and immunologic function. Therefore, the study of precancerous lesion is of great importance to cancer's prevention and control.

Third. More than one third of cancers can be prevented.

The tumor formation is a long process with several factors and stages. Precancerous lesion is of reversibility, so cancer is preventable.

The several factors, steps and stages of tumor formation have the following features.

The generation and growth of tumor can be roughly divided into several stages of initiation, promotion, metastasis and others. Cellular canceration induced by chemical carcinogen is a multistage process. The chemical carcinogenesis process of Experimental animals and the generating process of human tumors (such as colon cancer) have a series of changes, which are hyperplasia → pathological changes → benign tumor → malignant tumor → tumor metastasis, etc. The whole change process is complicated with multiple stages of initiation, promotion and evolution, etc. It often takes a long cytometaplasia time to change from normal cells to the tumor that can be detected clinically, which is a long cumulative process.

(1) Two-stage theory of tumor formation: In 1942, Beremblum carried out the experimental study of mouse's skin canceration induction, in which he used benzoapyrene

to treat mice's skins for about one year, and only three out of one hundred and two mice suffered from skin tumors. If mice's skins were treated with benzoapyrene for several months and then treated with the tumor promoter-croton oil, thirty-six out of eighty-three mice suffered from skin cancers, whose incidence rate was ten times higher than that of using benzoapyrene alone. If mice's skins were first treated with croton oil for several months and then treated with a carcinogenic substance, there would be no induced tumor. If mice's skins were only treated with croton oil for a long time, whose incidence rate of tumor would be lower than that of using benzoapyrene alone (1/106).

On the basis of this study results, Beremblum and Subik have proposed that cancerous process contains two different but intimate stages. One is a specific provocation stage. Small dosages of carcinogenic substance induce normal cells to become potential cancer cells. The other is nonspecific promoting stage. Potential cancer cells are further promoted to suffer from mutation and evolve into tumor under the action of tumor promoters, such as croton oil and others.

People hold that provocation process refers to the process that normal cells change into potential cancer cells under the action of carcinogenic substances. The time of promoting process is fairly short and generally irreversible. While promoting process is the process that potential cancer cells change into cancer cells under the action of tumor promoters. The early promoting stage is reversible but the late stage is irreversible.

Carcinogenic substance is a kind of mutagen, which plays a decisive role in canceration process. While cancer promoters do not have the mutagenicity, which can only promote potential cancer cells to have a further proliferation change and gradually evolve into cancer cells. During these two processes of provocation and promoting stages, induced cells grow out of control, escape from the host's immune surveillance, gradually form tumor cells with malignant phenotype and then evolve into tumor cells with infiltration and metastasis. This theory recognizes that tumor generation is quite a long process (months, years and even more than ten years) and will be impossible through a single factor or stage, which is very important to cancer prevention and control. It prompts that people have enough time to build up cancer-fighting ability, strengthen immunity, change life style and improve environmental pollution to prevent cancer. Intervention measures should be emphasized to tackle the reversible stage of cancer promoting.

(2) Multi-factor and multi-stage model of tumor formation: Vogelstein proposed the multi-stage model of genetics of colon cancer and histological change, which makes people get a better idea of the formation of human colon tumor and molecular events happening in the process of development. It proves that the synergic action between

424

cancer gene and cancer suppressor gene is the key factor for cellular canceration. The study conclusion is that canceration process of colon is a process with multiple involving genes and developing stages (Fig. 1).

Carcinogenic action

Genetic change Variance of cancer suppressor gene

Genetic change Oncogene abnormality

Genetic change Oncogene abnormality Abnormality of cancer suppressor gene

Cloning expansion

Genetic change Oncogene abnormality Abnormality of cancer suppressor gene

Normal cells transformed cells precancerous lesion malignant cells clinical diagnosis of tumor metastatic tumor

Initiation stage promoting stage evolutional stage metastatic stage

Fig. 1 Multi-factor and multi-stage model of tumor formation

Fourth. Anti-cancer method lies in prevention.

For almost half a century, human spectrum of disease has undergone a drastic change. Most communicable diseases have been effectively controlled. Chronic diseases, such as cardiovascular diseases and malignant tumors have been the most serious diseases threatening human health.

Cancer has become the most serious public health problem in the world. Compared with other chronic diseases, cancer's prevention and control face a greater challenge.

Over the last thirty years, the fatality rate of cancer in China is on an obvious rise, which has occupied the number one in causes of death of urban and rural residents. On average, one out of every four deceased persons dies from cancer.

Cancer not only seriously threatens human health but also causes the rapid rise of hospitalization costs. The direct costs of cancer treatment in China are about one hundred billion RMB every year, which makes patients and the whole society bear a huge economic burden.

Although each country inputs a large number of funds to treat cancer patients, the five-year survival rate of some common cancers has no obvious improvement in the recent twenty years. For instance, during the years from 1974 to 1990 in USA, the five-year survival rate of esophagus cancer only rose from 7% to 9%, stomach cancer from 16% to 19%, liver cancer from 3% to 6%, lung cancer from 12% to 15% and that of pancreatic cancer remained the same as 3%.

What's to be done? Anti-cancer method lies in prevention. Prevention and intervention is the most important thing in the field of public health.

As for the malignant cancer, prevention outweighs therapy. Worldwide tumor researchers have reached a consensus of adjusting public health resources and policies, shifting strategic focus from therapy to prevention, and carrying out positive and effective studies of pre-warning, early diagnosis and intervention to lower tumor incidence rate and raise curative rate.

The evidence in Cancer Report provided by World Health Organization proves that up to one thirds of cancers can be prevented. As long as every national government, medical workers and the common people actively take actions and shift the research emphasis of tumor prevention and treatment to tumor prevention, they can prevent above one thirds or even about half of the cancers.

Chapter 13: Suggestions on the Cultivation of Scientific and Technological Innovation Talents and the Transformation of Scientific Research Achievements

The first section To overcome cancer the scientific and technological talent is the key

First, To building the innovative countries the first should be prosperity and technological innovation

National Science and Technology Innovation Conference deepened the reform of science and technology decision 2020 into the ranks of innovative countries and the goal is to achieve scientific breakthroughs in key areas of science; strategic high-tech fields achieve leapfrog development; a number of areas of innovation go into the forefront of the world; Scientific quality generally improve into the ranks of innovative countries.

How to build an innovation-oriented country? Innovation-oriented countries should not only be prosperous and independent innovation, but also prosperous original innovation, not only should catch up with the international advanced level, but also the international leading level.

What is independent innovation? Independent innovation is the product of others, we also have, do not rely on other people's design, but our own design; the independent innovation is that our own design is better than others, but also superiority to have competitiveness.

What is the original innovation? Original innovation is that others do not have, or the world does not, which is my unique invention, not to learn other people, but people learn from us.

Innovation is not only the product innovation, but should be based on theoretical innovation, theoretical innovation is the greatest achievement. Scientific development is based on the basic theory of innovation, this is the largest invention, discovery of new theories, new laws, such as: Einstein Of the theory of relativity, Newton's law.

In order to establish the scientific and technological innovation-oriented countries, we must prosper the achievements of scientific and technological innovation, not only the results of independent innovation, but also must have the original results of innovation.

How can we have scientific and technology innovation, talent is the key. Talent standards must be true talent, both ability and political integrity. Whether it is not true ability or not must be able to obtain scientific research achievements, scientific and technological innovation achievements.

How can we have innovative results? Construction of the corresponding laboratory equipment is the key, with a good laboratory, there is the basic conditions for research, through experimental research, in order to innovate.

How can we have innovative results? Training personnel, building laboratories, are not the purpose of all scientific research; the goal of scientific research is to obtain the ultimate goal of scientific research.

To the outcome of the hero is from the results; to discuss the contribution is from the result; to evaluate the academic level is from the original innovation results; the original innovation results must be confirmed by the new agency.

How can we have technological innovation?

First of all, to cultivate scientific thinking, scientific mind, have academic atmosphere, ask some questions about why? Poor end, first ask questions, study the problem, and then solve the problem. Why do you want to ask more Why and how to do? What to do? To have a scientific and innovative atmosphere should be cultivated from the young people to.

Teachers at all levels must have scientific thinking, academic atmosphere, to train students to ask why? More using brain and thinking, analysis of problems, teachers are human soul engineers, to improve the quality of teaching, we must first raise the level and quality of teachers, improve the academic atmosphere of teachers, scientific and technological innovation thinking and academic standards. If the teacher does not have enough knowledge, he or she is afraid that the student ask why.

Second, how to train scientific and technological innovation talent

Talent training should walk on two legs:

1 First, attracting talent, recruiting talent and sending staff to study abroad, visiting scholars, to be returned after learning to participate in construction and technological innovation, this is an important way to cultivate talent, but this is only temporary, only catch but it will be difficult to suppress. The use of these talents and development of these talents need to pay attention to the following points: ① should have a better laboratory, to enable a group of people to lead a group of people. Should be used to train personnel, train a batch of China's own scientific and technological personnel, because please come in, or will go, should be used for incubation of talent, to help our country to train scientific and technological personnel. If it is Talent, it should have the result.

The other is to cultivate talent based on their own, the key is to build a good laboratory, in the long run, this is the root cause. It can not rely entirely on foreign training and should rely on their own training. After liberation, China's medical personnel are relying on their own training. How to cultivate their own, that is, run a large laboratory, through animal experiments, clinical research and work to achieve scientific and technological innovation, so as to original innovation, to go beyond.

After the liberation of new China's medical development, from scratch, is to go this road self-reliance, relying on their own talent, pioneering work.

For example, open heart surgery after cardiopulmonary bypass both the early years after the liberation failed to study, visit, exchange, no foreign medical journals, publications; in the late 50s of last century, in the early 60s, Xi'an, Tianjin, Shanghai, Wuhan, Nanjing, etc each city has several large hospitals to form a cardiopulmonary bypass open heart surgery animal experimental research group. Every group is done hundreds of dogs in cardiopulmonary bypass open heart surgery animal experiments,; after the successful operation in animal experiment it was applied for the clinical. Tianjin group also created the cardiopulmonary bypass half body cycle. I participated in the Wuhan animal experimental research group, and set up a group to visit Tianjin, Nanjing, Anyang for the study of animal experiments. China's cardiopulmonary bypass open heart surgery is through the dog's animal experiments to explore the experience of training their own talent started.

For example, liver transplantation surgery in the late 1970s has not yet established diplomatic relations with the United States, both failed to study, visit, exchange, nor foreign medical journals, publications, Shanghai Ruijin Hospital Dong Fang,

Lin Yanzhen, Wuhan Tongji Hospital Qiu Fazu, Xia Suisheng established liver Transplanted animal laboratories, were also carried out hundreds of dogs in liver transplantation animal experiments, both through the animal after the clinical trial in Shanghai, Wuhan, two groups of two groups of liver transplants have been carried out by animal experiments after the successful clinical liver Transplantation in Wuhan. In the 1980s when the conference confirmed the results of open liver transplantation, two groups Shanghai and Wuhan of animal experiments go hand in hand, but the Wuhan group 3 day earlier clinical than in Shanghai group, clinical liver transplant patients survival more than 3 days, Accordingly, the Ministry of Health will focus on Wuhan liver transplantation and establish organ transplantation Institute. At that time I was an expert evaluation head for the outcome of liver transplantation drafting and witnessed the beginning of China's liver transplantation surgery by animal experiments and the exploration of their own experience in training their own talent.

Third, the establishment of personnel training system and training institutions

The requirements of modern high-tech talent training mechanism should keep up with the development of modern high-tech; meet the needs of innovative countries and internationalization.

The scientific community predicted that 21st century leadership science will be based on molecular biology as the core of the life sciences; computer-centric information science and environmental science.

Pedagogy should keep pace with the development of the times and pedagogy should be applied in practice.

The current educational content can not keep up with the development of the times for the development of modern high-tech disciplines, must have a good laboratory, but the current shortage of laboratory personnel, the status is a lot of doctors or nurses; who can catch mice and do experiment is very little. It is not a lack of university graduates and graduate students, but the lack of laboratory experiments of modern high-tech intermediate professionals. To establish the innovative countries we must vigorously build science and technology innovation center and build a good laboratory, the construction laboratory must first train the laboratory Talent and must be trained from young people because since ancient times the hero is out of juvenile.

Therefore, the proposed: the establishment of the 21st century modern high interest and technical experimental intermediate personnel institutions so that the construction of laboratories provides personnel.

1 The establishment of modern high-tech life science and technology college (secondary, three-year system) for the tertiary institutions enrich the establishment of laboratory talent; Modern life science and technology progress quickly; genetic engineering, molecular biology, and cell genetic rapid develop.

2 founded the modern high-tech environmental science and technology college (secondary, three-year system); environmental science has attracted worldwide attention which will be emerging disciplines, new industries, the current energy-saving emission reduction. To set up two types of society, we must carry out a large number of research projects, to use modern high-tech pollution prevention and control technology, ecological balance, food hygiene supervision, etc. to cultivate a large number of environmental science, modern high-tech intermediate talent.

More than 80% of cancer are caused by environmental factors or closely related, therefore, the current energy-saving emission reduction, pollution prevention and pollution control, creating a "two-oriented society", is anti-cancer, anti-cancer primary prevention measures. Hope government support for the construction of "two-oriented society" to cultivate a large number of environmental protection science intermediate professionals.

3 founded modern high-tech information science and technology college (secondary, three-year system)

It is to enrich the construction of laboratories of corresponding universities and colleges. The quality and quantity of information professionals can represent a country's competitiveness and creativity.

Section II to establish a good laboratory

With the talent, it does not mean that there is a result; with talent, it does not mean that you can prosper scientific and technological innovation because the hero must have its place; scientific research design and scientific research assumptions must have laboratory experiments in order to draw conclusions.

Therefore, scientific and technological innovation must be a good laboratory, laboratory is the key. If no good laboratories, although the talent, there are issues, even if the project to get hundreds of thousands of dollars, if not experimental, it can only be utopian, empty talk and can not produce results.

First, the construction of a good equipment laboratory is essential for training for talent

The author is the first batch of college entrance examination after the liberation of college students, did not study specially, but also did not study aboard, but I made a number of international level results, the key is that I have a good laboratory. In the 60 years of the 20th century I participated in CPB animal laboratory and established the liver cirrhosis ascites laboratory; in the early 90s I established the Experimental Surgery Institute to capture cancer as the main direction; my animal laboratory equipment is better, there are mice, rats, the Netherlands pigs, rabbits, dogs, Monkeys and other animal experiments, a better animal sterile operating room which can make dog chest, abdominal major surgery, and animal observation of the ward, it can achieve results or conclusions from my design and program through experimental operation.

Many colleges and universities in China, subordinate, provincial universities are equipped with a number of teaching and research group, also cultivate a large number of graduate students, but some teaching and research group do not have laboratory or research room. Strictly speaking, it should only be called teaching group, teach and not research. No laboratory or research room, how can the research be carried out? Recruited a large number of graduate students, how to train and guide graduate students to do experiment and research for the problem? Teaching and research group does not have laboratory or laboratory and professors can only prepare lessonsl and ectures, and can not do experiments or Research topics. University professors should not only talk about the known knowledge of textbooks, but also should talk about today's new progress, the development of new trends, new achievements and unknown knowledge. There is no laboratory or research laboratory, the teacher cannot do research; they don't their own place to do experiments, how can they guide graduate students to do experiments?

Now a mentor may recruit a few graduate students to guide students how to choose topics, how to design, how to experiment operation, scientific research process to obtain results or conclusions. However, there are many teachers of the teaching and research group has no laboratory, no research, how to guide graduate students in the experimental operation and other research? Logically speaking, a mentor should have a good laboratory, it may guide graduate students to conduct scientific research, writing papers, the development of science.

It is therefore recommended that:

1. subordinate institutions of higher learning should have 1-3 national key laboratories

2. provincial institutions of higher learning should have 1-3 provincial key laboratories

3. municipal institutions of higher learning should have 1-3 municipal key laboratories

Laboratory rating according to the level of the talent and the results:

National key laboratories should be the leading international or international advanced level of results, a research leader, a master of science; the results must be identified and be rated; the original results must be verified at the provincial level of the new agency verification and higher authorities acceptance.

Three years can not have an international level results, the level should be reduced until the corresponding results after recovery.

Provincial key laboratories should have the leading domestic or domestic advanced level of scientific research and strive for the international advanced level results; must be identified rating, higher authorities acceptance. Municipal laboratories and provincial laboratories are basically similar.

The construction of laboratories should be done so that talent can work; make products of scientific research to have the land of the innovation; people have the land to cultivate.

Second, the laboratory is the incubator of innovative scientific and technological achievements

The laboratory is an incubator of scientific research personnel training, incubation pool of scientific and technological innovation results. The author experiences that experimental surgery is extremely important in the development of medicine and it is a key to open the medical restricted area. Many disease prevention methods were gained through that after many animal experiments in the laboratory the stability of the results obtained, then clinically validated, and finally applied for clinical so that patients benefit.

If no laboratory it cannot cultivate outstanding scientific and technological talent; if there is only the talent and is not a laboratory, it is also very difficult to scientific and technological innovation fruit. General master Yang Zhenning, Ding Zhaozhong had excellent laboratory equipments and won the Nobel Prize in Physics.

Therefore, if there is no laboratory through the experiment, it can only design, vision and is impossible to obtain scientific research and the idea will not become a reality.

Section III The scientific and technological achievements will be timely applied

Built innovation-oriented country, and a scientific and technological innovation center, independent innovation or the original results of the numerous innovations, how to timely transformation, development, application, so that the people benefit.

The purpose of scientific and technological innovation is one of the results of innovation, with the results, should identify the acceptance, through the results or the results will be identified or results of the council will be identified, the results of the level of acceptance, the original innovation results should check the new verification.

Project is not equal to the results - the current number of university promotion, promotion, graduate students pay attention to the project, which should be, but this understanding is not enough because the project is not equal to the results. With the project it does not necessarily achieve results; Only when the project has achieved results can be on behalf of the academic level and scientific research achievements. The project should not be the hero, but should be the results of academic standards and scientific research and the contribution of scientific research.

At present, some research institutes of universities and colleges only attach importance to scientific research projects, funds, and do not attach importance to the acceptance of scientific research results, many projects have not yet reached the end of scientific research results; every year the county hastily put a lot of national research funding in universities so it should be cherish and be sure to obtain the appropriate results, should be strictly enforced and give the results by due date; scientific research results should be appraisal, verified, and particle return warehouse to achieve scientific research; achievement should be acceptance and do achievement rating so that research should work vigorously, annual innovation and the results should be accumulated.

First, attention should be paid to scientific research achievements

How should the results of scientific research or scientific and technological research report be evaluated?

There should be a certificate of scientific research achievements or certificates; should be scientific research results or scientific and technological research report; should have more scientific research projects or research papers at home and abroad academic exchanges and academic impact at home and abroad; or have research papers published in magazines, or publishing research monographs.

The identification or evaluation of scientific research, should not be bundled "shelf", or locked in the "purdah" should go down the shelf, out of purdah, transformation, development and application.

The current situation, many of my college professors have scientific research results or quasi-results, I have a series of achievements in hand, there is no intermediary, no broker, no one matchmaking, I do not know how to attract foreign investment, there is no scientific research into, The development of mechanisms and institutions, I do not know what level of government to request guidance and support. Scientists, scientific research personnel can not be used on the results, nobody cares, beam "shelf"; entrepreneurs want results, can not be found This is a prominent social contradiction.

Second, how to transform and use

I suggest: government-led, matchmaking, government-led, investment.

Under the guidance of the government, the scientific research achievements transformation and development working committee shall be set up. Under the transformation and transformation work center and the transformation work office, the transformation work mechanism and the transformation work organization shall be established. The products will be promoted by the chamber of commerce.

In this way, scientists and entrepreneurs will be able to combine, transform, re-development, scientific research play a role, resulting in economic and social benefits.

Now the talent → laboratory → results → transformation, the development of benign relations list as shown below.

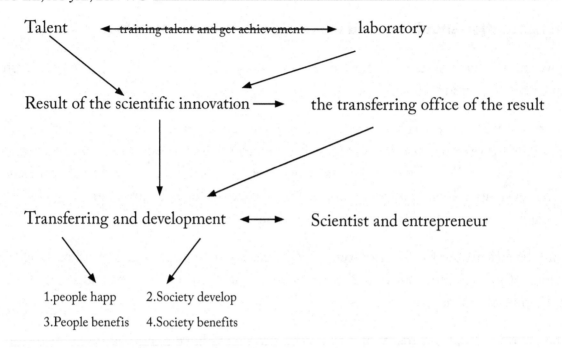

The relationship graph of Talent → laboratory → results

Chapter 14 Adhering to the new road of anti-cancer with Chinese characteristics

At present the country is implementing the spirit of the 18th National Congress to ensure the 2020 national goal of building a moderately prosperous society. National is building an innovation-oriented country, prosperity and scientific and technological innovation. General health awareness and scientific literacy are generally improved. Government at all levels governances environment promotes energy-saving emission reduction, pollution prevention, and pollution control whose excellent situation is very conducive to carry out anti-cancer, cancer control work for our cancer research and has created a major opportunity.

As we all know, the relationship between environment and cancer is great. As early as the 1980s many experts and scholars believe that more than 80% of cancer is caused by environmental factors, protect and restore a good environment, and is an important part of cancer prevention.

1. Attaching importance to environmental protection is conducive to anti-cancer, cancer control work

1). The environmental pollution and cancer

People's living environment includes natural environment and social environment. Natural environment refers to various natural factors around people. For instance, everyone has to breathe air, drink water and eat food. These common physical environments are called the big environment.

Everybody is engaged in one kind of work and adopts a certain life style, such as occupation, life habit and hobbies make up one kind of living environment, which is called the small environment.

No matter the big environment or small environment, both of them are external environments upon which mankind depends for survival and activities.

The physiologic condition of human body is the internal environment.

Materials in external environment become closely related to internal environment through the body's ingestion, digestion, absorption, metabolism and excretion, and then have a tremendous impact on human body.

In the anti-cancer, anti-cancer work, improving the living environment and improving living habits are one of the most important preventive measures. Therefore, the relationship between environment and cancer should be studied first:

Human beings rely on the survival of the air, water, soil and food, and bacteria, viruses, harmful chemical toxins, radiation pollution, not only can cause the various diseases, epidemic spread of infectious diseases, damage to people's health, but also lead to cell variation, causing cancer.

1))The relation between the environment and cancer

1. Air pollution and cancer

Human beings have developed thousands of tons of coal, oil and natural gas as fuels and energy sources, such as thermal power, smelting steel, automobiles and airplanes around the clock a large number of tar, kerosene, dust and other harmful gases To air pollution, air pollution can lead to many diseases, the most serious is lung cancer.

2. Water pollution and cancer

Water pollution, mainly industrial and agricultural production and urban sewage caused.

3. soil pollution, food chain and cancer

Human large-scale industrial and agricultural production activities, so that a large number of industrial waste water and pesticide fertilizer into the soil, so that deterioration of soil quality, human health threat, is also carcinogenic factors.

China's industrial development has made great contributions to China's economic development. However, in industrial development it has also brought environmental pollution problems, and must take active measures to strictly control pollution control.

Building a resource-saving and environment-friendly society on the industrialization and modernization of the prominent position of the development strategy should implement each unit and each family. Environment-friendly society is an important action to highlight environmental protection and is to curb environmental degradation priority.

①As to how to prove the relation between environmental pollution and cancer, many demonstrations have been given in history.

In 1775, English doctor Pott proved that cleaners of chimney have higher risk of suffering from scrotal skin cancer, as they always contact coal tar, which was the first historical case that combined cancer with environmental factors.

After 100 years, Germany doctor Volkman also recognized that the high rate of suffering skin cancer for workers was possibly related to the contact with coal tar.

In 1907, some scholar found that exposure to sunlight is related to skin cancer and reported firstly the epidemiologic research on sunlight and skin cancer. Researchers found that crews were always exposed to solar radiation that led to chronic skin diseases, which was often seen. Later, researchers proved that sunlight and ultraviolet rays were likely to result in skin cancer with animal model.

In 1915, the first animal model of inducing tumors by chemical agents was established. Besmearing tar repeatedly could make rabbits suffer from skin cancer, which provided experimental reasons for the theory of chemical carcinogenesis based on that cleaners of chimney were easy to suffer from carcinoma of scrotum in 1775. Later, people confirmed that and got the effective constituent by abstraction, named coal tar.

In the 1920s, bladder carcinoma was popular with the workers who produced alpha naphthylamine, ethyl naphthalene and benzidine dye. Almost all the workers who had done this suffered from bladder carcinoma later.

In 1930, the first chemical carcinogen, benzopyrene was abstracted from coal tar. The known substance of carcinogenic environment, coal tar was separated into different constituents, which were confirmed that they could result in cancer by experimental analysis with animal model.

In 1938, according to researches, it could be found that the process of chemical carcinogenesis was divided into two stages, the stage of activation and the stage of promotion. Non-specific stimulators could activate and promote the occurrence of cancer under small dose of carcinogen like besmearing tar or mastoid tumorous virus.

In 1940, researchers discovered that limitation of heat could reduce the occurrence of tumors for mice. It was proved that the intake of heat could encourage the occurrence of several kinds of tumors like breast carcinoma, liver cancer and skin cancer induced by benzoapyrene. Until today when obesity is popular worldwide, this project is attached with importance again by people.

In 1950, research on epidemiology discovered that smoking was related to lung cancer. By reviewing the lung cancer sufferers with the habit of smoking, it could be proved that smoking had close relation to lung cancer. Later, from the research on the obvious relation between smoking and the mortality of lung cancer among male doctors, it has been proved that smoking is a dangerous factor for many kinds of cancer and it can increase the mortality of cancer by 30%.

In 1958, it was been proved that food additive forbidden by reforming organization for food additive could induce the occurrence of cancer for human beings and animals.

In 1964, American surgeon Luther L Terry proposed that smoking was connected to lung cancer.

Until 1974, scientists found vinyl chloride was the major raw material of plastic industry, which was a potential strong carcinogen and could cause liver cancer.

In recent decades, according to epidemiologic research, it can be found that if workers in many occupations contact the carcinogens in manufacturing environment, the incidence rates of some parts will greatly increase. Elimination or avoiding these contacts can reduce the incidence rates gradually or even make them disappear, which plays an important role in the occurrence of tumors.

Various environmental factors outside human bodies are the major reasons resulting in the occurrence of cancer. Therefore, it is necessary to reduce the effects of these environmental, living and behavior factors to human bodies so as to get away from cancer.

The following is talking about the severe cancerogenic effects of environmental pollution like air pollution, water pollution and soil pollution, etc. to human beings.

②Air pollution and cancer: Human being can not survive without air even for only a minute. Therefore, air pollution can result in the occurrence of many diseases, especially respiratory diseases including the most severe one lung cancer.

At the beginning of 20th century, lung cancer mainly happened in such occupational environments like mines, exploitation and smelting. After world war one, the morality of lung cancer began to increase. In late 1930s, with the development of modern industry air pollution, occupational carcinogens and the consumption and production of tobacco and cigarette increased greatly. Meanwhile, the morality of male who suffered from lung cancer in western industrial developed countries rose rapidly. In the UK, the death rate of lung cancer was 10/100,000 in 1930, 53/100,000 in 1950, 99.7/100,000 in 1966 and 120.3/100,000 in 1975. From 1930 to 1975, it has an increase of twelve times in 45 years.

During 1934 to 1974, lung cancer rose from the fifth to the number one place in causes of death of American male. Its mortality rate rose from 3.0/100,000 to 54.5/100,000, up 17 times as compared with before. Female lung cancer went up from the eighth to the top three. Its mortality rate rose from 2.0/100,000 to 12.4/100,000, up 5.2 times as compared with before.

In the early 1980, lung cancer in 24 countries and regions involving UK, France, Netherlands, Germany and USA and others generally occupies the number one in the cause of death of malignant tumor patients. Since the mid-20th century, the tendency of high incidence of lung cancer in western industrial developed countries has been rising.

Dangerous gases in industrial developed countries, produced from power generation, steel-making, cars, planes, fuels, energy sources and volumes of smoke, are emitted into the atmosphere and pollute air. Human respiratory tract is irritated by breathing into polluted air, which causes the continuing rise of the incidence rate and mortality rate of lung cancer.

③ Water pollution of environmental pollution and cancer: Human activity in production and life depend on water at all times. Water quality pollution is mainly caused by industrial and agricultural production as well as urban pollution discharge. In China, township enterprises are having a fast development, which worsen industrial pollution. According to the survey, many major rivers are facing a serious pollution increasingly. Fertilizers, farm chemicals and pesticides in agricultural production lead to the serious pollution of water quality.

Some rural areas of China have a habit of using pond water. The research of Qidong County in Jiangsu Province has found that the high incidence of liver cancer in this area is related to drink pond water. Fusui County in Guangxi Province also has the similar report. All of these explain that water pollution is relevant to the incidence of liver cancer. Haining County in Zhejiang Province also finds that people drinking pond water are over seven times easier to suffer from colon cancer than people drinking well water.

In recent years, due to the advance of analysis technology of water quality, more than 100 different kinds of organic substances in water are found to have actions of carcinogenesis, cancer-promoting and mutagenesis. Animal experiments have proved that drink water mixed with the following chemical compounds can cause liver cancer, such as benzene hexachloride, carbon tetrachloride, chloroform, trichloroethylene, perchlorethylene, and trichloroethane, etc. Furthermore, there are some limnetic algae toxins, such as blue-green algae has an obvious action on the promotion of liver cancer.

Mulberry fish pond area of Shunde in Guangdong Foshan is low lying and easy to generate water-logging and water accumulation, so the water quality pollution is more serious. The incidence of liver cancer of local population is higher. While neighboring residents in Siping drink deep phreatic water. The water quality is good, so the incidence of liver cancer is lower. According to the research data of WHO and International Association for Cancer Research, drinking off-standard water can induce or promote the generation of cancer. The test indicates that drink water with a large amount of nickel is easy to induce oral cancer, throat cancer and carcinoma of large intestine; water with more cadmium is easy to induce esophageal carcinoma, laryngeal carcinoma and lung cancer; water with more plumbum is easy to induce stomach cancer, intestinal cancer, oophoroma and all kinds of lymph cancer; water with more iron and zinc is easy to induce esophageal carcinoma.

④ Environmental chemical pollution and cancer——chemical carcinogenesis: Chemical carcinogen refers to chemical substances that can induce the generation of tumor.

In the mid-20th century, the problem of chemical carcinogenesis attracts widespread attention, mainly because modern tumor incidence rate and mortality rate continue to rise. The age of suffering from cancer has a younger tendency. Environmental chemical pollution is also found to have a close relation to the incidence rate of tumor. World Health Organization also indicates that 80%~90% of human cancers are relevant to environmental factors, which are mainly chemical factors.

The following chemical substances have been studied and proved to have carcinogenic action.

Chloroethylene: In 1974, people began to realize that this substance is the cause of professional cancer. Experimental study has found liver cancer, brain cancer, renal carcinoma, lung cancer and cancer of lymphatic system in experimental animals exposed to Chloroethylene. But the related personnel cannot timely realize the hazardness of these substances from experimental results. Therefore, they fail to take measures to protect workers in time. Until recently, workers start to stop using the spraying agent of Chloroethylene; and plastic factory also change manufacturing technique to prevent workers from exposure.

Here to point out that Chloroethylene is an important raw material for record, packaging material, Medical test tube, household appliances, bathroom equipment and other kinds of plastic products. Plastic products themselves have no risk, but the liver cancer risk of workers in Chloroethylene factory is 200 times higher than that of common people.

Benzene: It is a kind of harmful chemical material, which can destroy the hematopiesis of marrow. If exposed in the environment filled with benzene, people may suffer from aplastic anemia that can change into leucocythemia after a long period. The first case of "leucucythemia led by benzene" was discovered in 1928.

Researches from other countries have also proved that benzene is a sort of harmful material with occupational hazards. Italian scientists have reported before 200 years that the risk of suffering from leucocythemia for the workers in printing houses and shoemaking factories was 20 times higher than that of others.

Some activities and addictions in daily life are usually related to environmental cancerogen palycyclic aromatic closely. Palycyclic aromatic produced by smoking is the key factor of inducing lung cancer for human beings. Meanwhile, palycyclic aromatic with carcinogenicity produced in cooking foods of oil and fat including frying, grilling and smoking, etc. are threatening extremely the health for human beings, which should be attached with great importance.

In addition, benzoapyrene in asphalt and hot-mix asphalt is closely related to the high risk of cancer occurrence for roadmen and worker dealing with the water proofing of roof. Farm labors often contact several kinds of pesticides, herbicide and chemical fertilizers which contain some known carcinogens and some that can induce cancer in experimental animals and others that are proved to be mutagenic agents after short-term test. And the pesticides can enter food chain and accumulate in biological system.

⑤ The physical factors in environmental pollution and cancer—ionizing radiation: With the development of technology, frequent nuclear tests, the applications of nuclear energy and radioactive nuclides are increasing, so as the radioactive substance poured in human environment. Therefore, people pay increasingly more attention to environmental pollution by ionizing radiation.

The ionizing radiation means the rays radiated by some radioactive substance in the process of transmutation. This kind of rays can give the absorbed substance adequate energy to divide ionize molecules and atoms. Some ionizing radiations are electromagnetic radiations like X-ray and γ-ray.

The sources of artificial radiation include nuclear tests which increase the radioactive environmental pollution, the exploitation, processing and retreat of nuclear fuel, for instance, in the exploitation of mineral radon gas and radioactive dust can pollute atmosphere. As the sources of energy in the world are less and less, more and more nations have been beginning to build nuclear power stations currently. This nuclear power industry can all discharge radioactive waste gas, water and residue which will pollute environment if mishandled.

Although radioactive nuclide can be applied extensively in industry, agriculture and medicine, the radioactive waste can still pollute environment.

The major effects of ionizing radiation to human bodies are body damages including chronic radiation diseases, malignant tumors, cataract, and decrease in the capacity to bear children, etc; radiation carcinogensis with longer delitescence like leucocythemia, skin carcinoma, lung cancer and osteocarcinoma; and hereditary damages which make descendants possessed with hereditary disease.

(6)carcinogens that enter foods from environmental pollution: With the development of technology, food processing has become increasingly industrialized. So both external environment and food processing itself can bring various external substance including chemical and biological carcinogens and pollute foods.

In the processing of raw material, adding manmade additions or using smoking, frying, baking, etc. to cook may result in the production of cancerogenic farrago in foods.

Usually finished food products are sent to customers after preservation and transportation which provide another source of carcinogens to pollute foods.

It is important to research on the sources of pollution to human foods and how to eliminate the pollution.

2>> The environmental pollution increased the incidence of cancer

With the development of modern industrialization a lot of energy consumption, a large number of production and life of the process of day and night kept a lot of tar, soot, dust and other harmful gases into the atmosphere, air pollution, water pollution,

444

soil pollution, food Pollution, occupational carcinogens soared. In recent decades of western developed countries the incidence of lung cancer and mortality rates increases rapidly, such as the British lung cancer mortality in 1930 to 10.0 million, in 1975 up to 120.3 / 10 million, 45 Year growth of 12 times. In the United States from 1934 to 1974, male lung cancer mortality increased from 3 .0/10 million to 54.5 / 10 million, an increase of 17 times the above data is very alarming. If no energy saving, it will be a lot of emissions Pollution, greatly harm human health, promote cancer incidence and mortality rate of rapid growth. Energy-saving emission reduction is for the healthy development of industrialization, continue to leap.

Because of environmental pollution and being harmful to society and harmful to human life, improving the environment, prevention and control of pollution, safeguard health are conducive to the construction of a healthy, happy, harmonious and environmentally friendly society. Therefore, what is the risk of environmental pollution? The most fear is that environmental pollutants contain many carcinogens causing people to increase the incidence of cancer, such as the Japanese nuclear power plant damage, leading to radiation material concentration greatly increasing in the surrounding air, water, soil, food nuclear to promote high incidence rate such as leukemia and cancer, not only curse contemporary and endanger future generations.

2). The treatment of environmental pollution is an important measure for cancer prevention

At present, we are carrying out resource-saving and environment-friendly society building a comprehensive test of supporting energy-saving emission reduction and sewage treatment. This policy and work have a great relevance to cancer prevention.

1. Human carried out extensive exploration and had accumulated a wealth of knowledge in the search for cancer etiology and occurrence of factors. The most prominent is that more than 80% of cancer is caused by environmental factors. Control of environmental pollution will greatly reduce the air, water, food contaminants and carcinogens.

2. Environmental factors and improper social behavior are risk factors for cancer, but these factors can be avoided or intervened. Therefore, the United Nations Health Organization proposed: 1/3 of cancer can be prevented; 1/3 of cancer can be treated by early treatment; 1/3 of the cancer can be effectively treated to alleviate the symptoms and prolong life.

Therefore, we must improve the environment, prevention and control of pollution, building an environment-friendly society, be fully aware of the importance of cancer prevention, environmental pollution and other carcinogenic factors for effective interventions to reduce the incidence of cancer.

Anti-cancer strategy is to prevent cancer, control of cancer, the use of I-level prevention, II level of prevention, III level prevention. The current pollution abatement are pollution control are a fundamental anti-cancer measures (I level of prevention).

I have been engaged in the basic research and clinical practice of tumor surgery for half a century. If we want to achieve the purpose of cancer prevention and control, we must be involved in China government-led, experts, scholars, mass participation, mobilization, thousands of households. Building an innovative country, building a moderately prosperous society are involved in the work of the government-led, mass participation, mobilization, thousands of households, which will be able to raise the awareness of anti-cancer, cancer prevention and to reduce ancer incidence rate.

In the construction of a moderately prosperous society and rural urbanization work, we formulate anti-cancer, anti-cancer outline, formulate anti-cancer, anti-cancer measures, formulate new towns, new rural cancer prevention and control plan and measures to carry out cancer prevention and cancer control and take the Chinese characteristics of anti-cancer, cancer control innovation path, overcome cancer, to build a well-off society, everyone's health, away from cancer.

1. I think that the current energy-saving emission reduction, pollution prevention and control in fact is the cancer prevention level I of the prevention and treatment of cancer. Its purpose and effect can achieve the role of cancer prevention class I. This is a golden opportunity and must seize this golden. I have been engaged in the basic experimental research and clinical practice of tumor surgery for half a century, I know that in order to achieve the purpose of cancer prevention and control we must have government-led, experts and scholars working hard, Mass participation, mobilization, thousands of households involved in the work in order to improve people's awareness of anti-cancer, to prevent cancer, cancer control and to reduce the incidence of cancer effect.

2. To carry out anti-cancer and cancer control, so far there is no practical way, not only from the technical and tactical, but from a strategic focus, the implementation of people-oriented, fundamentally stressed the harmony between people and the environment. It must do scientific research and must explore and innovate. Science is an endless frontier, scientific research is endless. With the developing vision, forward vision, under the guidance of the scientific concept of development, for energy conservation, pollution

prevention, treatment and anti-cancer, control cancer and reducing the incidence the cancer-related scientific research should be done, which will produce a lot of knowledge which is not yet known, and even the original innovation of scientific research and produce new disciplines, new industries.

Energy-saving emission reduction, pollution prevention and pollution control in essence contain significance and effect of anti-cancer and cancer control.

Cancer prevention and anti-cancer work are a hard nut to crack, but it should continue to bite down. Because cancer is a major human disease, cancer prevention and anti-cancer are the work of mankind. I know that it is not possible to do this work well if it is only dependent on the individual efforts of scholars; it must be under the guidance of the government, mobilize the masses, mobilization in order to do.

3). Insisting on building the innovation way of cancer prevention and cancer control with a moderately prosperous society of Chinese characteristics

China's energy-saving emission reduction, pollution prevention and pollution control and building a moderately prosperous society through the efforts will inevitably achieve great results while reducing the incidence of cancer, which is the characteristics of anti-cancer and cancer control in socialist countries, which is building a moderately prosperous society with chinese characteristics, which is cancer prevention and cancer control innovation path; the success of the work experience after 3-5 years can introduce this ways of building a moderately prosperous society with cancer prevention and control of the Chinese characteristics of innovation in our province and city to the country and the world.

Because more than 80% of cancers are associated with environmental pollution, improving environmental pollution may be a role in preventing cancer and controlling cancer. Control of pollution may prevent or control the entry of carcinogens into the environment. The improvement of the big environment and the small environment both can reduce, prevent or control environmental carcinogens into the human body or environmental carcinogens affect on the human body.

The current situation is a good opportunity to carry out energy-saving emission reduction, is also a good opportunity to carry out anti-cancer, cancer research. In the past it also was realized the importance of anti-cancer and cancer control ; however it was just discussed in the paper and just for the scientific education. Now under the specific practice with bluiding the rich country, anti-cancer and controlling can be a great time and can be achieved to reduce the incidence of cancer. Everyone should be aware of their responsibilities on the shoulders. In this excellent situation, it uses this situation best, do a good job of anti-cancer to improve people's awareness of anti-cancer, and change some living habits, and improve some living environment, and have environment friendly and harmonious life so that people will be healthy, happiness, longevity, away from cancer.

Appendix

Our experiment:

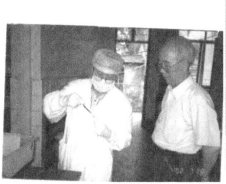
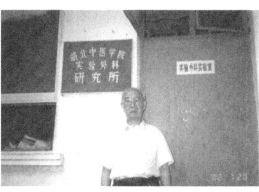

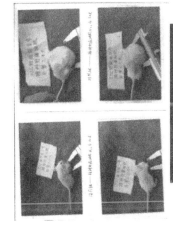
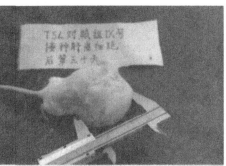
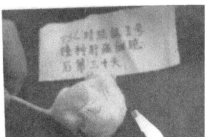